CANCER ETIOLOGY, DIAGNOSIS AND TREATMENTS

OSTEOSARCOMA

SYMPTOMS, DIAGNOSIS AND TREATMENT OPTIONS

Cancer Etiology, Diagnosis and Treatments

Additional books in this series can be found on Nova's website under the Series tab.

Additional e-books in this series can be found on Nova's website under the e-book tab.

CANCER ETIOLOGY, DIAGNOSIS AND TREATMENTS

OSTEOSARCOMA

SYMPTOMS, DIAGNOSIS AND TREATMENT OPTIONS

EDWIN CHOY
EDITOR

New York

For permission to use material from this book please contact us:
Telephone 631-231-7269; Fax 631-231-8175
Web Site: http://www.novapublishers.com

Library of Congress Cataloging-in-Publication Data

ISBN: 978-1-63321-052-3

LCCN: 2014939981

Published by Nova Science Publishers, Inc. † New York

Contents

EDITOR'S NOTE

Edwin Choy, MD PhD
Assistant Professor, Harvard Medical School
Massachusetts General Hospital Center for Sarcoma and Connective Tissue Oncology

Before the use of chemotherapy, the treatment of localized osteosarcoma often involved amputation for local control of the disease. But even after definitive local control, the majority of patients would ultimately develop metastasis and die of this disease. Then, in 1974, Norman Jaffe, Emil Frei [1] , James Holland [2], Gerald Rosen [3,4], and others published reports demonstrating improved survival with adjuvant chemotherapy, given either before or after surgery. Since then, with the increased use of adjuvant chemotherapy, the prognosis for patients improved until the 1990s, when the majority of patients diagnosed with nonmetastatic osteosarcoma were being cured. However, the prognosis for osteosarcoma when diagnosed today is still not significantly improved when compared to the 1990s. Additionally, for the 30-40% of patients who either present with metastatic disease or develop metastasis after initial surgery, the prognosis remains quite poor. We know that cytotoxic therapies, as a tool, are now being maximized. Additional cytotoxic therapy, either as dose dense or high dose chemotherapies or additional agents, do not seem to offer additional benefits above the standard regimens of "MAP" (methotrexate, adriamycin, cisplatinum) and "IE" (ifosfamide, etoposide). Therefore, new strategies to systemically treat osteosarcomas are still in great need despite the huge advances that were made in the 1970s.

This book is intended to give readers both a state of the art overview of the use of surgery and radiology in the treatment and diagnosis of osteosarcoma as well as an exploration of the frontiers of osteosarcoma research. By no means did we intend to offer a comprehensive review of all of the research and experimental strategies to improve osteosarcoma. We do not discuss in depth Mifamurtide (liposomal muramyl tripeptide phosphatidylethanolamine; L-MTP-PE), which is approved for commercial use in Europe. We also do not offer an extensive review of Samarium-153 lexidronam (153Sm-EDTMP), which is sometimes used to treat metastatic osteosarcoma, albeit with great toxicities. Both of those topics are already heavily reviewed and the reader will easily find sufficient literature to read about them. Rather, we sought to focus most of our chapters on the fringes of translational osteosarcoma research – topics that are promising but not completely in vogue -- in hopes that we could stimulate interest and conversation in fields within the osteosarcoma research community that may open doors for additional collaborations and research.

References

[1] Jaffe N, Frei E 3rd, Traggis D, Bishop Y. "Adjuvant methotrexate and citrovorum-factor treatment of osteogenic sarcoma." *N Engl J Med.* 1974 Nov 7;291(19):994-7.

[2] Cortes EP, Holland JF, Wang JJ, Sinks LF, Blom J, Senn H, Bank A, Glidewell O. "Amputation and adriamycin in primary osteosarcoma." *N Engl J Med.* 1974 Nov 7;291(19):998-1000.

[3] Rosen G, Suwansirikul S, Kwon C, Tan C, Wu SJ, Beattie EJ Jr, Murphy ML. "High-dose methotrexate with citrovorum factor rescue and adriamycin in childhood osteogenic sarcoma." *Cancer.* 1974 Apr;33(4):1151-63.

[4] Rosen G, Tan C, Sanmaneechai A, Beattie EJ Jr, Marcove R, Murphy ML. "The rationale for multiple drug chemotherapy in the treatment of osteogenic sarcoma." *Cancer.* 1975 Mar;35(3 suppl):936-45.

In: Osteosarcoma
Editor: Edwin Choy

ISBN: 978-1-63321-052-3

Chapter 1

OSTEOSARCOMA: AN INTRODUCTION

Alessio Biazzo[1,*], Massimiliano De Paolis[1], Nikolin Ali[1], Carlo Romagnoli[1] and Davide Maria Donati[1]

[1]Oncologic Orthopaedic Department,
Rizzoli Orthopaedic Institute,
Bologna, Italy

ABSTRACT

This chapter is a broad introduction and overview of the clinical aspects of osteosarcoma. This includes an overview of classical osteosarcoma and its epidemiology, localization, symptoms, and methods of diagnosis. We then discuss details of osteosarcoma staging according to the Enneking's classification. We use the World Health Organization (WHO) nomenclature to discuss the histopathologic features, focusing on microscopy findings, differential diagnosis, and biology of classical osteosarcoma. All three main modalities of treatment are discussed, including surgery, chemotherapy and radiation-therapy. We then offer a brief overview of the less common variations of osteosarcoma that may be seen in the clinic. This overview is meant to offer a survey of osteosarcomas and clinical approaches, and serves as an introduction to the other chapters in this book.

---

* E-mail: ale.biazzo@yahoo.it.

INTRODUCTION

Osteosarcomas (OS) are malignant bone tumors composed of mesenchymal cells producing osteoid and immature bone [1]. OS is the most frequent nonhaematologic primary malignant bone tumor. There are several varieties of OS which can be divided into two subgroups: high-grade and low-grade. The last one are very different in their clinical, pathologic and therapeutic-prognostic features and are classified as separate entities (periosteal OS, parosteal OS, low-grade central OS).

High grade OS can be divided into different subtypes: classic OS, teleangiectatic OS, secondary OS, small cell OS, high grade OS of the surface, multicentric OS, intracortical OS and OS of jaw bones (table 1). According to the cellular differentiation, we can describe three varieties of classic OS: osteoblastic OS, chondroblastic OS and fibroblastic OS [1].

CLASSIC OSTEOSARCOMA

Epidemiology and Localization

Classic OS is the most frequent variety and the most frequent primary malignant tumor of bone, excluding myeloma, considered a systemic neoplasm. Its prevalence is of 2/3 cases/million/year (only 0,2% of all malignancies). There is a predilection for male sex at a ratio of 1,5-2:1 because of the skeletal growth period is longer in males than females. OS has a bimodal age distribution, with a first peak during the second decade of life and a second peak in older adults. In 75% of cases it is manifested between 10 and 30 years of age. Other cases of OS can be observed during advanced age but they are usually secondary to other conditions, such as Paget's disease, irradiated bone, chronic osteomyelitis, bone infarct and dedifferentiated chondrosarcoma. Very rare cases are reported to be related to benign conditions, such as Giant Cell Tumors (GCT), chondromas, non-ossifying fibromas [2].

OS has no forbidden areas. Nonetheless, there are skeletal areas where there is strong predilection and others where the tumor is exceptionally rare. The areas of predilection are, in this order: the distal femur, the proximal tibia, the proximal humerus, the proximal femur, the diaphysis of the femur and the pelvis (figure 1). Fifty % of OS are localized around the knee [3]. However, OS can also occur in the axial skeleton, most commonly in the pelvis [4].

Table 1. Incidence of different subtypes of OS. From Rizzoli Institute

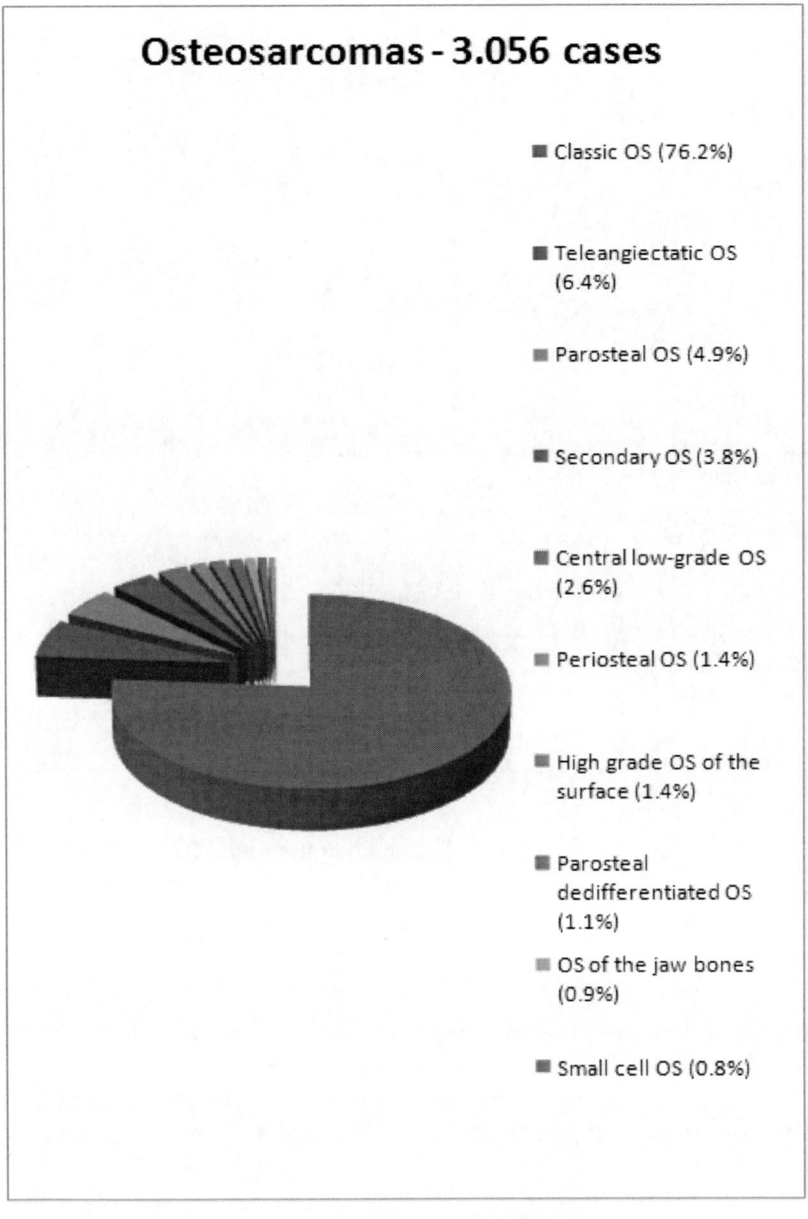

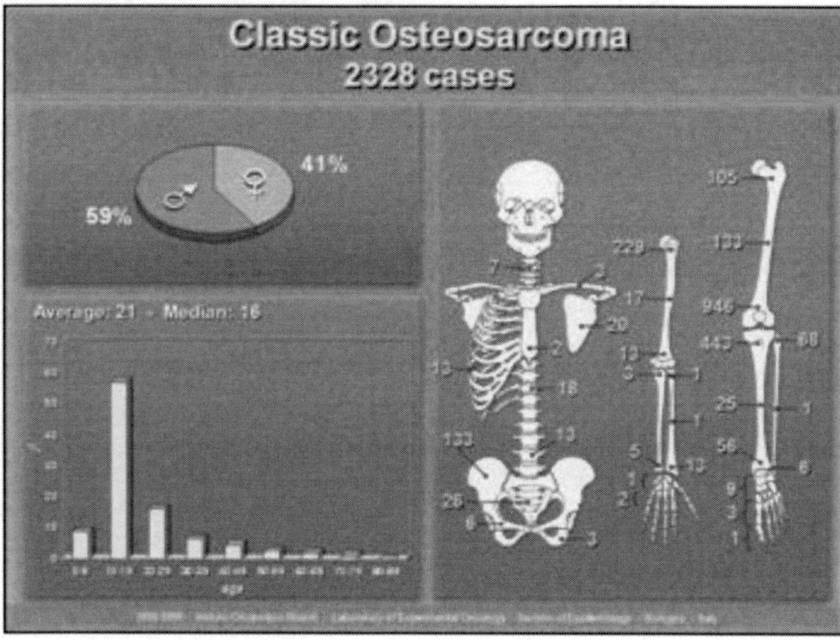

From Rizzoli Orthopaedic Institute [5].

Figure 1. Sex prevalence, age prevalence and localization of OS.

In the long bones there is predilection in the metaphysis and metadiaphysis. The growth cartilage represents an important obstacle to the invasion of the epiphysis.

Symptoms and Diagnosis

Patients usually have symptoms for several months (rarely exceeding 6 months) before a diagnosis is made. Pain is usually the first symptom, often referred to trauma. In few weeks it increases and painful swelling appears. Physical examination may reveal the presence of a tender and firm soft tissue mass at the primary site. The skin above the tumor tends to be warm and palpation is painful. High temperature and limited joint motion are advanced signs. Pathologic fracture may occur in osteolytic forms.

The regional lymph nodes are not enlarged, except in advanced phase. The correct diagnosis of OS can be achieved through a correct approach to the disease and the combination of clinical and radiographic aspects. The final step to confirm the hypothesis is the biopsy.

The most important clinical aspects are the age of the patient and the site of the neoplasm. The amount of time between the first symptoms and diagnosis is generally less than 6 months.

The radiographic aspect of OS is that of a malignant tumor that starts intra-medullary, breaches the cortex, surpasses the periosteum and expands in the soft tissues.

It is usually a combination of radiolucency and radiodensity, sometimes completely eburneous in osteogenetic forms or completely radiolucent in osteolytic ones [1] (such as teleangiectatic OS). At the periphery of the area the new periosteal formation and elevation of the cortex can create the so-called Codman's triangle (Figure 2).

Ossification in the soft tissue in a radial or "sunburst" pattern is classic for OS but is neither a sensitive nor specific feature.

Defining the local tumor extent with MRI and CT has been shown to be an accurate predictor of tumor extent determined at the time of surgical resection [6-7].

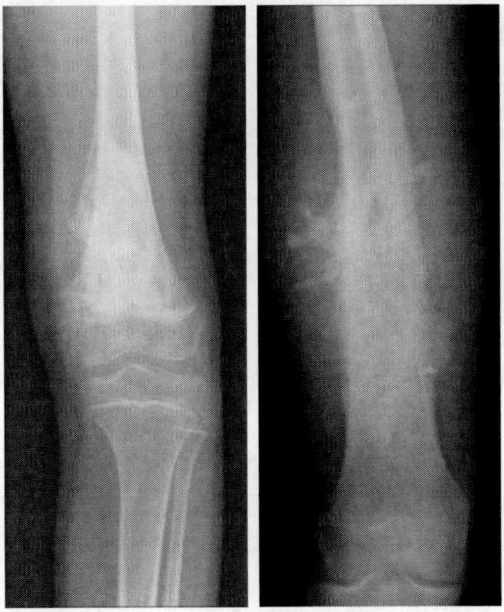

Figure 2. On the left: osteoblastic OS of the distal femur in a 12 year-old boy. On the right: osteolytic-osteoblastic OS with sunburst aspect.

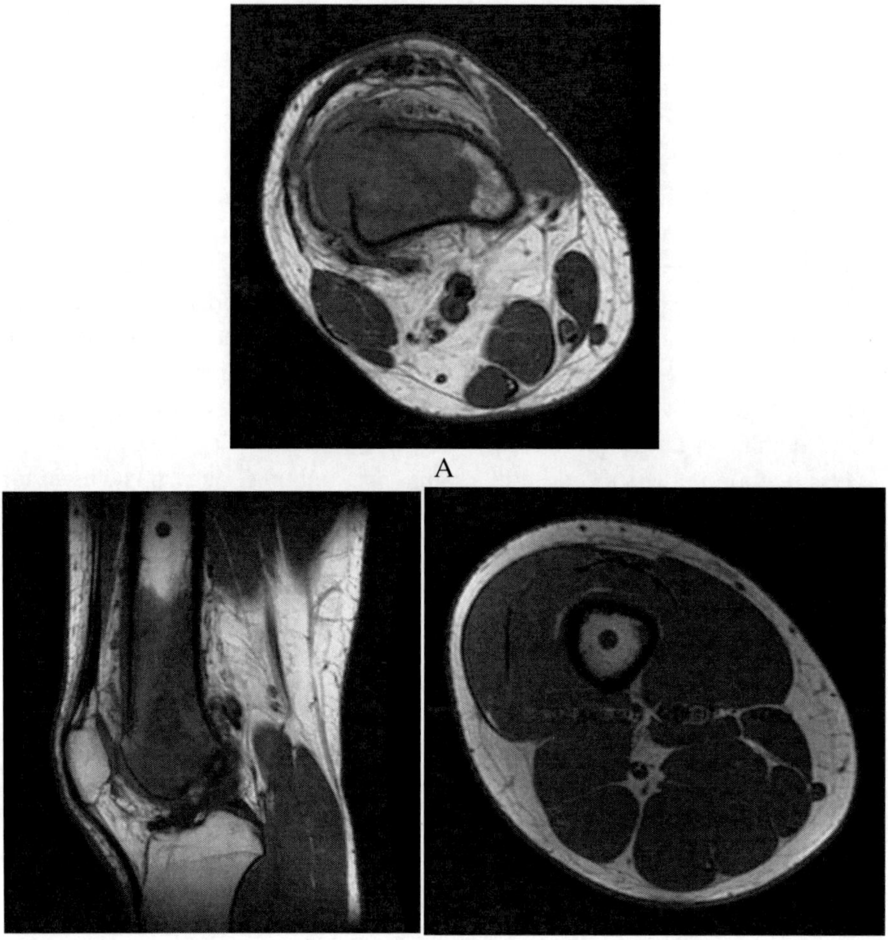

Figure 3. Seventeen year-old boy with classic OS of the distal femur. A: MRI shows local extension of the tumor, which breaks the lateral cortex (stage IIB). B-C: skip metastases.

MRI is useful to determine the intra- and extraosseous extent, soft tissue, contiguous structure involvement of the tumor and skip lesions (Figure 3).

CT is useful to study the relationship of the tumor with large vessels or internal organs and invasion of the joint. Chest-C is crucial to detect pulmonary metastasis and bone scan is useful to determine bone metastasis.

Tissue biopsy of OS must be obtained to confirm the diagnosis even when clinical and radiographic aspects are highly suggestive. It should be performed with a needle biopsy and when necessary CT-guided. When a needle biopsy is not diagnostic or technically not possible, an incisional biopsy should be performed.

STAGING

OS is staged according Enneking's classification [8] (table 2). This system categorizes localized malignant bone tumors by grade and by the local anatomic extent. The compartimental status is determined by whether or not the tumor extends through the cortex. Patients with distant metastases are staged III.

At presentation 80% of OS are stage II-B; only 5% are stage II-A, because most high-grade OS break through the cortex early in their natural history. About 15% of OS are stage III [9]. Virtually all patients are presumed to have subclinical microscopic metastases [10]. The most frequent site for metastatic presentation is the lung, but respiratory symptoms develop with extensive involvement [11].

Table 2. Enneking's classification. G1: low- grade; G2: high grade; T1: intracompartimental; T2: extracompartimental; M0: no distant metastases; M1: distant metastases

Stage	Grade	Site	Metastases	Definition
IA	G1	T1	M0	Low-grade A Intracompartimental
IB	G2	T2	M0	Low-grade B Extracompartimental
IIA	G1	T1	M0	High-grade A Intracompartimental
IIB	G2	T2	M0	High-grade B Extracompartimental
IIIA-B	G1-G2	T1-T2	M1	Metastatic Either low-high grade Either A or B

However metastases can also occur in other bones and soft tissues. Maybe, presentations with multiple bone metastases may represent multifocal primary tumors [11], but Errani's studies [12] have already demonstrated that in epithelioid emangioendothelioma with multiple nodules there is a single gene mutation, which is WWTR1-CAMTA1. Thus, it seems to be more probable that multicentric OS does not exist and it's a metastatic spread of a single neoplastic cellular line.

Before the use of chemotherapy, 80-90% of patients with OS died of metastases. So, indirectly, it can be said that micrometastases are present at the onset in 80-90% of patients.

Death from OS is usually the result of progressive pulmonary metastases with respiratory failure due to widespread disease [13].

In addition to imaging the primary bone tumor various other radiological studies help to determine the extent of disease at presentation. These include a radionuclide bone scan with methylene diphosphonate labeled with technetium-99m, which helps defining the extent of the primary tumor [14] (Figure 4).

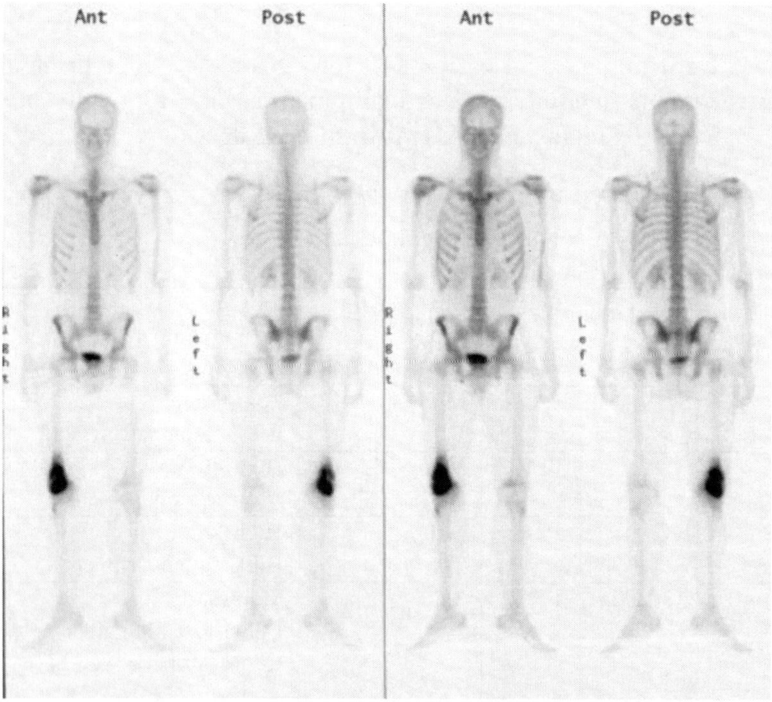

Figure 4. Isotope bone scan of localized OS of the distal femur.

Radionuclide bone scanning is also useful to detect "skip" lesions within the same bone and distant bone metastases [15].

Postero-anterior and lateral radiographs of the chest allow detection of lung metastases in most cases but the CT of the lungs is more sensitive and has become the imaging procedure of choice [16] (Figure 5).

Eighteen-fluorodeoxy-glucose positron emission tomography (18FDG-PET) is also being increasingly used in the initial staging and treatment monitoring.

HISTOPATHOLOGIC FEATURES

The current World Health Organization (WHO) classification of OS recognizes three major subtypes of classic OS: osteoblastic, chondroblastic and fibroblastic, according the predominat type of matrix in the tumor [17]. Osteoblastic OS has osteoid or bone as predominant type of matrix. Chondroblastic OS has predomimance of chondroid matrix, whereas fibroblastic OS is composed of malignant spindle cells with only scant osteoid.

The presence of osteoid, even if minimal, distinguishes the chondroblastic and fibroblastic subtypes of OS from chondrosarcoma and fibrosarcoma/malignant fibrous histiocytoma, respectively, with which they may be histologically confused.

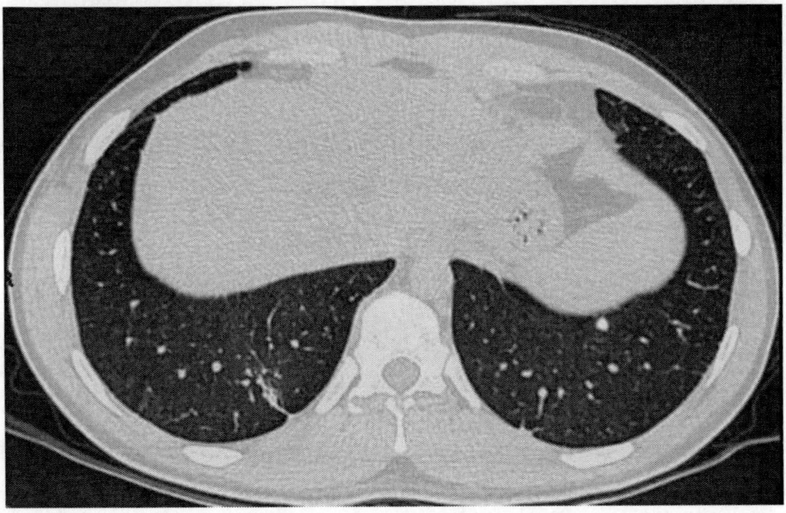

Figure 5. Arrow: metastatic nodule in a 17 year-old boy with OS of the distal femur.

Moreover, there is no convincing evidence of a difference in clinical behavior or outcome based on histological subtype.

From a macroscopic point of view, the tumoral tissue, which is generally compact, tends to be whitish or rose-colored. The presence of neoplastic osteoid and bone gives it a harder consistency. The sclerosing areas are characterized by eburneous hardness. As ossification increases vascularity decreases, so that the harder or more eburneous areas are also those which are whiter [1] (Figure 6).

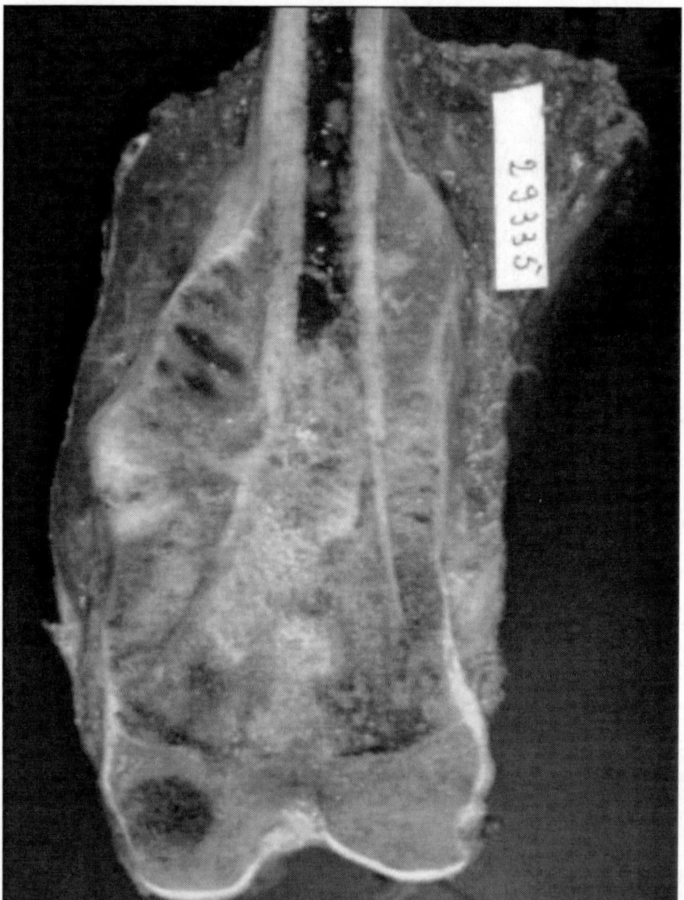

Figure 6. Specimen of OS of the distal femur. The lesion breaks the medial and lateral cortex (IIB). The tumor does not surpass the growth cartilage.

In OS, hemorrhagic areas, yellowish dry areas of necrosis, cystic cavities are frequently observed. If cartilaginous component is present as in chodroblastic type or in dedifferentiated OS, whitish-translucent or mucoid areas may be present.

Rarely, it's possible to observe intramedullary neoplastic nodes which are separated from the main tumor (skip metastases. Figure 7).

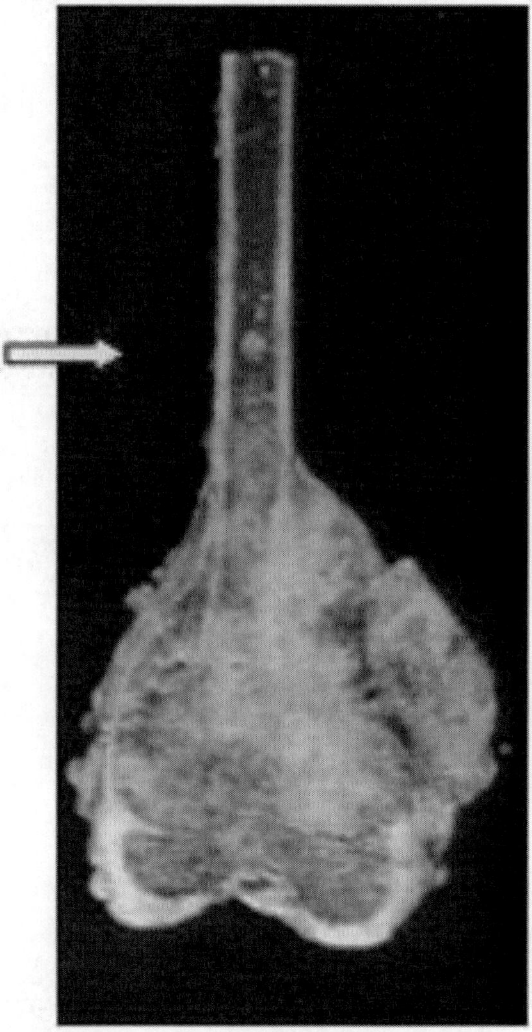

Figure 7. The arrow indicates a skip metastases.

When growth cartilage is still present, often is not surpassed by the tumor (Figure 6). In more aggressive forms, the cartilage may be destroyed with neoplastic invasion of the epiphysis.

From a histological point of view, OS consists of a sarcomatous tissue which produces osteoid matrix and bone.

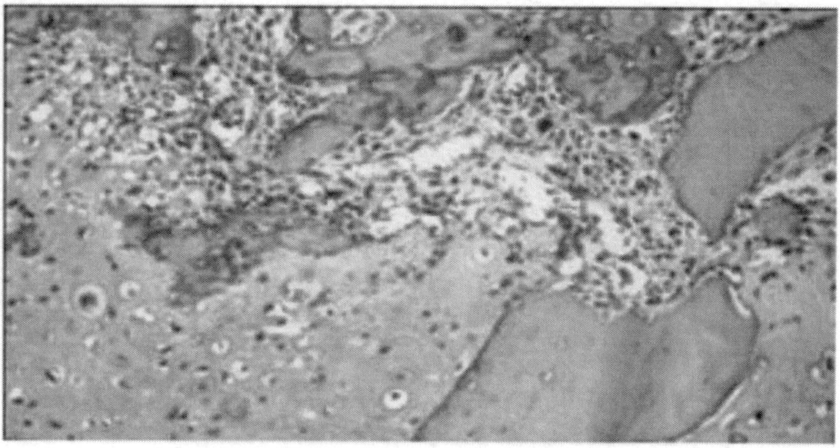

Figure 8. Sarcomatous tissue with cells producing osteoid and bone. Neoplastic osteoid and osseous material are shaped with an absolutely anarchical architecture.

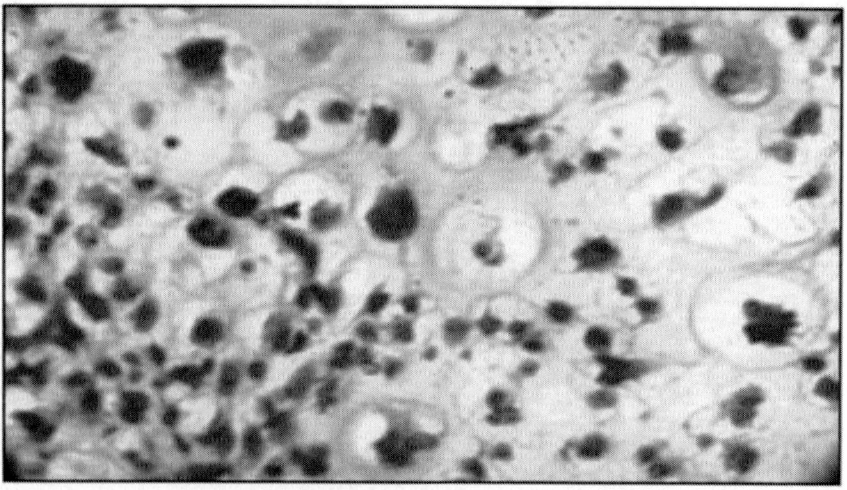

Figure 9. The aspects of the high-grade malignancy are fairly evident: large, pleomorphic and hyperchromic cells are seen.

Usually, the more peripheral areas of the tumor are those which are less ossified, while the central ones are more ossified (Figure 8).

Often OS is classified as grade 4, characterized by large cells, atypia, hyperchromia, frequent and atypical mitotic figures (Figure 9).

The deposit of osteoid matrix and bone is shaped with an anarchical architecture.

In osteogenetic forms, the cells, incarcerated in the abundant neoplastic bone, become scattered and scarce, their volume decreases, their nuclei become small and with very dense chromatin up to pyknosis.

In eburneous or devitalized areas of OS, evident aspects of cellular malignancy may be searched for in vain. In these forms, there are two important diagnostic elements: the structural disorder of the new bone matrix and the fact that the neoplastic bone permeates the medullary spaces of the host bone [1].

Giant cells are frequently found in OS. They may be gigantic neoplastic cells with one or more monstruous nuclei, that is, sarcomatous giant cells. In other cases there are multinucleate giant cells with no nuclear atypia, identical to osteoclasts.

If OS surpasses the cortex and perforates the periosteum, there is a mixture of neoplastic osteogenesis and reactive bone, which contributes significantly to the image of Codman's triangle.

Regarding to the genesis, it's now clear that OS originates from intraosseous mesenchimal cells which tend to an osteoblastic differentiation.

Some data suggest that OS is more likely to originate in areas of lively bone production: in fact the higher incidence of OS during the growth age and in areas where this growth is more intense, the incidence in boys with high stature, the insurgence in pagetic bone (where bone turnover is elevated and persistent for many years), support these data.

DIFFERENTIAL DIAGNOSIS

The differential diagnosis depends on the radiological aspects at the onset and includes infections, benign tumors (aneurysmal bone cyst, giant cell tumor) and malignant tumors (Ewing's sarcoma, lymphoma and metastatic carcinoma). The location of the tumor within the bone and the skeletal location help to distinguish OS from Ewing's sarcoma, the second most frequent type of bone tumor in this age group. Metastatic bone disease from other primary bone tumors, such as lymphoma, neuroblastoma and rhabdomyosarcoma, although not frequent in this age group, is also part of the differential diagnosis.

BIOLOGY

We have a very limited understanding of the etiology of OS. We know that the peak incidence coincides with a period of rapid growth, suggesting a correlation between rapid bone growth and the evolution of OS [18]. Other evidence supports this relationship, such as the higher incidence in tall people than in short people. However, OS can arise in many patients before and after the adolescent growth spurt. Radiation exposure is one of the few documented risk factors for OS [19].

The molecular pathogenesis of OS is characterized by a complex pathway, involving impairment of P53 and/or RB1 functions. This genetic feature originates from the high instability of OS cells, which can lead to multiple cell populations within the same tumor, with consequent changes in cell behavior that can be responsive of unresponsiveness to chemotherapy.

The p53 gene product in normal cells increases in response to DNA damage and directs the cell to either stop progression through the cell cycle or undergo apoptosis [20]. The Rb gene product likewise regulates cell cycle progression [21]. Although germline mutations of either p53 or Rb gene are rare, these genes are altered in the majority of OS tumor samples [22].

There are other altered oncogenes in OS tumor cells. These includes amplifications of the product of the murine double minute 2 (MDM2) gene, amplification of cyclin dependent kinase 4 (CDK4), and overexpression of human epidermal growth factor receptor 2 [18].

The complex unbalanced karyotypes that caractherized OS can be the result of telomere dysfunction. Telomeres are nucleoprotein structures that cap chromosome ends and serve at least three protective functions: preserving recognition of chromosome as damaged DNA, preventing chromosomal end-to-end fusions and recombinations, and accommodating the loss of DNA that occurs with each round of replication. Normal human somatic cells have a finite proliferative capacity and telomere length is one of the checkpoints that determine when a cell stops dividing [23]. As cells divide, the telomere length gradually decreases to a critical size, at which point senescence is triggered by a p53-dependent process. Human cells may bypass this checkpoint by inactivating the p53 pathways. About 85% of cancers activate an enzyme called telomerase, which lengthens telomeres [24] and at least 50% of OS are dependent upon the alternative telomere-lengthening mechanism to maintain telomeres [25].

Other authors have suggested that OS can have a viral etiology, based on the fact that bone sarcomas can be induced in selected animals by viruses [26]. However, there is no convincing data that viruses are a major etiologic factor in OS.

TREATMENT

Patients with low-grade osteosarcoma do not require chemotherapy, and the survival of such patients is rarely affected by the disease. In contrast, high-grade tumors tend to metastasize and are routinely treated with chemotherapy in addition to surgical resection, with a survival rate of approximately 70% (Figure 10). The use of surgery alone can result in a probability of survival below 20%, while the use of chemotherapy alone can result in a probability of survival less than 10% [5].

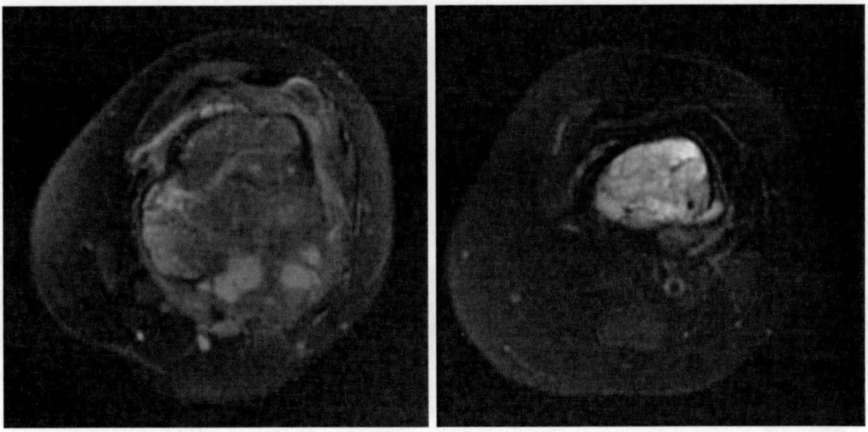

Figure 10. Fourteen year-old girl with teleangiectatic OS of the distal femur. On the left: pre-chemotherapy. On the right: post-chemotherapy.

Chemotherapy

Two different studies definitively proved the need for adjuvant chemotherapy to improve outcome for patients with localized extremity OS [10, 27].

The most active agents include cisplatin, doxorubicin, ifosfamide and high-dose methotrexate. Etoposide has little activity in OS when used as single agent and its use has been proposed in combination with ifosfamide.

In the early 1980s, investigators at the Mayo Clinic carried out the first randomized trial of adjuvant chemotherapy for OS [28]. In that study, following surgical resection, patients were randomly assigned to either observation or chemotherapy.

There was no difference in outcome between the two groups, and the disease-free survival rate was 40%, suggesting that the nature history of the disease had changed and that this accounted for the difference in outcomes observed in the adjuvant chemotherapy trials. Two subsequent randomized studies clarified this controversy. Link et al. [10] developed a randomized study of observation and adjuvant chemotherapy. Patients treated with surgery alone had a 2-year relapse-free survival probability of 17%, versus 66% for those receiving adjuvant chemotherapy. Eilber et al. [27] reported similar results, definitively proving that adjuvant chemotherapy produced higher disease-free survival rates for patients with non-metastatic OS.

Rosen et al. [29] introduced the concept of chemotherapy administration prior to definitive surgery. This approach offered the opportunity to develop a custom-made prostheses for limb-salvage procedures and the theoretical advantage of early treatment of micrometastases while facilitating the surgical procedure. It also provided the opportunity to examine the histological response of the tumor to chemotherapy and assess its effectiveness. A strong correlation between the degree of necrosis (Huvos grade) and subsequent disease-free survival was observed. A theoretical problem with this type of approach is that the delay in removal the tumor could lead to the emergence of chemotherapy resistance. However, a prospective Pediatric Oncology Group trial demonstrated no difference between treatment using immediate definitive surgery and treatment with neoadjuvant chemotherapy followed by definitive surgery [30].

The identification of the prognostic value of necrosis degree following chemotherapy led to the suggestion that chemotherapy could be modified for patients with less necrosis (currently, poor responders are those patients with less than 90% of necrosis) in an attempt to increase the probability of disease-free survival. Investigators at Memorial Sloan-Kettering Cancer Centre reported an improved outcome for patients with poor histological responses following a change in postoperative therapy [31].

Nowadays, the standard postoperative-chemotherapy for poor-responders is based on the combination of ifosfamide and etoposide, useful also in metastatic patients.

Most recent studies performed by the German-Austrian-Swiss Cooperative Osteosarcoma Study Group (COSS) demonstrated that best results can be achieved by the combination of preoperative administration of methotrexate, cisplatin, doxorubicin and ifosfamide, with a 10-year survival rate of 71% [32].

The Scandinavian Sarcoma Group (SSG) has also performed various nonrandomized neoadjuvant chemotherapy trials for high-grade OS. They used a three-drug combination of high-dose methotrexate, cisplatin and doxorubicin up front and replacement with ifosfamide and etoposide for poor responders, resulting in a 5-year over-all survival rate of 74%.

Also an italian study performed at the Rizzoli Institute confirmed that the use of ifosfamide and etoposide for poor-responders resulted in an improved outcome [33].

In 2005 the Children's Oncology Group (COG), Cooperative Osteosarcoma Study Group (COSS), European Osteosarcoma Intergroup (EOI) and Scandinavian Sarcoma Group (SSG) designed a study (EURAMOS) to determine whether altering postoperative therapy based on histological response improved the outcome.

The study design includes a backbone of 10 weeks of preoperative therapy using MAP (methotrexate, adriamycin and cisplatin). Following surgery, patients are stratified according to histological response. Patients classified as "good responders" (>or=90% necrosis) are randomized to continue MAP or to receive MAP followed by maintenance pegylated interferon, while "poor responders" (<90% necrosis) are randomized to either continue MAP or to receive MAPIE [34] (MAP+ifosfamide, etoposide). Two-thousand and sixty patients were enrolled in the study, which actually is the largest osteosarcoma study conducted (Figure 11). The first results will be available in 2014 and 2015.

Although adjuvant chemotherapy is effective in the setting of localized OS, the outcome for patients with clinically detectable metastases at diagnosis continues to be suboptimal [35, 36]. The standard management of these patients follows the same principles as the management of those patients who present with localized disease and, with this approach, a small subset of patients achieves prolonged disease-free survival [35,36]. There is no standard treatment for recurrence of OS; usually these patients underwent amputation and postoperative chemotherapy.

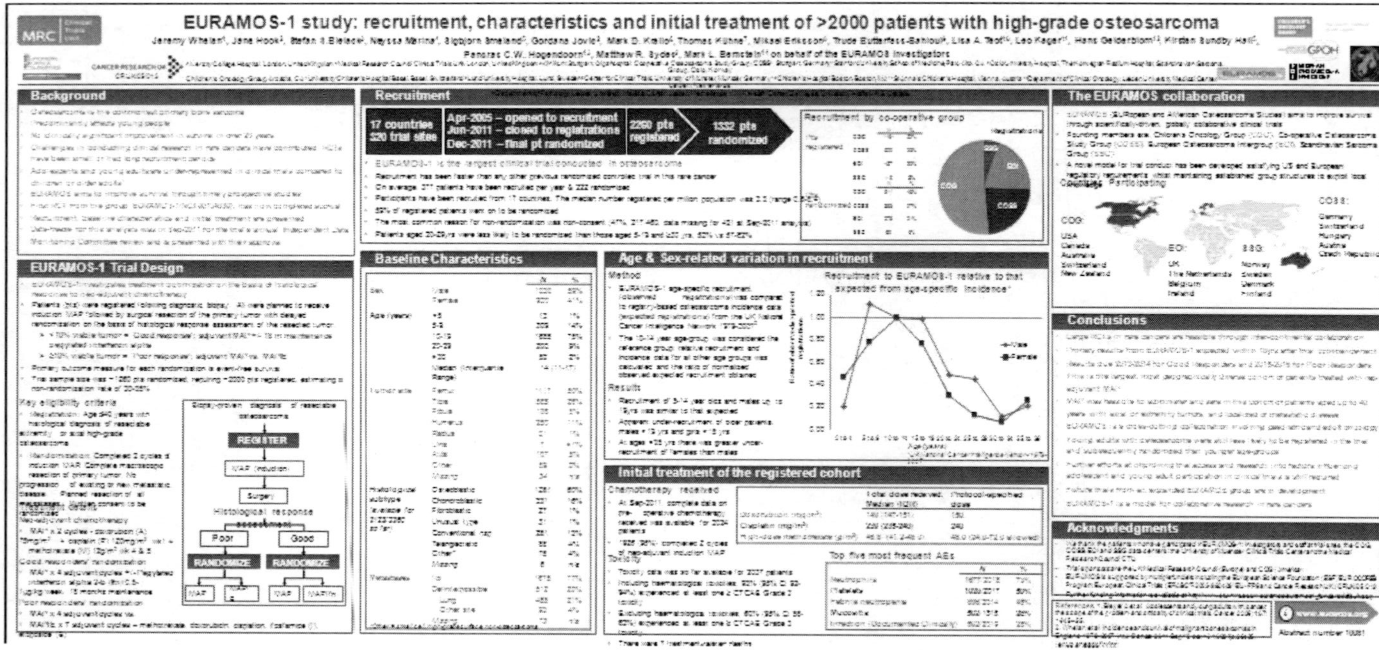

Figure 11. The preliminary results of the EURAMOS protocol presented in 2012.

Unfortunately, the use of chemotherapy is associated with acute and long-term toxicities, such as hearing loss [37] and hypomagnesemia [38] associated to cisplatin, anthracycline-induced cardiomyopathy [39], nephropathy due to methotrexate and sterility.

Since doxorubicin appears to be an important component of the chemotherapy, methods to minimize the potential for cardiotoxicity are under evaluation.

These include the use of dexrazone [40] and pegylated liposomal doxorubicin associated to continuous-infusion of doxorubicin: in fact, seems to be that they can minimize the toxicity related to anthracyclines, but there is limited information about their long-term efficacy.

The first informations that emerged from clinical studies are that the major cause of failure of the current neoadjuvant chemotherapy protocols for OS is the natural or acquired drug resistance, which occurs in 35-45% of patients. Although several studies have been reported in the past 10 years, a clear picture of molecular determinants of drug resistance in OS is still far to be determined.

SURGERY

The goal of any malignant tumor operation is to perform a complete en bloc removal of the lesion with adequate margins. The use of neoadjuvant chemotherapy along with advances in imaging techniques has enabled the oncologic surgeon to obtain local control rates equivalent to amputation using limb-salvage surgery. Therefore, limb-salvage has become the standard of care, except in situations where it may compromise oncologic outcome [18].

After tumor removal, there are different reconstructive techniques, such as autogenous bone grafts, structural bone allografts (intercalary or osteoarticular) and metallic endoprostheses. The choice of the procedure depends on the location of the tumor and the age of the patient.

Autogenous bone grafts can be non-vascularized (from the pelvis or other sites) or vascularized (fibula). They have the advantage of high incorporation rate but potential donor site morbidity. Vascularized fibula is an important option in femoral, tibial and humeral intercalary resections and in failure limb reconstructions as salvage technique.

Structural allografts have no donor site morbidity. The major problem is the difficulty of the graft incorporating with the host bone (nonunion) and the fracture. Their advantage is that they are a biologic solution and, if they heal and do not fracture, may last the patient's lifetime. Intercalary allografts spare the epiphysis and growth plate and preserve bone stock for future reconstructions (Figure 12). Osteoarticular allografts may be used in the reconstruction of the proximal humerus, distal femur and proximal tibia as well as potentially any joint. Infection can occur in 10-15% of allograft reconstructions [41] and nonunion at the osteosynthesis can occur in another 10-25% [42]. Infection often requires graft removal, while nonunion can be managed by revision fixation and autogenous bone grafting. Both these complications are more likely in patients receiving chemotherapy. Augmentation of the allograft with a vascularized fibula may facilitate osseous integration of the allograft and prevent some complications, such as nonunions and fractures [43].

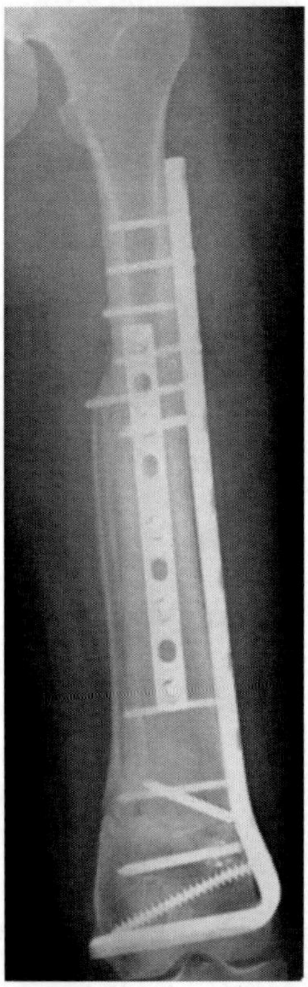

Figure 12. Intercalary allograft reconstruction with massive bone graft and vascularized fibula in 18 year-old girl.

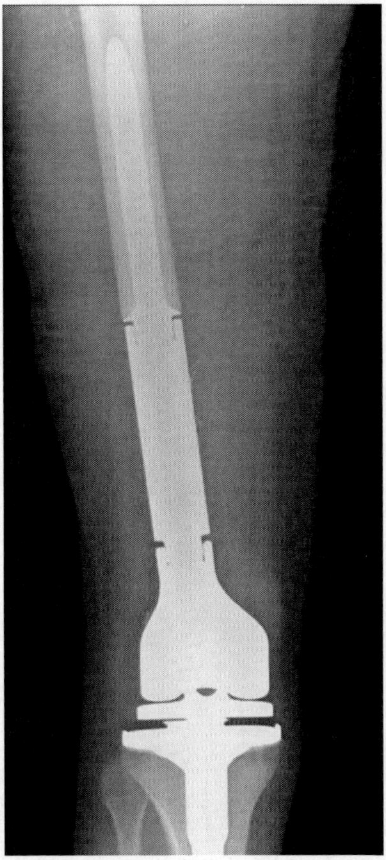

Figure 13. Reconstruction of the distal femur using modular prostheses in a 22 year-old man with OS.

Metallic modular endoprostheses provide an immediate stable reconstruction, but they present some problems, such as loosening and mechanical failure (Figure 13). Among complications, infections are the most likely, with rates ranging from 0% to 35% [44-46]. The durability of the prostheses is influenced by many factors, such as tumor site, type of prostheses, patient's weight and life-style. Prosthetic reconstructions of the proximal humerus tend to be more durable since they are not subjected to weight-bearing stresses.

Allograft-prosthetic composites (APC) are another alternative for limb-salvage surgery [47]. Their advantage is the hybridization of a more conventional arthroplasty with the potential incorporation of an allograft for future bone stock (Figure 14).

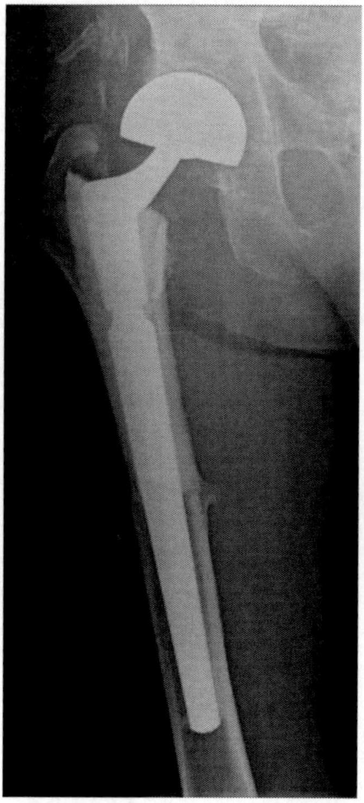

Figure 14. Reconstruction of the proximal femur with APC in a 21 year-old man with OS.

Special considerations can be made for periacetabular pelvic lesions. In fact, due to the complex anatomy of this region and to the presence of important neurovascular structures to preserve, reconstructions can be a challenge and outcomes can be unsatisfactory. Saddle prostheses, APC and complete endoprostheses have all been performed with different results and each one with disadvantages and complications. Nowadays, saddle prostheses are used only as salvage technique for failure of previous reconstructions. Several papers [48-51] have already demonstrated that allograft reconstructions for periacetabular lesion are those with better results and low rate of complications, but should be performed by expertise surgeons and in centers of reference.

Special considerations can be made also for immature patients. The skeletally immature patient represents a particular challenge and reconstructions must be dynamic in order to accommodate future growth. In girls, the growth spurt occurs in pre- and early adolescence (12-14 years), while in boys it happens 1-2 years later (14-16 years). Most of the growth in the lower extremity occurs at the physes around the knee joint (distal femur 40%, proximal tibia 30%) while the upper femur and the lower tibia have contributions of about 15% each other. Since limb-sparing procedures usually result in resection of a major growth center, other alternatives need to be considered in skeletally immature patient. These include expandable prostheses and limb lengthening via distraction osteogenesis.

PALLIATIVE THERAPY FOR ADVANCED OSTEOSARCOMA

Advanced bone OS has two distinct clinical forms: it may be either locally advanced or metastatic in various organs.

Locally advanced OS usually necessitates a life-threatening or highly mutilating surgical procedure. The symptoms might include severe pain, sepsis, tumor fungation, hemorrhage, thrombosis, pathologic fractures, radiation-induced necrosis and severe functional impairment. The tumor tends to be chemoresistant and requires salvage amputation for a potential cure and, even after radical amputation, metastases are common [52].

Diffuse metastatic OS is usually regarded as an incurable condition that requires palliation. Metastatic disease may be the first presentation but is usually a late evolutionary phase of a formerly localized tumor that failed to respond to induction chemotherapy, limb-sparing surgery and adjuvant chemotherapy [52].

Numerous drug combinations have been assessed in treated and untreated metastatic disease. The most effective of these contained cisplatin, doxorubicin and high dose methotrexate plus leukovorin either as a two- or three-drug regimen.

Radiation therapy can be used as second-line palliative approach because it has a limited role in the management of OS due to the relative tumor radioresistance and the need for large dose of radiation (>70Gy) to achieve clinical response.

As second-line palliative approach, it is common practice to prescribe the same agents that were used for induction but with a higher dose. For example, doxorubicin can be administered in higher dose in association to cardioxane, a cardioprotector agent. High dose methotrexate and folinic acid rescue is commonly used for metastatic OS, but this approach is associated with substantial morbidity because of renal toxicity. Ifosfamide may be given as a single agent or in combination with etoposide.

Amputation surgery is generally not performed in advanced disease, but according to Malawer et al. [53] there are some indications that are: involvement of the proximal limb or a major joint, accompanied by intractable pain, sepsis, tumor fungation, hemorrhage, vascular thrombosis, pathologic fractures, radiation-induced necrosis; or a limb with severe functional impairment.

Pulmonary metastasectomy should be considered in patients with four or fewer pulmonary nodules, unilateral pulmonary metastases or longer intervals between primary tumor resection and metastases.

Radiotherapy

Radiotherapy along with surgical resection is generally used to treat lesions situated in inaccessible sites. Preoperative radiotherapy could be given before surgery to increase the success rates of limb-amputation techniques and reduce the risk of tumor recurrence. High-dose photon irradiation (50-70 Gy) can be used in combination with aggressive chemotherapy when tumors are located in inaccessible sites such as the pelvic bone, vertebral column and base of the skull. This irradiation is also useful in patients who do not consent to surgery [54].

An innovative approach of carrying out intraoperative extracorporeal irradiation to the bone was recommended by Anacak et al. [55]. The affected bone was irradiated at 50 Gy and was then reimplanted into the body. No local recurrence or symptoms or graft failures were observed in the irradiated bone during follow-up.

Prognosis

The most important prognostic factor at diagnosis is the presence of clinically detectable metastases, which confers an unfavorable prognosis [56]. The histologic response to induction chemotherapy is the second prognostic factor but cannot be assessed at the time of the diagnosis. The third important prognostic factor is represented by the site of the primary tumor, with axial lesions having an inferior outcome [57]. Also serum LDH and alkaline phosphatase levels correlate with outcome [10, 58].

Other Histotypes

Teleangiectatic Osteosarcoma

This is the second variety of OS (about 6% of all OS). It's completely osteolytic, with a sponge-like structure filled of blood, a scarce, immature osteogenesis. Sex, age and localization are the same as in classic OS.

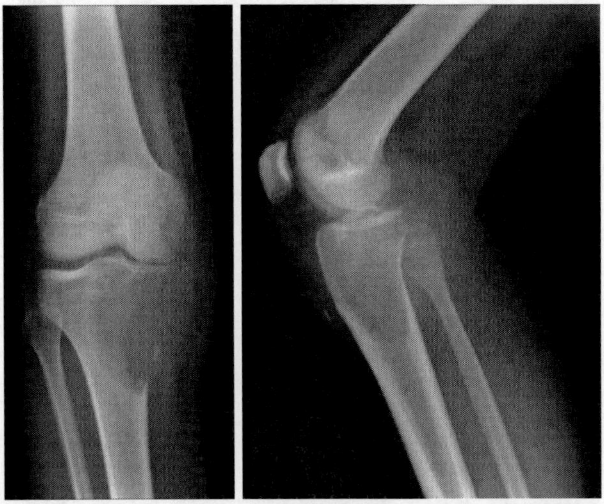

Figure 15. Teleangiectatic OS of the proximal tibia in a 20 year-old girl.

Clinically it has an aggressive course, usually staged IIB. Imaging shows an osteolytic lesion with ill-defined limits and fluid levels (Figure 15). Treatment and prognosis are the same as for classic OS. Some data suggest that response to preoperative chemotherapy is particularly good, which can be explained by the rich vascularity of the tumor.

Secondary Osteosarcoma

These OS occur in cartilage tumors (dedifferentiated chondrosarcoma), Paget's disease, fibrous dysplasia, bone infarct, GCT, chronic osteomyelitis, radiated bone and exceptionally non-ossifying fibroma [2]. Most of cases are observed in advanced age (Figure 16).

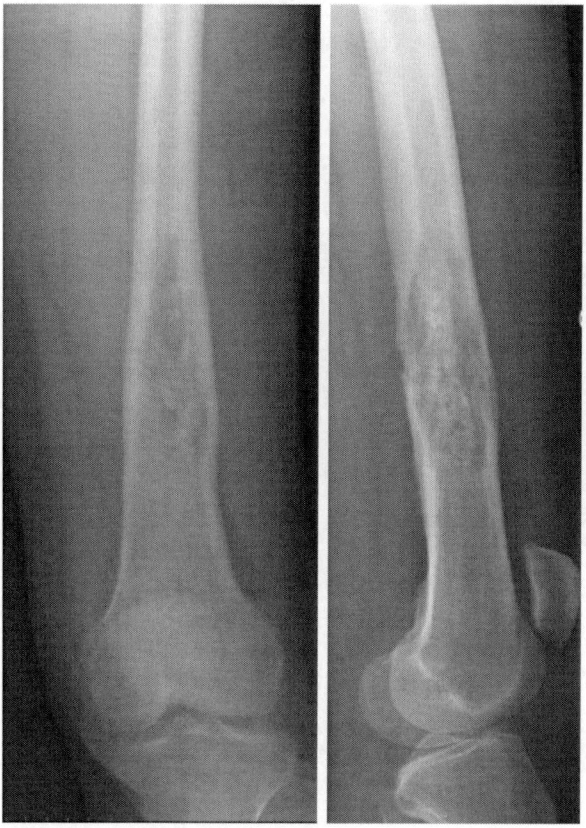

Figure 16. Secondary OS of the distal femur in a 59 year-old man.

Treatment is the same as for classic OS, except for the fact that the patient age often contraindicates the use of chemotherapy. In this group we usually used EUROBOSS protocol (European Bone Over 40 Sarcoma Study), that is a combination of cisplatin, ifosfamide, doxorubicin and high dose of methotrexate only in poor responders. Prognosis is generally worse as compared to primary OS.

Small Cell Osteosarcoma

This is a very rare variety (1-2% of all OS). Clinical presentation and imaging are not different from usual OS. Histologically, the tumor is composed by small cells, similar to Ewing's sarcoma, but producing bone (and sometimes cartilage) matrix and without the immunohistochemical positivity to Ewing's specific antibodies. The prognosis is worse as compared to classic OS.

High Grade Osteosarcoma of the Surface

Very rarely a high grade OS presents at the bony surface, with minimal involvement of the underlying cortex. Apart from this, it does not differ from usual intramedullary OS in age, site and histology. Imaging shows mixed non-mineralized and mineralized tumor matrix and some degree of periosteal reactive osteogenesis, but not the features specific of periosteal or parosteal OS. Treatment and prognosis does not differ from classic OS.

Periosteal Osteosarcoma

It is a predominantly chondroblastic OS of intermediate malignancy, originating from the periosteum usually in long bone diaphyses. It is rare (1-2% of all OS), it has preference for male sex with a wide range of distribution, with prevalence in the second decade of life. The imaging shows a periosteal, fusiform, radiolucent mass, with well-defined borders (Figure 17). It usually contains speculated radiodensities perpendicular to the cortex that is either intact or superficially eroded, sometimes with a Codman's triangle. Typically, the medullary canal is uninvolved.

The tumor tissue is mainly chondroblastic, being more cellular at the periphery, more chondroid at the centre of the lobuli. Lace-like osteoid among malignant osteoblasts is present, and defines this tumor as OS. It generally grows slower than classic OS, but much less slow than parosteal OS. Treatment consists of en bloc resection with wide margins. Metastases have been observed in about 15% of cases. Therefore, prognosis is good, after wide surgery and without chemotherapy. Cesari et al. [59] reported the Rizzoli Institute's experience with periosteal osteosarcoma, with a ten-year overall survival rate of 84% in a series in which all patients but one were managed with resection. The overall survival rate for patients managed with chemotherapy and resection did not differ from that for patients managed with resection alone.

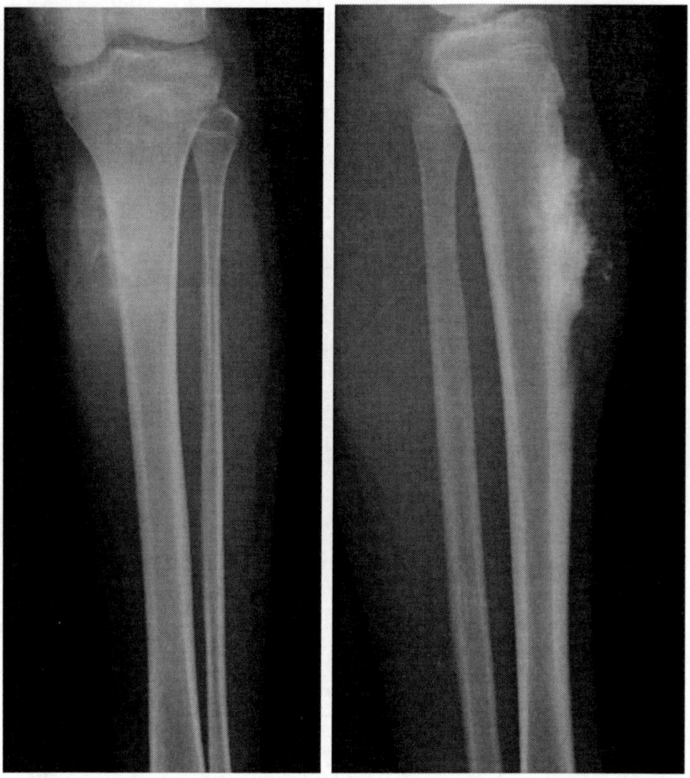

Figure 17. Periosteal OS of the proximal tibia in 17 year-old boy.

PAROSTEAL OSTEOSARCOMA

This OS originates at the surface of the bone, with abundant production of dense bone and low-grade anaplasia. It is infrequent (5-6% of all OS) with slight preference for female sex. Usually it appears between 20 and 50 years.

Almost exclusive of the long bones, it originates from the metaphysis. The most typical site of origin is the distal metaphysis of the femur in its posterior aspect (60% of cases).

Clinically it's often asymptomatic, with a bony hard mass. Duration of symptoms can be 1-2 years or even 5 years.

Due to slow growth, parosteal OS is usually seen when it's large. It is a lobulated mass of osseous radiodensity, fused to the cortex with a broad base of implant. Towards the diaphysis, the medullary canal is usually not involved.

From a histological point of view, parosteal OS is composed by spindle cells and collagen fibers embedding osseous trabeculae, generally not bordered by osteoclasts (differential diagnosis with fibrous dysplasia). Bone matrix is formed by metaplasia from tumor cells and trabeculae are not rimmed by osteoblasts. The majority of parosteal OS is grade 1 or 2 but it may progress in malignancy and transform into high-grade OS.

The course is usually slow. The stage is IA or IB. Treatment of choice is represented by surgical excision with wide margins and without chemotherapy. Hemicylindric resection is usually possible in the popliteal region, through a double approach (medial and lateral). More often, a complete segmental resection of the affected bone is needed. Metastases may be present in grade 2.

In rare cases, the presence of lytic areas at imaging can be found and it corresponds to a possible dedifferentiation. Dedifferentiated parosteal OS is as malignant as classic OS.

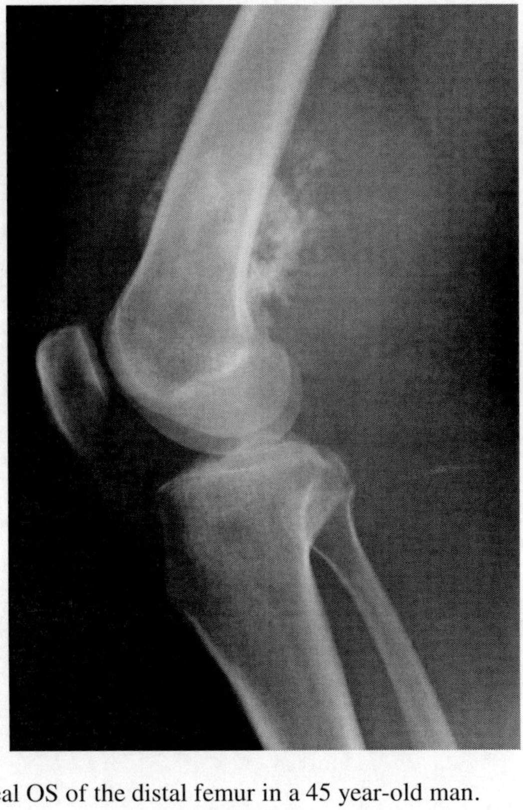

Figure 18. Parosteal OS of the distal femur in a 45 year-old man.

CENTRAL LOW-GRADE OSTEOSARCOMA

It is an intramedullary, bone producing tumor with a low-grade (1-2) of anaplasia. It has been suggested to represent the counterpart of parosteal OS.

It's rare (2-3% of all OS) and without no prevalence for sex. Age ranges from 10 to 70 years, with a mean age around 30 years. Preferred site are long bones, particularly distal femur and proximal tibia. It is usually centered in the metaphysis.

Clinical course is often of long duration due to mild pain and moderate swelling. Imaging shows a lytic or sclerotic lesion with in some cases well-defined borders. In half of the cases a soft tissue mass can be present.

From a histological point of view the tumor is composed of spindle cells producing collagen and bone. The tumor closely mimics the histological pattern of parosteal OS.

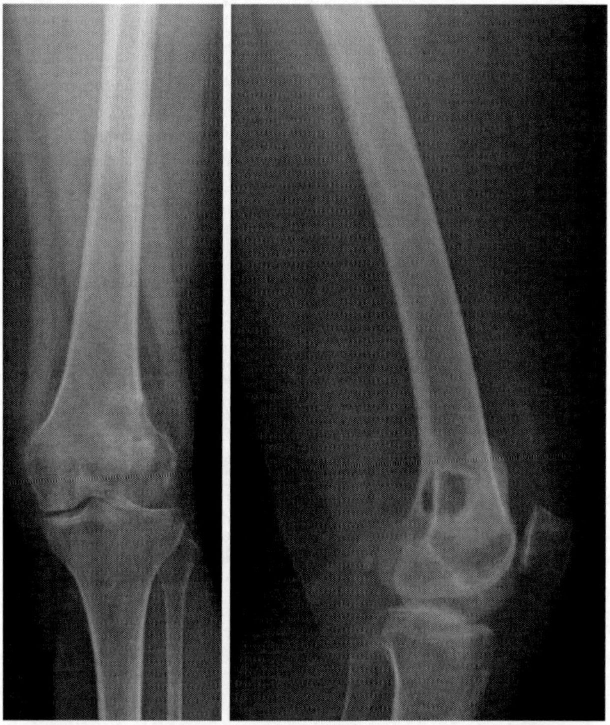

Figure 19. Central low-grade OS of the distal femur in a 45 year-old woman.

When osteogenesis is scarce, the tumor is similar to desmoid tumor and low-grade fibrosarcoma. The cells demonstrate slight atypia with few mitotic figures. The grade is either 1 or 2. The course is slow. In 15% of patients the tumor shows a progression of malignancy, transforming into high-grade OS. The stage is IA or IB.

Treatment of choice is represented by surgical resection of the affected bone segment with wide margins and without chemotherapy. Metastases to the lungs are reported in 10% of cases, and mostly in tumors that progressed in malignancy. Prognosis is good, unless the tumor becomes a high-grade OS.

REFERENCES

[1] Campanacci Mario. Bone and soft tissue tumors. Piccin editore, 1999.

[2] Biazzo A., Errani C., Gambarotti M., De Paolis M., Donati D. M., Giannini S. Spindle cell sarcoma of bone arising from a non-ossifying fibroma: a case report. *Journal of Clinical Orthopaedics and Trauma,* 2013 June;4(2):80-84.

[3] Dahlin D. C., Coventry M. B. Osteogenic sarcoma. A study of six hundred cases. *J. Bone Joint Surg. Am.*, 1967 Jan.;49(1):101-10.

[4] Estrada-Aguilar J., Greenberg H., Walling A., Schroer K., Black T., Morse S. et al. Primary treatment of pelvic osteosarcoma. Report of five cases. *Cancer*, 1992 Mar. 1;69(5):1137-45.

[5] Rizzoli Syllabus. Atlas of musculoskeletal tumors and tumorlike lesions. Bologna, 2011-2012.

[6] Gillespy T. 3rd, Manfrini M., Ruggieri P., Spanier S. S., Pettersson H., Springfield D. S. Staging of intraosseous extent of osteosarcoma: correlation of preoperative CT and MR imaging with pathologic macroslides. Radiology, 1988 Jun.;167(3):765-7.

[7] Panicek D. M., Gatsonis C., Rosenthal D. I., Seeger L. L., Huvos A. G., Moore S. G. et al. CT and MR imaging in the local staging of primary malignant musculoskeletal neoplasms: Report of the Radiology Diagnostic Oncology Group. *Radiology,* 1997 Jan.;202(1):237-46.

[8] Enneking W. F. A system of staging musculoskeletal neoplasms. *Clin. Orthop. Relat. Res.*, 1986 Mar.;(204):9-24.

[9] Kaste S. C., Pratt C. B., Cain A. M., Jones-Wallace D. J., Rao B. N. Metastases detected at the time of diagnosis of primary pediatric extremity osteosarcoma at diagnosis: imaging features. *Cancer,* 1999 Oct. 15;86(8):1602-8.

[10] Link M. P., Goorin A. M., Miser A. W., Green A. A., Pratt C. B., Belasco J. B. et al. The effect of adjuvant chemotherapy on relapse-free survival in patients with osteosarcoma of the extremity. *N. Engl. J. Med.*, 1986 Jun. 19;314(25):1600-6.

[11] Fitzgerald R. H. Jr., Dahlin D. C., Sim F. H. Multiple metachronous osteogenic sarcoma. Report of twelve cases with two long-term survivors. *J. Bone Joint Surg. Am.*, 1973 Apr.;55(3):595-605.

[12] Errani C., Sung Y. S., Zhang L., Healey J. H., Antonescu C. R. Monoclonality of multifocal epithelioid hemangioendothelioma of the liver by analysis of WWTR1-CAMTA1 breakpoints. *Cancer Genet.*, 2012 Jan.-Feb.;205(1-2):12-7.

[13] Meyers P. A., Gorlick R. Osteosarcoma. *Pediatr. Clin. North Am.*, 1997 Aug.; 44(4):973-89.

[14] McKillop J. H., Etcubanas E., Goris M. L. The indications for and limitations of bone scintigraphy in osteogenic sarcoma: a review of 55 patients. *Cancer,* 1981 Sep. 1;48(5):1133-8.

[15] Enneking W. F., Kagan A. "Skip" metastases in osteosarcoma. *Cancer*, 1975 Dec.;36(6):2192-205.

[16] Neifeld J. P., Michaelis L. L., Doppman J. L. Suspected pulmonary metastases: correlation of chest x-ray, whole lung tomograms, and operative findings. *Cancer,* 1977 Feb.;39(2):383-7.

[17] Raymond A. K., Ayala A. G., Knuutila S. Conventional osteosarcoma. In: Kleihues P., Sobin L., Fletcher C. et al., eds. WHO Classification of Tumours: Pathology and Genetics of Tumours of Soft Tissue and Bone. Lyon, France:IARC Press, 2002:264-270.

[18] Marina N., Gebhardt M., Teot L., Gorlick R. Biology and therapeutic advances for pediatric osteosarcoma. *Oncologist,* 2004;9(4):422-41.

[19] Weatherby R. P., Dahlin D. C., Ivins J. C. Postradiation sarcoma of bone: review of 78 Mayo Clinic cases. *Mayo. Clin. Proc.*, 1981 May;56(5):294-306.

[20] Lane D. P. Cancer. P53, guardian of the genome. *Nature,* 1992;358: 15-16.

[21] Huang H. J., Yee J. K., Shew J. Y., Chen P. L., Bookstein R., Friedmann T. et al. Suppression of the neoplastic phenotype by replacement of the RB gene in human cancer cells. *Science,* 1988 Dec. 16;242(4885): 1563-6.

[22] Miller C. W., Aslo A., Tsay C., Slamon D., Ishizaki K., Toguchida J. et al. Frequency and structure of p53 rearrangements in human osteosarcoma. *Cancer Res.*, 1990 Dec. 15;50(24):7950-4.

[23] Harley C. B. Telomere loss: mitotic clock or genetic time bomb? Mutat. Res., 1991 Mar.-Nov.;256(2-6):271-82.

[24] Shay J. W., Bacchetti S. A survey of telomerase activity in human cancer. Eur. J. Cancer, 1997 Apr.;33(5):787-91.

[25] Sangiorgi L., Gobbi G. A., Lucarelli E., Sartorio S. M., Mordenti M., Ghedini I., Maini V., Scrimieri F., Reggiani M., Bertoja A. Z., Benassi M. S., Picci P. Presence of telomerase activity in different musculoskeletal tumor histotypes and correlation with aggressiveness. Int. J. Cancer, 2001 May 20;95(3):156-61.

[26] Friedlaender G. E., Mitchell M. S. A virally induced osteosarcoma in rats. A model for immunological studies of human osteosarcoma. *J. Bone Joint Surg. Am.*, 1976 Apr.;58(3):295-302.

[27] Eilber F., Giuliano A., Eckardt J., Patterson K., Moseley S., Goodnight J. Adjuvant chemotherapy for osteosarcoma: a randomized prospective trial. *J. Clin. Oncol.*, 1987 Jan.;5(1):21-6.

[28] Edmonson J. H., Green.S. J., Ivins J. C., Gilchrist G. S., Creagan E. T., Pritchard D. J. et al. A controlled pilot study of high-dose methotrexate as postsurgical adjuvant treatment for primary osteosarcoma. J. Clin. Oncol., 1984 Mar.;2(3):152-6.

[29] Rosen G., Murphy M. L., Huvos A. G., Gutierrez M., Marcove R. C. Chemotherapy, en bloc resection, and prosthetic bone replacement in the treatment of osteogenic sarcoma. *Cancer,* 1976 Jan.;37(1):1-11.

[30] Goorin A. M., Schwartzentruber D. J., Devidas M., Gebhardt M. C., Ayala A. G., Harris M. B. et al. Presurgical chemotherapy compared with immediate surgery and adjuvant chemotherapy for nonmetastatic osteosarcoma: Pediatric Oncology Group Study POG-8651. *J. Clin. Oncol.*, 2003 Apr. 15;21(8):1574-80.

[31] Rosen G., Marcove R. C., Caparros B., Nirenberg A., Kosloff C., Huvos A. G. Primary osteogenic sarcoma: the rationale for preoperative chemotherapy and delayed surgery. *Cancer,* 1979 Jun.;43(6):2163-77.

[32] Fuchs N., Bielack S. S., Epler D., Bieling P., Delling G., Körholz D., Graf N., Heise U., Jürgens H., Kotz R., Salzer-Kuntschik M., Weinel P.,Werner M., Winkler K. Long-term results of the co-operative German-Austrian-Swiss osteosarcoma study group's protocol COSS-86 of intensive multidrug chemotherapy and surgery for osteosarcoma of the limbs. *Ann. Oncol.*, 1998 Aug.;9(8):893-9.

[33] Bacci G., Picci P., Ferrari S., Ruggieri P., Casadei R.,.Tienghi A. et al. Primary chemotherapy and delayed surgery for nonmetastatic osteosarcoma of the extremities. Results in 164 patients preoperatively

treated with high doses of methotrexate followed by cisplatin and doxorubicin. Cancer, 1993 Dec. 1;72(11):3227-38.

[34] Marina N., Bielack S., Whelan J., Smeland S., Krailo M., Sydes M. R., et al. International collaboration is feasible in trials for rare conditions: the EURAMOS experience. *Cancer Treat. Res.*, 2009;152:339-53.

[35] Bacci G., Briccoli A., Ferrari S., Saeter G., Donati D.,.Longhi A. et al. Neoadjuvant chemotherapy for osteosarcoma of the extremities with synchronous lung metastases: treatment with cisplatin, adriamycin and high dose of methotrexate and ifosfamide. *Oncol. Rep.*, 2000 Mar.-Apr.;7(2):339-46.

[36] Kager L., Zoubek A., Pötschger U., Kastner U., Flege S., Kempf-Bielack B. et al. Primary metastatic osteosarcoma: presentation and outcome of patients treated on neoadjuvant Cooperative Osteosarcoma Study Group protocols. *J. Clin. Oncol.*, 2003 May 15;21(10):2011-8.

[37] Brock P. R., Bellman S. C., Yeomans E. C., Pinkerton C. R., Pritchard J. Cisplatin ototoxicity in children: a practical grading system. *Med. Pediatr. Oncol.*, 1991;19(4):295-300.

[38] Hayes F. A., Green A. A., Senzer N., Pratt C. B. Tetany: a complication of cis-dichlorodiammineplatinum(II) therapy. *Cancer Treat. Rep.*, 1979 Apr.; 63(4):547-8.

[39] Krischer J. P., Epstein S., Cuthbertson D. D., Goorin A. M., Epstein M. L., Lipshultz S. E. Clinical cardiotoxicity following anthracycline treatment for childhood cancer: the Pediatric Oncology Group experience. J. Clin. Oncol., 1997 Apr.;15(4):1544-52.

[40] Wexler L. H., Andrich M. P., Venzon D., Berg S. L., Weaver-McClure L., Chen C. C. et al. Randomized trial of the cardioprotective agent ICRF-187 in pediatric sarcoma patients treated with doxorubicin. *J. Clin. Oncol.*, 1996 Feb.;14(2):362-72.

[41] Lord C. F., Gebhardt M. C., Tomford W. W., Mankin H. J. Infection in bone allografts. Incidence, nature, and treatment. *J. Bone Joint Surg. Am.*, 1988 Mar.;70(3):369-76.

[42] Gebhardt M. C., Jaffe K., Mankin H. J. Bone allografts for tumors and other reconstructions in children. In: Langlais F., Tomeno E., eds. Limb Salvage-Major Reconstructions in Oncologic and Nontumoral Conditions. Berlin, Germany:Springer-Verlag, 1991:561-572.

[43] Manfrini M. The role of vascularized fibula in skeletal reconstructions. *Chir. Organi. Mov.*, 2003 Apr.-Jun.; 88(2):137-42.

[44] Grimer R. J., Belthur M., Carter S. R., Tillman R. M., Cool P. Extendible replacements of the proximal tibia for bone tumours. *J. Bone Joint Surg. Br.*, 2000 Mar.;82(2):255-60.

[45] McDonald D. J., Capanna R., Gherlinzoni F., Bacci G., Ferruzzi A., Casadei R. et al. Influence of chemotherapy on perioperative complications in limb salvage surgery for bone tumors. *Cancer,* 1990 Apr. 1;65(7):1509-16.

[46] Malawer M. M., Chou L. B. Prosthetic survival and clinical results with use of large-segment replacements in the treatment of high-grade bone sarcomas. *J. Bone Joint Surg. Am.*, 1995 Aug.;77(8):1154-65.

[47] Hejna M. J., Gitelis S. Allograft prosthetic composite replacement for bone tumors. *Semin. Surg. Oncol.*, 1997 Jan.-Feb.;13(1):18-24.

[48] Donati D., Di Bella C., Frisoni T., Cevolani L., DeGroot H. Alloprosthetic composite is a suitable reconstruction after periacetabular tumor resection. *Clin. Orthop. Relat. Res.*, 2011;469:1450-1458.

[49] Delloye C., Banse X., Brichard B., Docquier P. L., Cornu O. Pelvic reconstruction with a structural pelvic allograft after resection of a malignant bone tumor. *J. Bone Joint Surg. Am.,* 2007;89:579-587.

[50] Bell R. S., Davis A. M., Wunder J. S., Buconjic T., McGoveran B., Gross A. E. Allograft reconstruction of the acetabulum after resection of stage IIB sarcoma. Intermediate-term results. *J. Bone Joint Surg. Am.,* 1997;79:1663-74.

[51] Guest C. B., Bell R. S., Davis A., Langer F., Ling H., Gross E. et al. Allograft-implant composite reconstruction following periacetabular sarcoma resection. *J. Arthroplasty*, 1990;5 Suppl:S25-34.

[52] Merimsky O., Kollender Y., Inbar M., Meller I., Bickels J. Palliative treatment for advanced or metastatic osteosarcoma. *Isr. Med. Assoc. J.*, 2004 Jan.;6(1):34-8.

[53] Malawer M. M., Buch R. G., Thompson W. E., Sugarbarker P. H. Major amputations done with palliative intent in the treatment of local bony complications associated with advanced cancer. *J. Surg. Oncol.,* 1991;47:121-30.

[54] Dai X., Ma W., He X., Jha R. K. Review of therapeutic strategies for osteosarcoma, chondrosarcoma, and Ewing's sarcoma. *Med. Sci. Monit.*, 2011 Aug.;17(8):RA177-190.

[55] Anacak Y., Sabah D., Demirci S., Kamer S. Intraoperative extracorporeal irradiation and re-implantation of involved bone for the treatment of musculoskeletal tumors. *J. Exp. Clin. Cancer Res.,* 2007;26:571-74.

[56] Bielack S. S., Kempf-Bielack B., Delling G., Exner G. U., Flege S., Helmke K. et al. Prognostic factors in high-grade osteosarcoma of the extremities or trunk: an analysis of 1,702 patients treated on neoadjuvant cooperative osteosarcoma study group protocols. *J. Clin. Oncol.*, 2002 Feb. 1;20(3):776-90.

[57] Ozaki T., Flege S., Kevric M., Lindner N., Maas R., Delling G. et al. Osteosarcoma of the pelvis: experience of the Cooperative Osteosarcoma Study Group. *J. Clin. Oncol.*, 2003 Jan. 15;21(2):334-41.

[58] Levine A. M., Rosenberg S. A. Alkaline phosphatase levels in osteosarcoma tissue are related to prognosis. Cancer, 1979 Dec.;44(6):2291-3.

[59] Cesari M, Alberghini M, Vanel D, Palmerini E, Staals EL, Longhi A, et al. Periosteal osteosarcoma: a single-institution experience. Cancer. 2011 Apr 15;117(8):1731-5.

In: Osteosarcoma
Editors: Edwin Choy
ISBN: 978-1-63321-052-3

Chapter 2

SURGICAL TREATMENT OF OSTEOSARCOMA IN THE EXTREMITIES

Santiago A. Lozano-Calderón, M.D., Ph.D.
Department of Orthopaedic Surgery, Musculoskeletal Oncology Service, Massachusetts General Hospital, Harvard Medical School, Boston, MA, US

ABSTRACT

Treatment of osteosarcoma of the extremities is challenging. The introduction of adjuvant and neoadjuvant chemotherapy has been crucial in improving patient survival. However, local control is also key for cure. With the advent of better imaging, earlier detection and chemotherapy protocols, local control and survival rates of patients undergoing to limb-preserving surgery are comparable to those receiving amputation but with improved functional outcome. Currently, 80 to 90% of patients with osteosarcomas of the extremities undergo limb-salvage surgery.

The following is a review of the history and development of surgical treatment for local control of osteosarcoma of the extremities. A particular emphasis is given to the goals of surgical treatment and preoperative planning. Subsequent discussion of the different modalities of treatment is done through this chapter, analyzing the indications, pitfalls, outcomes and complications of different surgical treatment options including amputation, rotationplasty and limb-sparing surgery.

There is no surgical standard treatment for all patients, but there is a best treatment for each individual patient. It is the surgeon's duty to select the surgical treatment alternative that will benefit the patient the most.

The physician should approach this decision making holistically, taking into consideration biological, technical, demographic, functional and psychosocial variables.

HISTORY OF SURGICAL TREATMENT

The term sarcoma derives from the Greek Sarx, which means flesh. [1] The term "osteosarcoma" was introduced first by Alexis Boyer (1757-1833).[2] The first large clinico-pathological correlation of bone sarcomas (165 cases) was by Samuel Weissel Gross in 1879. [3] He noticed the tendency of these tumors to spread haematogenously to the lung, the occurrence of "skip areas" and the low incidence of local lymphatic involvement. Because of the presence of these "skip lesions", Weissel Gross recommended amputation at a high level for successful treatment. [3]

In 1940, Albert Ferguson [4] reported 258 cases of osteogenic sarcoma treated by amputation taken from the American Bone Sarcoma Registry, this investigation was for many years the main determinant of sarcoma treatment [4]. In his series, he reported a survival rate of 8% when the amputation was performed within 6 months of diagnosis vs. 28% when performed 6 months after. Therefore, he recommended local control before definitive amputation including modalities of treatment such as radiation therapy, tumor excision and implantation of bone grafts [4]. Many challenged Ferguson's findings as it was considered that patients surviving longer than 6 months could potentially have a diagnosis different than osteosarcoma [5]. MacDonald and Budd [5] among others shared this view. In 1943, both authors reported that only 18% of the 118 five-year survivors in the American Bone Sarcoma Registry actually had bone-producing sarcomas [6]; almost 80% of the cases appeared to be fibrosarcomas or chondrosarcomas. Other authors such as Coley and Harold reported similar findings in 1950. [7]

Part of the confusion in determining the proper treatment originated from the lack of consensus definining osteosarcoma. [8] Some considering tumors producing bone osteosarcomas [5, 9-14] whereas others give the term to different tumors arising from bone. [6, 8, 15] Optimal treatment remained controversial until the early 1970s.

Primary surgical ablation was recommended by many authors. [9, 11, 16-19] However, due to high mortality rates, many proposed high-dose radiation plus/minus delayed surgery. [20-24] In 1955 Cade et al. [20], reported their outcomes with 70 to 90 Gy of radiation followed by 6 months of observation and delayed amputation if pulmonary metastasis did not developed in that period of observation. With this approach, ablative surgery was avoided in patients with poor prognosis. This modality of treatment became the standard in different countries including the Netherlands and the UK. [12, 24, 25] Some suggested this approach (only with radiation) to be curative. [22, 26] However, the main limitation of this protocol was the lack of local control. The majority of these patients developed chronic pain, pathological fractures, significant functional limitation, tumor fungation and chronic depression among other complications. [6, 21, 23, 27, 28] Most of these tended to occur months before metastasic pulmonary disease developed. Therefore, amputation was used as a palliation treatment. Furthermore, additional investigations demonstrated subsequently that radiation with delayed amputation did not improve the 5-year survival rates when compared to immediate amputation. Survival rates were even lower with radiation alone. [9, 11, 12, 19, 23, 27-31]

The overall 5-year survival rate in patients with non-metastasic osteosarcoma of the extremities at that time was between 15 to 20%. [5, 9, 10, 12, 16, 19, 23, 28-34] These poor rates suggested that 80% of the patients had microscopically disseminated disease at the time of surgery. [34] Even though early and radical surgery proved to be essential for local control, it proved to be insufficient for systemic treatment and subsequent cure. Most of these patients died of pulmonary metastasis and evident recurrent disease. [5, 10, 16, 28, 30]

In the early 1970's, the introduction of effective chemotherapy changed the course of the disease increasing the overall and disease free survival. In 1972 Cortes reported tumor regression in metastatic disease of the lungs in 41% of patients with osteosarcoma treated with Adriamycin. [35] In the same year Jaffe reported similar response (40%) in children treated with Methotrexate. [36] Since then chemotherapy was developed and evaluated in structured clinical research. Multiple investigations contributed to the current protocol of adjuvant and neoadjuvant chemotherapy combined with surgery, which has improved the survival rates up to 70% at 5 years. [37-40] Protocols using mainly four medications: Doxorubicin, cisplatin, Ifosfamide and high-dose Methotrexate, have proved in non-randomized studies to improve the percentage of patients suitable for limb-sparing surgery. [41, 42] Recent literature reports that 80% of patients who present with osteosarcoma of the extremities are candidates for limb-salvage surgery. [41, 42] Multiple single institution investigations have not found differences in terms of survival and recurrence in patients treated with amputations vs. those treated with limb salvage. [42-50]

GOALS OF SURGERY FOR OSTEOSARCOMA OF THE EXTREMITIES

The main goal of surgery when treating osteosarcoma in the extremities is to obtain local control of the disease. This implies an en bloc resection with tumor-free or negative margins. The ideal is a wide margin in which there are no tumor cells at the cut surface of the resected specimen. The resection should be out of the reactive tumor zone. (Figure 1).

The resection with satisfactory margins can be achieved through an amputation or a limb sparing procedure. As mesntioned before, different retrospective investigations have not demonstrated survival advantage of amputations over limb reconstruction. [42-50] Limb salvage surgery is more common now days as preoperative chemotherapy decreases peritumoral edema and increases mineralization of the mass, facilitating or making more feasible en bloc resections that allow subsequent reconstruction. [51]

The second objective of the surgery is to provide the best possible functional extremity to the patient based on the severity of the disease and functional necessities of each particular patient.

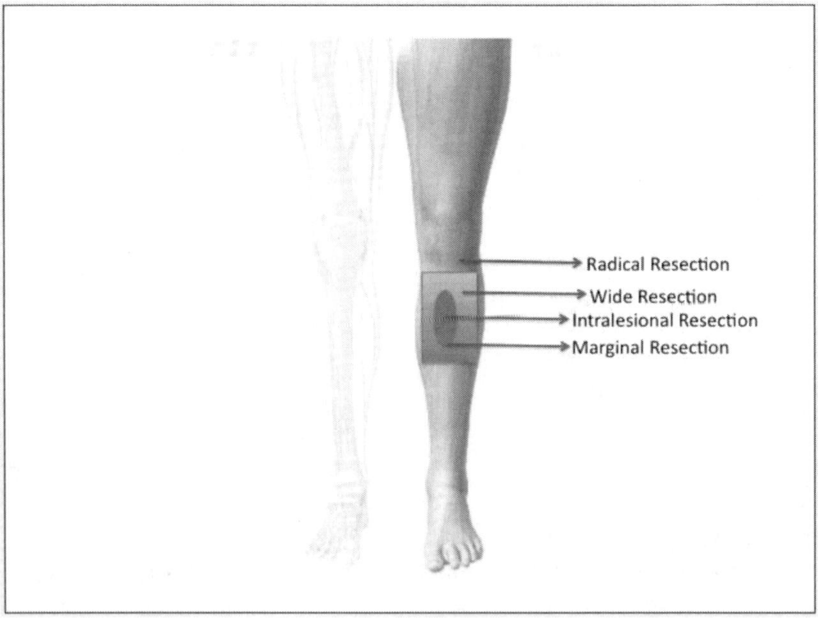

Figure 1. Margins of resection for tumor management.

It is key to have a detailed pre-operative conversation with the patient and assess his/her necessities and expectations in relation to the surgery. The patient and family should understand that the main and most important surgical objective is local control; function is secondary. The surgeon should be careful in not sacrificing a good margin aiming for possibly better function.

After the resection (amputation or limb-sparing surgery), comes the reconstruction. There are different alternatives in terms of prosthetics for patients who had undergone amputation. The variety of reconstruction techniques also applies to limb-sparing surgery in which allografts, metallic-endoprosthesis, allograft-prosthetic composites and rotationplasty are the main techniques.

In some cases, the tumor is located in a bone that is expendible (g.e. proximal or diaphyseal fibula, clavicle, ribs). In that case scenario, reconstruction is not necessary. (Figure 2)

The following sections describe different surgical techniques that musculoskeletal orthopaedic surgeons use for the treatment and local control of osteosarcoma, following the principles described above.

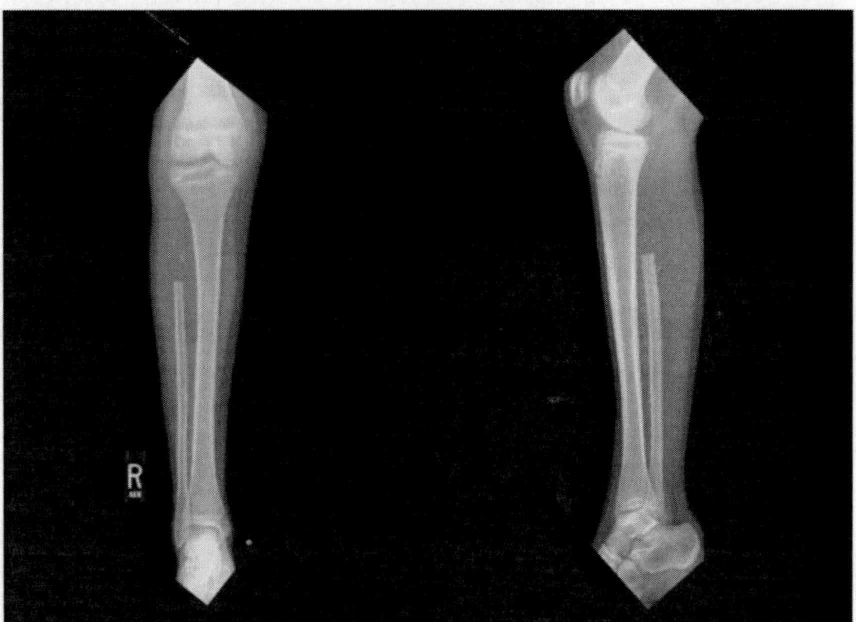

Courtesy of Francis Hornicek, MD, PhD.

Figure 2. AP and lateral radiographic views of a 13 year-old female patient with fibulectomy proximal fibula for management of osteosarcoma.

Preoperative Planning

Preoperative planning is a key component of the surgery. It starts with the re-staging studies after the patient has completed preoperative chemotherapy. It is very important to review these studies as the modality of surgery may change. Additionally, a closer interaction with other specialties might be necessary, as local control may need to be combined with the treatment of metastatic disease in the lungs for example. Sometimes, these procedures can be performed under a single anesthesia event but it is very important to take into consideration the patient health status, the complexity of the procedures to be performed and the feasibility of both surgical teams interacting in a single surgery.

Imaging studies are vital in preoperative planning. Every patient should have orthogonal full-length radiographic views of the entire affected bone as well as an MRI with and without contrast. The MRI is very helpful in identifying "skip metastasis". These are important to identify in order to obtain adequate local control and avoid leaving viable tumor after not determining correctly, the extent of the disease. In addition, the MRI provides information about peritumoral edema as well as the location of vital neurovascular structures in relation to the tumor.

Anatomic evaluation of the surgical site should be performed using radiographs and the T1 sequences of the MRI. In cases where the osseous anatomy is intricate like in the pelvis, CT scans or CT angiographies may be needed. (Figure 3)

Especific Modalities of Surgical Treatment

Amputation

It is one of the most radical resections. However, still is susceptible to local tumor recurrence in the stump if there is disease spread inside the osseous medullar space or if there are skip metastasis that were no identified preoperatively at the level of the resection.

This modality of treatment is used less frequently as it was few decades ago. [52] With the advent of chemotherapy and better imaging studies, more patients are suitable for limb salvage surgery. Functional outcome after amputation in the lower extremities is quite good with modern prostheses.

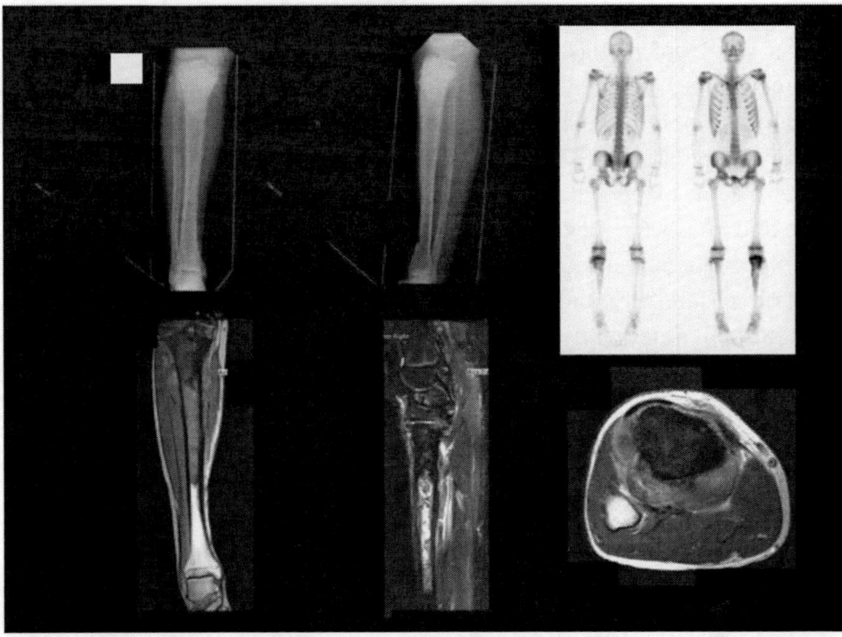

Courtesy of Mark Gebhardt, MD.

Figure 3. Proximal tibia osteosarcoma, Radiographic [1,2], MRI [3,4, 5] and bone scan [6] studies. MRI images T1 sequence for surgical planning.

Most patients can perform well even in many athletic activities in addition to the daily activity baseline. Results in the upper extremity are not as good as current prostheses are very limited in replacing hand function. [53] This occurs even with myoelectric prosthesis.

Common indications for amputation include tumor location affecting vital neurovascular structures for function and viability, tumor progression during chemotherapy, tumor recurrence and failure of limb reconstruction. [54]

Oncologic principles for this modality of treatment include adequate surgical margin in bone and soft-tissue. However, the skin and soft-tissue flaps should be planned and fashioned to obtain the longest residual limb as this will decrease the energy expenditure and improve functional outcome. Contrary to the non-oncologic amputations where the flaps are generally symmetric and uniform (g.e. fish-mouth, posterior or anterior based flaps), flaps in oncologic amputation are not conventional as they need to be modified according to the location of the tumor, presence of previous incisions or fungating masses, extend of edema, etc. It is key to consider and be aware of the vasculature of the patient pre-operatively. Most relevant pitfalls to avoid complications such as dehiscence or necrosis of the closing wound include transection of the muscle at the level of the skin and distal to the level of the osteotomy cut; Soft-tissue flaps should cover the osteotomy site with minimal tension; Lastly, the remaining bone in the residual limb should be smoothed to round edges in order to avoid pressure points when using a prosthesis. [54]

In terms of management of neurovascular structures, nerves should be isolated and dissected. They should be gently pulled into the wound and ligated. Subsequent transection with a cold scalpel over a flat surface should be performed carefully and as a single cut. Major vessels should be ligated with a double ligature with suture and/or clips.

Before final closure, adequate hemostasis should be achieved. Drains should be used to avoid hematoma formation if bleeding from the surgical bed is persistent. The exit point of any drain should be in line with the surgical incision.

Different pitfalls and recommendations are characteristic of each amputation/disarticulation depending on the level. Tables 1A and 1B are a summary of clinical characteristics, surgical pitfalls, functional outcome and energy expenditure at the upper and lower extremity respectively. Figure 4 describes the different levels of amputation in the upper and the lower extremity.

Reconstruction with prosthesis is very diverse and depends on many variables such as the level of amputation, age, co-morbidities and level of functionality of the patient. Table 2 is a summary of prosthetic modalities with their characteristics and indications for use.

Rotationplasty

This procedure was originally described in 1930 for the treatment of sequelae of tuberculosis affecting the bone such as knee ankylosis or limb shortening. [55] The also known Van Nes rotationplasty was later used as a treatment option in proximal femoral focal deficiency. [55, 56] The key concept in this surgical technique is to use the distal portion of the affected extremity to obtain a longer and more functional residual extremity. [55, 57, 58] Traditionally, the bone resection is done across the femur above the knee joint level. The remaining of the ipsilateral extremity is used to recreate a knee joint with the ankle joint. This is achieved by reattaching the distal extremity 180 degrees from the natural position. With this modality of surgery an above the knee amputation is converted to a below the knee amputation. [55]

This is advantageous when compared to an above the knee amputation as there is a longer lever arm that reduces the requirement of energy for ambulation, there is a knee joint, and there is a foot that tolerates better the socket than the stump in an above the knee amputation.

Functional outcome in activities of daily living and sports is satisfactory with this technique [59]. However, this is rarely used as a first option of treatment as more patients each year are candidates for limb-sparing surgery. There is also concern in terms of the psychological impact with this procedure. [58] Currently, the tendency is to use this as a salvage procedure. Figure 5 demonstrates a patient with osteosarcoma of the distal femur treated with a Van Nes Rotationplasty.

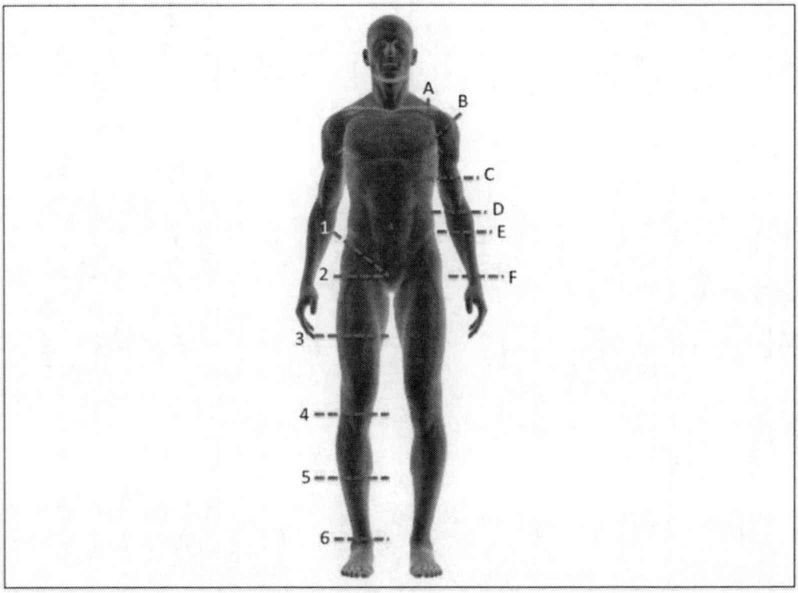

Figure 4. Levels of amputation for the upper and lower extremity. A: Forequarter Amputation upper extremity. B: Shoulder disarticulation. C: Transhumeral amputation (High and Low). D: Elbow disarticulation. E: Transradial Amputation. F: Wrist Disarticulation. 1: External hemipelvectomy. 2: Hip Disarticulation. 3: Above the knee amputation: (High/Medium and low transfemoral). 4: Knee Disarticulation. 5: Below the knee amputation: (High/medium and low transtibial amputation). 6: Syme amputation.

Table 1A.

Upper Extremity Amputations and Disarticulations			
Level	Indications	Pitfalls	Function and prostheses
Forequater Amputation	Brachial plexus involvement Direct extension to chest wall Glenohumeral joint involvement Pathologic fracture with significant displacement Poor biopsy technique	Lateral position Soft-tissue coverage is challenging May need coverage with free flap (fillet-technique) using tissue from distal portion of the amputated limb	No functional prosthesis available Cosmetic prosthesis for reconstruction of the shoulder profile Problems with balance during gait, and when standing or sitting
Shoulder Disarticulation	Involvement of the proximal humerus not affecting the glenohumeral joint Involvement of neurovascular bundle in the arm Diffuse involvement of soft tissue of the arm	Position in the lateral or supine position Preserve proximal musculature as much as possible	Cosmetic advantage over forequater amputation Preserve proximal musculature for myoelectric prosthesis Body-powered prosthesis are usually contraindicated
Above the elbow amputation Proximal Third Middle Third Distal Third	Tumors affecting the distal humerus/elbow Involvement of the neurovascular bundle Recurrent soft-tissue sarcoma Failed limb-salvage surgery	Position patient supine Try to maintain length in residual stump without sacrificing oncologic outcome Maintain muscle tension through myoplasty or myodesis	Proximal amputations function as shoulder disarticulations Distal amputations function as elbow dislocations Short arm amputations are not functional but offer good cosmetic result May use myoelectric or body-powered prosthesis The longer the residual stump the more effective energy scenario in body-powered prosthesis

Upper Extremity Amputations and Disarticulations			
Level	Indications	Pitfalls	Function and prostheses
Above the elbow amputation Proximal Third Middle Third Distal Third (Cont)		Myoplasty causes simultaneous co-contraction eliminating dual local muscle control Myodesis maintains isolated muscle contracture improving functional result as it preserves antagonistic muscle control	For transhumeral amputation prosthetic elbow center of rotation should match cotralateral elbow Humeral cut should be at least 5 cms shorter than elbow center of rotation to fit myoelectric prosthesis well In longer stumps suspended prosthesis above the elbow match very well contralateral center of rotation at the cost of cosmesis Function of prosthesis is limited.
Below the elbow amputation Proximal Third Middle Third Distal Third	Extensive soft-tissue tumors of the wrist or hand Masses affecting neurovascular bundle Recurrent tumors of the hands, wrist or distal forearm	Position patient supine Preserve ulnar and radial length but take into consideration size of myoelectric prosthesis if used. May use hand table	Myoelectric or body powered prosthesis can be used. Pronation and supination are lost in midlength and short trans-radial amputations Short transradial amputations need residual limb that can assist in carrying weight of the prosthesis Body-powered prosthesis may harnessed above the elbow using the distal humeral condyles
Wrist Disarticulation	Extensive soft tissue tumors of the hand	Place patient in the supine position Use hand table	Preferred over below the elbow amputation as pronation and supination can be maintained It has a better lever arm and increased power Prosthesis can be harnessed over distal styloid Wrist disarticulation prosthesis allow active pronation/supination Limb-length discrepancy can occur, some patients may prefer a higher amputation for cosmetic reason
Ray Amputations	Lesions confined in a metacarpal or within the finger in with phalanx or metarpal amputation may limit optimal function	Placed patient in the supine position Use a hand table Consider neurovascular structures	Offers good cosmetic result Amputation through carpal bone preserves wrist flexo/extension Bimanual activities can be performed without a prosthesis Prenhension can be achieved with a prosthesis Wrist prosthesis have an extra-articulation for hand placement in

Table 1A. (Continued)

Upper Extremity Amputations and Disarticulations			
Level	Indications	Pitfalls	Function and prostheses
Ray Amputations (Cont)		Try to maintain muscular balance May use index transposition to improve hand symmetry and function Do not use index transposition when: Manual labor Adductor pollicis resected with tumor In thumb and index amputation a post resection reconstruction is required	space For cosmetic reasons some patients may prefer wrist disarticulation Post reconstruction for index and thumb amputations is cosmetic and functional Lack of tactile feedback may lead to rejection or limited prosthesis use by the patient

Table 1B. Amputations of the Lower Extremities

Lower Extremity Amputations and Disarticulations			
Level	Indications	Pitfalls	Energy Expenditure
Hemipelvectomy External	Recurrent pelvis tumors Tumors affecting the sciatic notch Tumors affecting sciatic nerve	Bowel preparation even though peritoneum is rarely accessed Ureteral stent placement for easy identification of ureters Adequate arterial and venous access for hemodyanamic status and fluid resuscitation Bowel preparation even though peritoneum is rarely accessed Ureteral stent placement for easy identification of ureters Adequate arterial and venous access for hemodyanamic status and fluid resuscitation Positioning in sloppy lateral affected site tilted 45° Entire hindquarter is prepped and draped Anteriorly or posteriorly based flap depending on affected n/v bundle and soft tissue envelope Posterior flap depends on gluteus maximus Anterior flap based on quad muscle Posterior flap more commonly used Retract peroneal cavity gently in the medial direction Iliac vessels are identified and ligated. Be mindful of the inferior vena cava (IVC) in the right-sided amputations Resect psoas at the SI joint level Inguinal canal contents must be identified and divided within the pelvis Dissect bladder and urethra away from pubic symphysis	200% Most forces absorbed by lower back Lateral trunk shifting is required for forward propulsion of prosthesis Increased lumbar lordosis and transverse rotation of the lower spine are also required in the swing phase

Table 1B. (Continued)

Lower Extremity Amputations and Disarticulations			
Level	Indications	Pitfalls	Energy Expenditure
		Release sacrospinous and sacrotuberous ligaments before pelvic osteotomies If flaps cannot be developed the remaining of the extremity can be used as free fillet lower leg flap Obtain adequate hemosthasis Closure by layers Use drains	
Hemipelvectomy Internal	Recurrent pelvis tumors Tumors affecting the sciatic notch Tumors affecting sciatic nerve Involvement of hip joint Involvement of femoral n/v bundle Tumors that cross Sacro-Iliac joint and involve the sacrum Involvement of one neurovascular structure is not a definitive indication^	Bowel preparation even though peritoneum is rarely accessed Ureteral stent placement for easy identification of ureters Adequate arterial and venous access for hemodyanamic status and fluid resuscitation Bowel preparation even though peritoneum is rarely accessed Ureteral stent placement for easy identification of ureters Adequate arterial and venous access for hemodyanamic status and fluid resuscitation Positioning in sloppy lateral affected site tilted 45° Entire hindquarter is prepped and draped Be mindful of the inferior vena cava (IVC) in the right-sided amputations Resect psoas at the SI joint level Inguinal canal contents must be identified and divided within the pelvis Dissect bladder and urethra away from pubic symphysis Release sacrospinous and sacrotuberous ligaments	200% Most forces absorbed by lower back Lateral trunk shifting is required for forward propulsion of prosthesis Increased lumbar lordosis and transverse rotation of the lower spine are also required in the swing phase Abnormal forces in the spine are placed during heel strike when the hip and the knee joints need to be stabilized Patients usually require assistive device for ambulation In patients that depend on assistive devices sometimes ambulation is easier without prosthesis

Lower Extremity Amputations and Disarticulations			
Level	Indications	Pitfalls	Energy Expenditure
		before pelvic osteotomies Obtain adequate hemosthasis Closure by layers Use drains	
Hip Disarticulation	Tumors affecting proximal femur Extensive metastasic disease in the thigh Involvement of neurovascular bundle Acetabulum should be not affected Posterior soft tissue should be sufficient	Position patient in sloppy lateral, affected site at 45° posteriorly Use drains Post-operative compressive dressings Early prosthesis fitting	Close to 200% Incorporation of ischium in prosthesis allows to bear weight through ischium It secures prosthesis Acts as a fulcrum that helps to keep pelvis leveled during ambulation
Above the knee Amputation (AKA) Proximal Third Middle Third Distal Third	Distal femoral lesions Proximal tibia lesions with intra-articular extension	Place patient in the supine position Create the longest possible residual limb Preserve at least 5 cm in length measuring from lesser trochanter In keeping length is important to consider space for clearance of the prosthetic knee Match center of prosthetic and native knee Depending on soft-tissue and skin flaps thickness osseous femoral transection is usually 12-14 cm above the knee joint Resection should include edematous tissue To optimize stability and increase function performed adductor myodesis Attach over the quadriceps and the ischiotibialis muscles	65% Transfemoral prosthesis stabilize pelvis through: Ischial containment Ischial weightbearing Socket hydrostatic pressusres Higher Energy expenditure due to required adductor musculature action Gait is not fully physiologic and is characterized by lateral trunk lean Obtaining normal gait pattern requires significant strength and training It is difficult for socket to maintain adduction (adductor myodesis is key) Less energy expenditure when adduction is maintained as lateral lean decreases

Table 1B. (Continued)

Lower Extremity Amputations and Disarticulations			
Level	Indications	Pitfalls	Energy Expenditure
		Close the overlying fascia and skin Drains may or may not be used Immobilize patient in a splint keeping hip in neutral If no splint is used, keep patient in the prone position three times a day	Lack of adduction forces shift of weight over the prosthetic side during single limb stance and to maintain coronal stabiliy
Knee disarticulation	Mid-diaphyseal tibia lesions Proximal tibia lesions with no articular involvement Rarely used due to risk of articular contamination Careful selection of patients is key to avoid complications	Place patient in the supine position As adductor muscle group distal insertion is preserved, no myodesis is required Usually preferred in pediatric population as length of the femur can be controlled to match contralateral knee center of rotation Consider to shave distal femoral condyles to decrease bulky end of the stump Drains may or may not be used Obtain adequate hemostasis before closure Closure is performed attaching anterior elements such as capsule, patellar tendon and retinaculum are attached to posterior elements including gastronecmius complex Fascia and skin are the superficial layers Immobilize patient in a splint keeping hip in neutral If no splint is used, keep patient in the prone position three times a day	Between 40 and 65% Depends on body habitus of patient Difficult to match center of rotation of the knee with prosthesis, especially in adults If condyles left intact prosthesis can be held in suspension with compression socket above the condyles If condyles are shaved prosthesis can be stabilized with suction socket
Below the knee amputation (BKA) Proximal Third Middle Third Distal Third	Best in distal tibia metaphysis or epiphysis Hindfoot sarcomas	Place the patient in the supine position Evaluate XRs pre-operatively to determine optimal tibia length To maintain minimal function preserve at least 2.5 cms of tibia for every 30 cm of height in your patient	

Lower Extremity Amputations and Disarticulations			
Level	Indications	Pitfalls	Energy Expenditure
		Minimal length required length for function is 5 cm Placement of cut is usually at the myotendinous junction of the grastrocnemius muscle	
		Aim for a longer residual limb if possible Closing should be done by layers either by tension myodesis or myoplasty Tension myodesis implies to suture muscles to bone under physiological tension Myoplasty implies attachment of muscles to the opposing muscular group Avoid excessively thick posterior or anterior distal flap as this may affect stability of the socket in the future Avoid short flat and closure under tension to avoid blistering, necrosis and soft-tissue/wound complications May use or not drains Sterile coverage with compressive dressing and maintaining knee in extension with splint. May used U based ant/post splints	causing prosthesis instability
Syme's Amputation	Foot Sarcomas not affecting the heel pad and not involving the tibiotalar joint.	Place patient in the supine position Amputation is performed in through the tibio-talar joint Posterior flap contains the fat pad of and the heel's skin Durability depends on the flap's viability If there are complications with the fat pad or skin necrosis, a BKA is necessary as a salvage procedure Different techniques have been described for stabilization of the heel pad including casting, taping trough tibio-fibular holes and lastly keeping a calcaneal remnant to be fused to the distal tibia	15% of energy expenditure Key to maintain healthy and stable heel pad Residual limb has a weight-bearing distal end Start early weight-bearing with prosthesis Functional Cosmesis concern because of bulky appearance Limitations in prosthesis selection

Table 1B. (Continued)

Lower Extremity Amputations and Disarticulations			
Level	Indications	Pitfalls	Energy Expenditure
Pirogoff's Amputation	Foot Sarcomas not affecting the heel pad and not involving the tibiotalar joint. Hindfoot procedure	Position patient in the supine position Similar to Syme's Instead of disarticulation and subperiosteal dissection of the calcaneous and osteotomy perpendicular to the longitudinal axis of the calcaneous is performed Posterior flap contains the osteotomized calcaneous. The distal tibia and fibula are also osteotomized and bone fragments are pinned Heel pad migration is rare To obtain functional results fusion of the tibia to the calcaneous is required	15% of energy expenditure Residual limb has a weight-bearing distal end Start early weight-bearing with prosthesis Functional Cosmesis concern because of bulky appearance Limitations in prosthesis selection Risk of non-union and/or malunion is traded by heel pad stability
Transmetatarsal Amputation	Tarsal tumors, extracompartment al Usually implies resection of multiple metatarsals according to lesion	Position patient supine Significant soft-tissue loss Flap closure is usually required Vascularized free flaps do not tolerate weight bearing If soft-tissue closure is obtained modifications to shoe wear are required including full contact inserts, toe fillers, carbon plates, etc	Less than 15% No prostheses available May need shoe modification Alternatives of inserts include: Total contact insert Toe fillers Carbon plates (push off)
Midfoot amputations Linsfranc Chopart	Linsfranc: Tarsometatarsal joint Chopart: Midtarsal joint	Rarely used as equinus and equino-varus deformities form commonly Resultant foot offers limited functional benefits	Less than 15% Limited shoe modifications, prostheses

Lower Extremity Amputations and Disarticulations			
Level	Indications	Pitfalls	Energy Expenditure
Ray Resection	Tumor contained to metatarsal Metatarsophalangeal joint	Place patient in the supine position Good functional results, especially in lateral column Better functional result is obtained with metacarpal resection than with metatarsal osteotomy No need of metarcarpal transposition More impairment when 1st metacarpal is resected	Less than 15% More functional disturbance in first metacarpal resections Late stance and push-off affected with in this scenario Prosthesis consists on total contact shoe insert with a carbon plate Lateral resection require only total contact shoe insert
Phalangeal Resection	Tumor contained in phalanx	Patient is positioned supine	Minimal functional deficit, especially with lesser toes Amputation of greater toe requires prosthetic reconstruction with total contact shoe insert with a carbon plate to restore third rocker stand

^ If only femoral vessels are affected, these can be reconstructed. Patients with isolated deficit of the sciatic or the femoral nerves can compensate for function.

Table 2A. Prosthesis for upper extremity amputations

Types of Prosthesis Upper Extremity			
Type	Mechanism	Advantages	Disadvantages
Myoelectric Prosthese	Surface electrodes transmit electrical activity on residual limb musculature. Usually used in transradial amputations Types: <u>Two-site/Two function devices:</u> Separate electrodes for flexion and extension <u>One-site/Two function device:</u> One electrode for flexion and extension 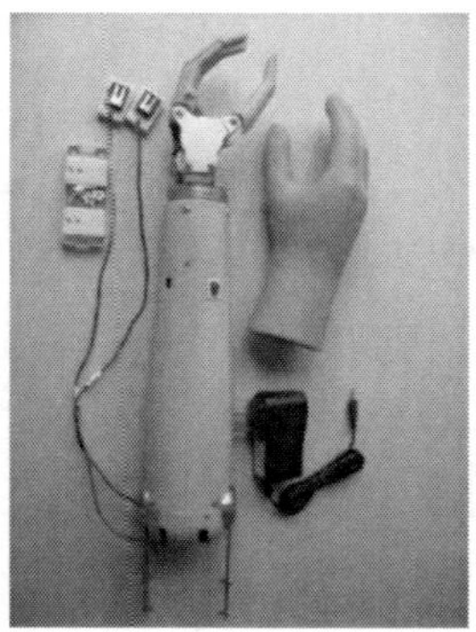	Good for sedentary work Allows overhead activities Better cosmesis Allows more proximal coverage	Heavier than body-powered prosthesis Higher costs Decreased sensory feedback Requires maintenance

Types of Prosthesis Upper Extremity			
Type	Mechanism	Advantages	Disadvantages
Body-powered Prosthesis	Terminal device activates with shoulder flexion and abduction Harness center off the midline of C7 towards non-amputated side 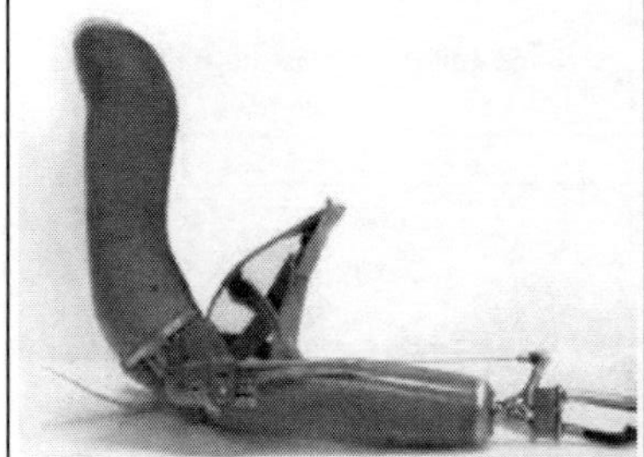	Excellent for heavy labor Moderate cost and weight Less maintenance required Higher sensory feedback	Poor cosmesis Requires preserved function of remaining upper extremity
Classification by Mechanism of Terminal Device			
Terminal Device	<u>Passive terminal device:</u> More cosmetic but less functional <u>Active terminal device:</u> More functional less cosmetic. Uses hooks or prosthetic hands with cables or myoelectric devices		

Table 2A. (Continued)

Types of Prosthesis Upper Extremity			
Type	Mechanism	Advantages	Disadvantages
		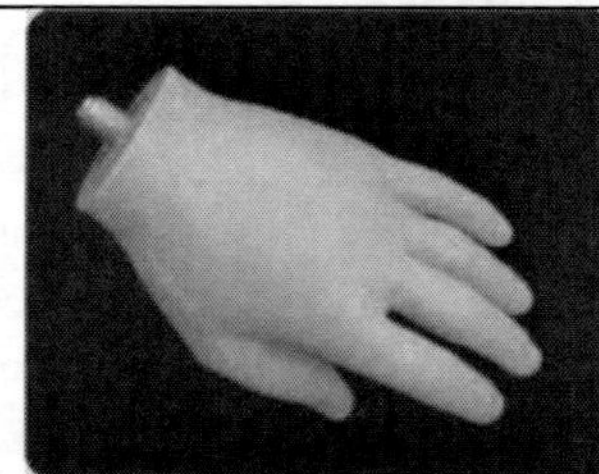	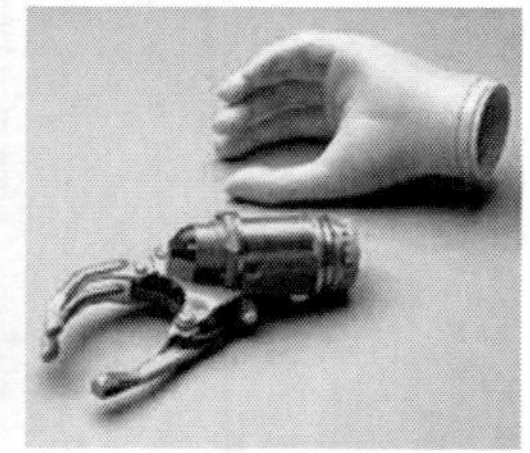
Classification by Grip Type			
Grip Type	Presicion Grip (pincer) Tripod grip (Palmar Grip, 3-jaw chunk pinch) Lateral Pinch Hook power grip Spherical grip	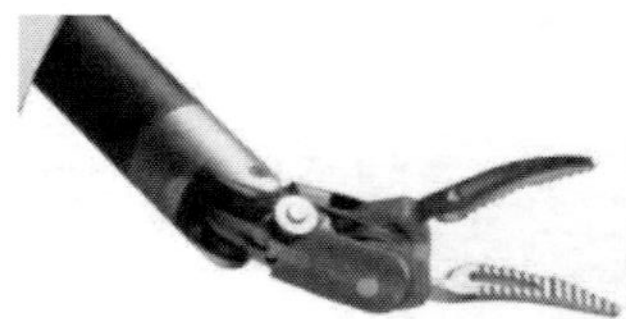	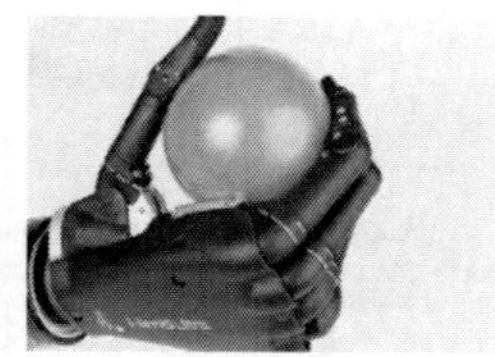

Classification by Prehension Devices			
Types of Prosthesis Upper Extremity			
Type	Mechanism	Advantages	Disadvantages
Prehension Device Types	**Hand-like Device** Thumb, index and long finger components Improved cosmesis using a glove Good choice for office work **Non-Hand Prehension device** Hook or two-finger pincer with parallel surfaces May use task-specific tools Good for physical labor **Myoelectric Device** Only to be use in clean environment free of dust, dirt, water or solvents	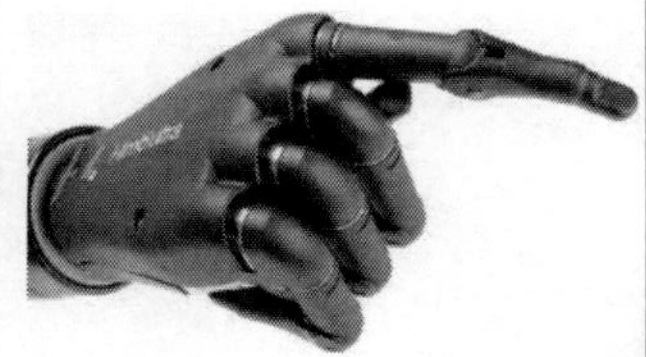 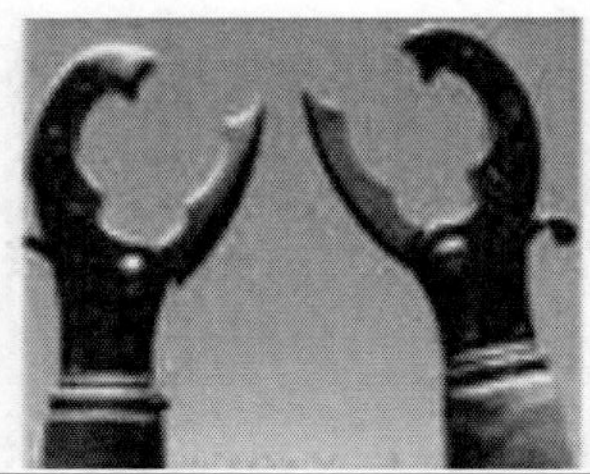	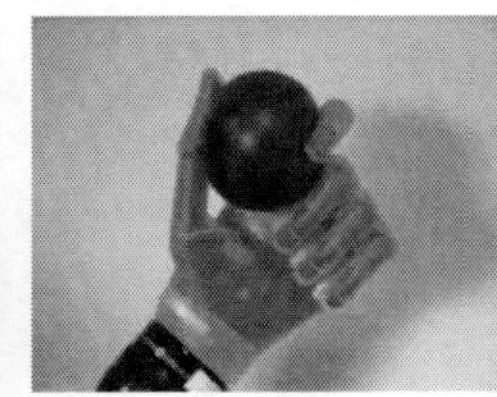
Classification by operation mechanism			
Voluntary Opening	Close at rest opens with activity More common than voluntary closing	N/A	N/A
Voluntary Closing	Open at rest Residual forearm flexors close device	N/A	Heavier Less durable and high maintenance

Table 2A. (Continued)

Types of Prosthesis Upper Extremity			
Type	Mechanism	Advantages	Disadvantages
Classification by Anatomic Location			
Wrist Units	Quick to disconnect Allows easy change with specialized function Locking wrist prevents rotation during grasping and/or lifting Wrist flexion unit: Used in long residual limb. Use in B/L amputees	N/A	N/A
Elbow Units	**Rigid Elbow Hinge:** Use in short trans-radial amputation with inability to pronosupinate with maintenance of elbow flexion **Flexible Elbow Hinge:** Use in wrist disarticulation or long transradial amputation with good pronation/supination and elbow flexoextension	N/A	N/A
Shoulder Units	Use for cosmetic reasons High Energy Expenditure Use in forequater or shoulder level of amputation	N/A	N/A

Classification by mechanism of action, mechanism of the terminal device, grip type, prenhension device type, patient operation mechanism and by anatomic location.

Table 2B. Prosthesis for lower extremity amputations

Types of Prosthesis Lower Extremity (Knee)			
Type	Mechanism	Socket	Suspension Systems
Knee Prosthesis	Used in above the knee amputations and knee disarticulations They provide controlled knee motion Alignment of prosthesis with weight-bearing axis of the patients knee is key Connected by a socket or suspension systems	Connects the stump and the prosthesis. Protect the stump Requires multiple adjustments as edema resolves Patellar tendon bearing prosthesis (Most common)	Attaches prosthesis to residual limb using belts, straps and suction. Suction/Suspension: Standard suction: Form-fitting rigid or semirigid socket that fits onto residual limb Silicon suction: Silicon based sock fits over stump and then it is inserted into socket. It provides airtight seal between prosthesis and stump
Classification by type of joint			
Type	Indications	Characteristics	Image

Table 2B. (Continued)

Types of Prosthesis Lower Extremity (Knee)			
Type	Mechanism	Socket	Suspension Systems
ycentric	Transfemoral amputation Knee disarticulation Bilateral amputations	Variable knee center of rotation Supports increased weight when compared to constant friction knee Controlled flexion Ability to walk at a moderate fast pace	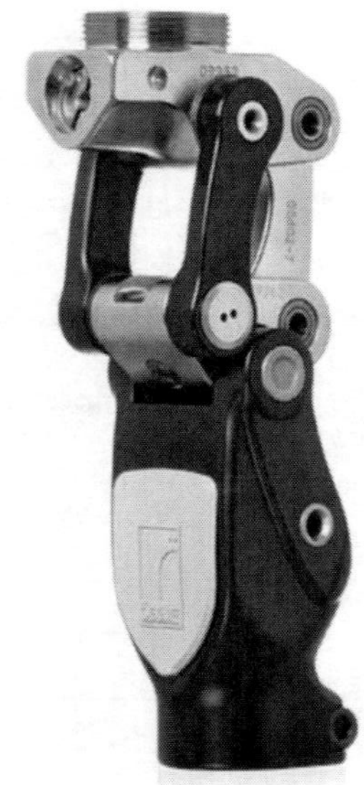

Types of Prosthesis Lower Extremity (Knee)			
Type	Mechanism	Socket	Suspension Systems
Stance-phase control knee	Proximal femur amputations in the elderly Patient that need to walk in uneven terrain	Constant friction of the knee in the swing phase Weighbearing through the prosthesis locks up through the high friction housing	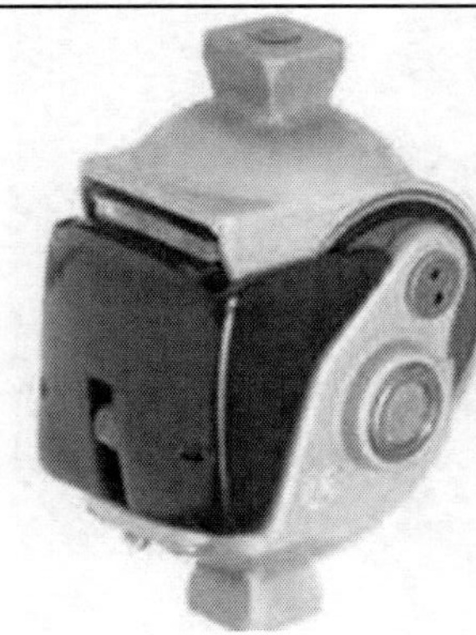
Fluid Control	Indicated in active patiens willing to sacrifice wearing a heavier prosthesis in exchange for utility and variability	Can be hydraulic or pneumatic Allows variable cadence through piston mechanism Prevents excessive flexion Extends knee earlier in gait cycle	

Table 2B. (Continued)

Types of Prosthesis Lower Extremity (Knee)			
Type	Mechanism	Socket	Suspension Systems
			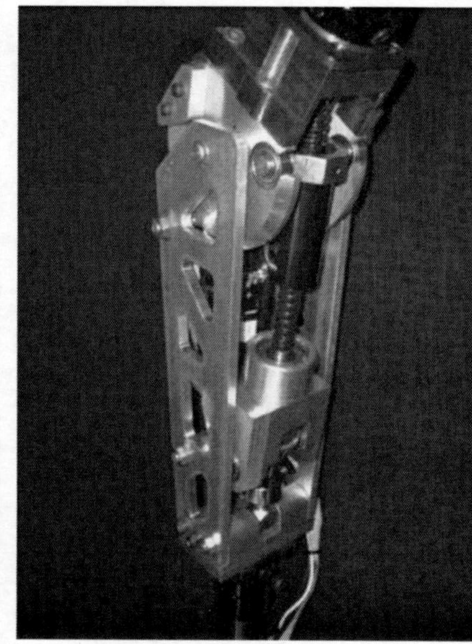

Types of Prosthesis Lower Extremity (Knee)			
Type	Mechanism	Socket	Suspension Systems
Constant Friction	General use Patients walking in even or uneven terrain Most common pediatric prosthesis Not recommended for older or weak patients	Hinge uses a screw or rubber pad to apply friction to the knee to decrease knee swing Allows only for single speed walking Depends on alignment for stability during stance phase	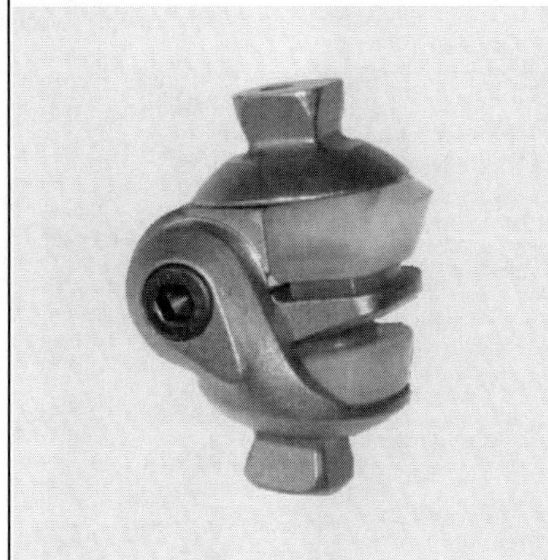
Manual locking knee	Constant friction hinge with an extension lock	Extension lock can be unlocked to allow knee to act like constant friction knee	

Table 2B. (Continued)

Types of Prosthesis Lower Extremity (Knee)			
Type	Mechanism	Socket	Suspension Systems
			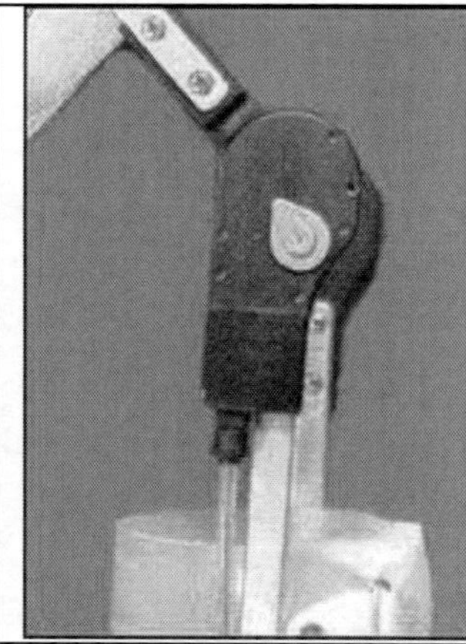
Other components of prosthesis: Pylon: Simple shell or tube that attaches the socket to the terminal device. New designs allow for axial rotation and absorb, store and release energy Exoskeleton: Soft foam designed to match the contralateral limb. It has an outer hard shell Endoskeleton: Internal metal frame with cosmetic soft covering Terminal device: Most commonly a foot but it may vary			
Types of Prosthesis Lower Extremity (Knee)			

Type	Mechanism	Socket	Suspension Systems
Types of Prosthesis Lower Extremity (Foot)			
Type	Indications/Mechanism	Advantages Disadvantages	Image
Single Axis Foot	Ankle hinge that allows plantar flexion and dorsiflexion	Poor durability Poor cosmesis	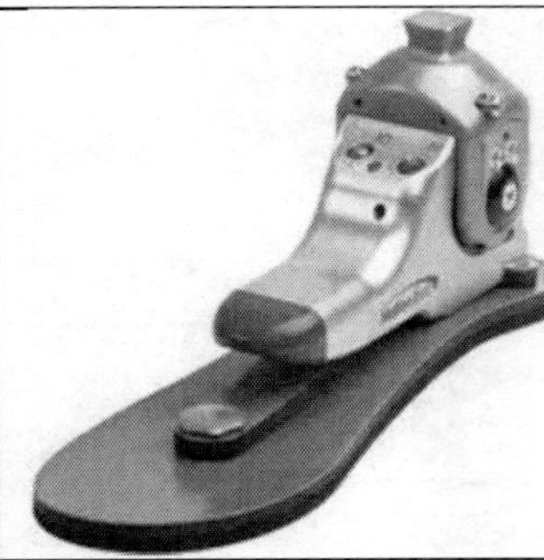
SACH (Solid Ankle Cushioned Heel) foot	General use in patients with low acitivity levels Use is being phased out	Overload of the contralateral foot	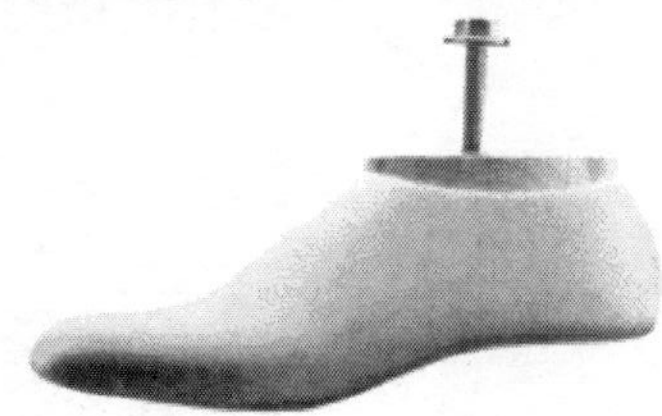

Table 2B. (Continued)

Types of Prosthesis Lower Extremity (Knee)			
Type	Mechanism	Socket	Suspension Systems
Dyanamic Response (Energy Storing) foot	General use for most activities Patients that ambulate over uneven surfaces Articulating: Patients walking in uneven surface Articulating: Indicated in higher demand activities Shorter keels are not as responsive and are indicated for moderate activity Longer keels indicated high-demand patients	Articulating: Allows inversion & rotation Absorbs loads and decreases shear forces Flexible keels that act as a spring to decrease contralateral loading Flexible keel provides push off Posterior projection of keel help with transition heel-strike Sagittal split allows inversion/eversion	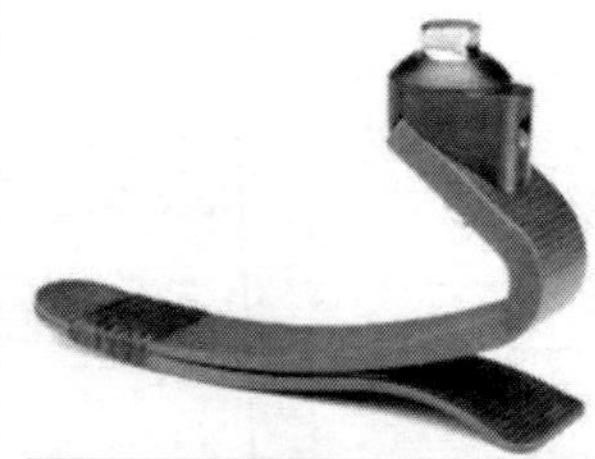 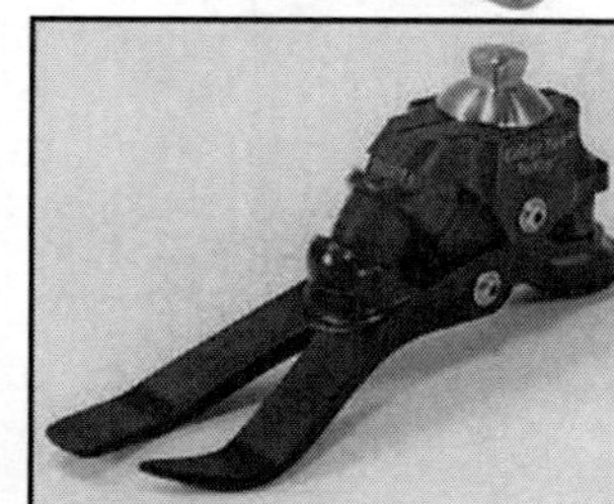

Classification by mechanism of action, type of joint, and anatomic location.

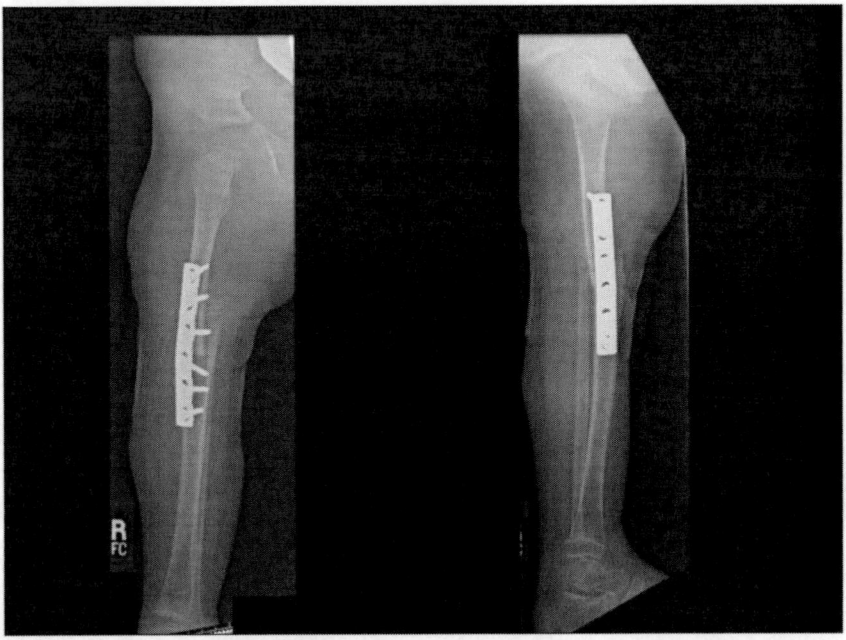

Courtesy of Megan Anderson, MD.

Figure 5. AP and Lateral Radiographs of a 3 year-old female patient with distal femoral osteosarcoma involving the growth plate treated with rotationplasty.

Limb-Sparing Surgery

As mentioned before, the success of surgical treatment in patients with osteosarcoma depends on the appropriate selection of patients for each particular procedure. Limb-sparing surgery is not the exception to this principle. Even though this type of interventions are an aim to maintain function, the oncologic objective is always more important and should not be sacrificed. There were some concerns with this modality of resections in terms of safety but this issue has been addressed several times in the published literature, making this technique a good alternative of treatment. [42-50] The goal with this technique is to resect the tumor completely with a good margin or cuff of healthy tissue surrounding the entire tumor.

In terms of final function, it remains unclear the difference between patients with amputation and those that undergo limb-preserving surgery as their comparison is not as simple as it may appear at first glance. Mavrogenis [60] demonstrated better functional outcome and similar survival rates in patients with osteosarcoma of the distal tibia that underwent limb salavage vs. those having amputations. However, these findings do not apply to every amputation and different types of limb reconstruction. [60] There is evidence demonstrating that oxygen consumption is higher in patients undergoing amputation than those with limb-preservation surgery. [49, 61] The higher the level of amputation is, the higher the energy expenditure. [62, 63] There is also proved psychological benefit in patients who had their extremity preserved. However, the rate of complications and number of subsequent surgeries is higher than in patients that underwent amputation. [49]

A controversial area in terms of indications for limb-sparing surgery is the presence of a pathologic fracture. [64-66] This situation may be a contraindication and the traditional teaching was to treat these patients preferably with amputations. However, multiple reports that demonstrated fracture healing during pre-surgical chemotherapy with subsequent limb-salvage surgery challenged this principle. Intuitively, most investigators recommended amputations in this scenario as an "unacceptable" high local rate of recurrence can be expected in patients with fractures treated with limb preservation. Scully in 2002 [67] reported the experience of 8 institutions comparing 52 patients with osteosarcoma and pathologic fracture to 55 osteosarcoma patients who did not present a pathologic fracture. Patients were followed for at least 2-years or until recurrence, metastasis or dead. The authors found that patients with pathologic fractures during preoperative chemotherapy had a higher local recurrence rate and decreased survival when compared to patients that did not have pathologic fractures in the setting of limb-reconstruction surgery. [67] However, there was and still there is a question after this investigation: At what extend the higher recurrence and lower survival rate depends on the tumor itself? A more aggressive malignancy that affects bone, severely, to the point of causing a pathologic fracture, is most likely a tumor that, regardless of the presence of a pathologic fracture, has a higher likelihood of local recurrence and lower survival. New investigations have helped to elucidate better what to do in the presence of pathologic fractures. In the case of non-displaced fractures in patients responding well to chemotherapy, there is evidence proving the safety of using limb-sparing surgery. [64, 66] In more complex fractures two recent investigations have further investigated the impact of pathologic fractures. Both of them concluded that the risk or recurrence is the same that in patients without fracture. However, there is a lower survival rate that correlates with the argument of these tumors being more biologically aggressive. [64, 66]

Limb sparing surgery as an alternative needs to be fully discussed with the patient and his/her family. There should be a complete understanding of the expected function, potential complications and risk of multiple surgical interventions. Patients performing high-impact activities and contact sports should be discouraged to return to this type of activity after limb-preserving surgery. Also patients need to know that rotationplasty and amputation still are options of treatment if there is failure of the initial reconstruction. Limb-sparing surgery may require multiple procedures related to revisions allografts or prosthesis and conversions from allografts to metallic endoprosthesis or allorgraft-prosthesis composites.

In every modality of treatment, life expectancy should be part of the equation. Limb salvage is not the exception. Traditionally, limb-sparing surgery is preferred in patients with low life expectancy. However, if the patient's survival outlives the reconstruction, subsequent revisions or ablative surgery are options for future management.

Limb salvage entitles osseous reconstruction and restoration of the soft-tissue envelope. Osseous reconstruction is commonly based on allograft/autograft reconstructions (biologic) or metallic endoprosthetic devices. Both techniques present advantages and disadvantages. The success of each technique depends extensively on the indications of use. Traditionally, allograft reconstructions preserve bone stock, allow reconstruction of the articular surface and recreate attachments for ligaments and tendons. However, complications such as fractures, non-unions and infections may be present during the clinical course of this modality of limb-sparing surgery. Endoprostheses on the other hand offer immediate mechanical stability, which allows early rehabilitation and ambulation. However, infection and lack of bone stock preservation, and failure of the mechanical components are some of the concerns with the use of this technique. The following is a description of each reconstruction modality in detail.

Endoprosthetic Reconstruction

The earliest endoprosthetic reconstruction occurred in 1940 when Drs. Austin Moore and Harold Bohlman used a vitallium proximal femoral prosthesis in a patient with giant cell tumor of bone. [68] In the early 1970's Drs. Francis and Marcove started the current era of endoprosthetic reconstruction characterized by radical resection with subsequent placement of the prosthesis.

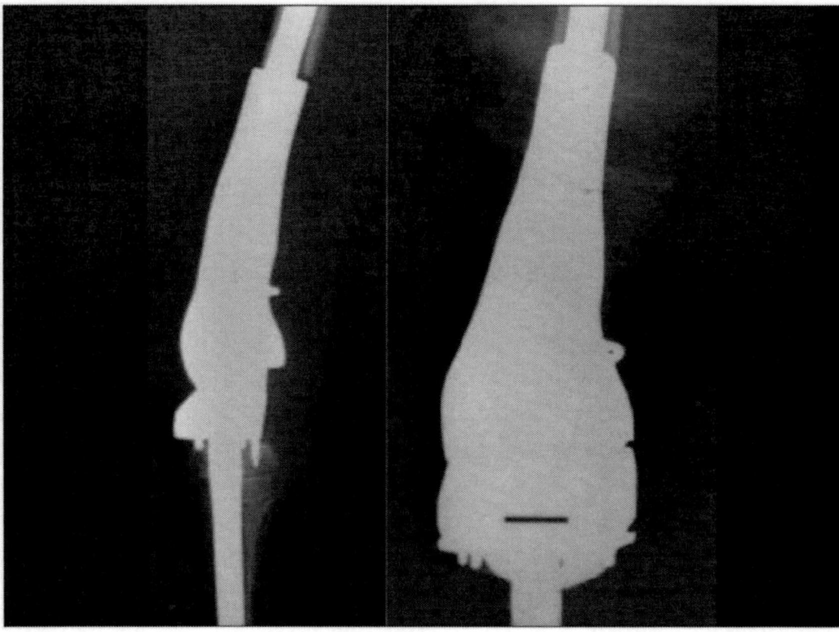

Figure 6. AP and lateral radiographs of the distal femoral replacement performed by Kenneth Francis at New York University in 1973 in a patient with osteosarcoma.

The former developed a distal femoral replacement for the treatment of osteosarcomas and the latter a total femur replacement. [69] (Figure 6).

At that time, patients had to wait a fair amount of time to have their prosthesis custom-made. Dr. Gerry Rosen introduced the concept of induction chemotherapy, which consisted in the use of Adriamycin and Methotrexate before the surgical resection. Eventually, the standard, as discussed in other sections of this chapter, became the use of neoadjuvant chemotherapy, surgery and adjuvant chemotherapy.

Current designs are based on modular systems. The second –generation universal system was originally named modular segmental replacement system (MSRS) but recently renamed to modular replacement system (MRS). This technology was introduced in 1988 (Howmedica Inc. Rutherford NJ, currently owned by Stryker) and was designed with the objective of providing modular replacements for the proximal humerus, proximal femur, total femur, distal femur and proximal tibia.

During the following years, evaluation of the mechanisms of failure of these prostheses has helped to make technological improvements that have increased implant longevity and decreased complications. Key changes include: availability of multiple stem diameters, which facilitates the use of the largest stem possible in each particular case. This is important as the larger the stem the lower the risk of stem fracture. In addition, the use of a facing reamer that matches the outer radio of the prosthesis, allows perfect sitting of the implant in bone and protects the stem from bending forces, reducing furthermore the risk of stem fracture.

The second change is the use of cemented stems. The experience in total joint replacements has a good record for approximately 25 years. There is enough literature demonstrating that cement is biologically well tolerated by patients. The cement functions as a grout and corrects any mismatches between the intramedullary anatomy and the stem shape. The loosening that was observed and attributed initially to the use of cement, known as "cement disease", has been proved to be related to the biologic response to polyethylene wear debris. Cemented stems ensure immediate stem fixation, facilitating early weight-bearing and early rehabilitation. Non-weight-bearing status length and the necessity to use braces post-operatively decrease substantially with the use of cemented constructs.

The third new development in modular prosthesis is the use of circumferential porous coating in the part where the stem attaches to the body of the prosthesis. This area allows ingrowth of bone graft placed at the prosthesis junction (extraskeletal fixation). This new bone protects the bone stem as it shares all the bending and loading stresses on the implant. This area also allows the growth of bone, which produces a seal between the fluid and polyethylene debris formed in the joint and the susceptible bone cement interface. This phenomenon, described by Ward in 1993 as the "interface nose", essentially eliminates the risk of osteolysis. [70] (Figure 7).

Lastly, specifically for restoration of the knee, the use of a rotating-hinged prosthesis facilitates reconstruction of a stable joint, independently of the soft-tissue deficiency that is typically seen after wide resection of tumors. This system also offers more mobility than the traditional hinged or highly constrained prostheses. A benefit of this design in decreasing aseptic loosening is the reduction of stress forces in the prosthesis/cement/bone or the prosthesis/bone interfaces that is responsible of this mechanical phenomenon.

In addition to changes to the prosthesis per se, there are also developments in the instrumentation and assembling of these systems, which facilitate surgery from the technical standpoint. Also a new emphasis has taken place in terms of reconstruction of soft-tissues. Newer designs have holes or porous surfaces that allow reinsertion or reconstruction of soft-tissues such as the extensor mechanism and patellar tendon in proximal tibia replacements.

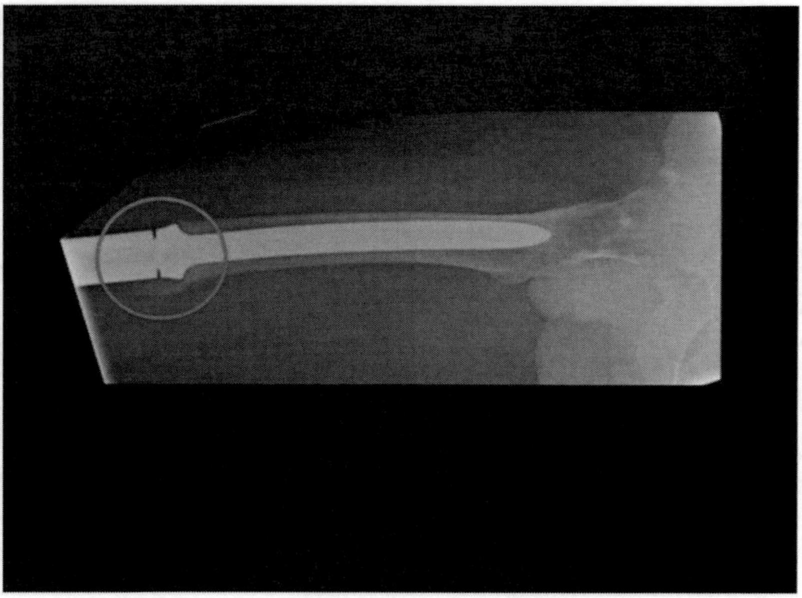

Figure 7. "Interface nose" in press-fit prosthesis, distal femoral replacement.

These features, despite not being optimal, facilitate the reconstruction of soft-tissues and improve function somewhat in this patient population. (Figure 8).

When compared to the traditional prosthesis used for the treatment of degenerative joint disease, the body of literature in oncologic prosthesis is limited as it is the number of studies and length of follow up as this is a relatively recent technology or modality of treatment. As malignant tumors are considerably more frequent around the knee –distal femur/proximal tibia-, most investigation focus in prostheses of this area.

Survival rates for distal femoral rcplacements have been assessed by different groups. In the mid 1990s cohorts form Chicago [42], England [71] and New York [72], reported survival rates of 66% at 10 years, 64% at 7 years and 59% at 10 years respectively. Survival rates are traditionally higher in proximal femoral replacements (89% at 10 years) and lower in the proximal tibia (54% at 10 years). Most recent investigations report a higher survival rate at 10 years, 75%. [73-84] Longevity is expected to continue to improve as remarkable improvement has been made in terms of polyethylene structure. The newer highly cross-linked polyethylene and newer methods of annealing and packing reducing free radicals is expected to continue decreasing failures related to polyethylene debris.

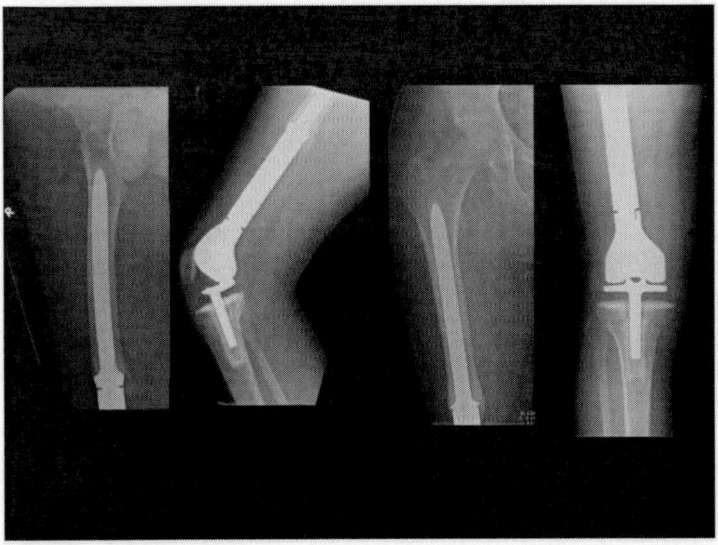

Courtesy of Mark Gebhardt, MD.

Figure 8A. AP and lateral radiographs of a distal femoral replacement, cemented tibia components and press-fit femoral component.

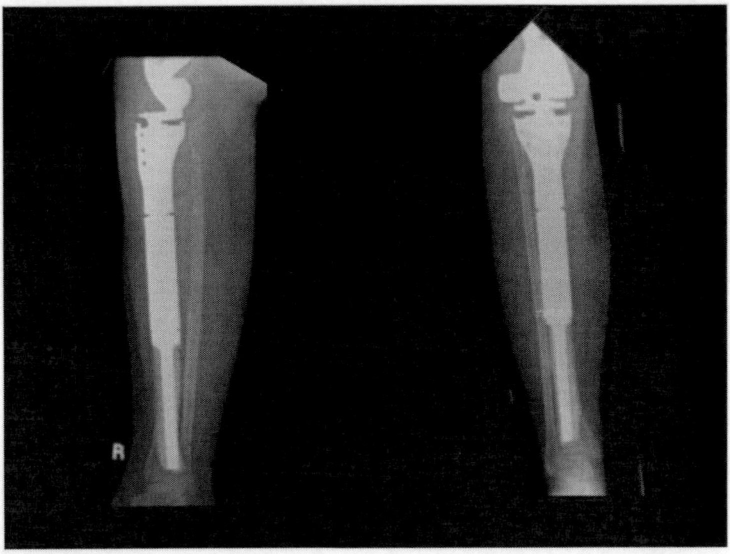

Courtesy of Mark Gebhardt, MD.

Figure 8B. AP and lateral radiographs of a cemented proximal tibia replacement. Notice the cemented tibial component.

Table 3 is a summary of the most important literature in oncologic endoprostheses longevity.

Despite of all the discussed mechanical and structural modifications, failure still is a problem as the survival of patients is improving with the current oncologic treatments based on systemic chemotherapy and radiation. This phenomenon is placing a higher demand in the longevity of prosthesis and therefore, a substantial current research is focused in the causes for endoprosthesis failure. Traditionally, mechanical reasons were considered the main reason for failure, as these designs have very high constraining forces when compared to the traditional total knee or total hip arthroplasties. Jeys et al. [85] reported the English experience with 661 patients followed at least for 10 years.

Table 3. Survival of Endoprosthetic Reconstructions

Group	Prosthesis type	Follow up	Survival rate
Horowitz, 1991	Distal Femur	10 years	59%
Roberts, 1991	Distal Femur	7 years	64%
Rougraff, 1994	Distal Femur	10 years	66%
Horowitz, 1991	Proximal Femur	10 years	89%
Horowitz, 1991	Proximal Tibia	10 years	54%
Capanna, 1994	Distal Femur	51 months	Not Reported
Morris, 1994	Total Femur	23 months	Not Reported
Malawer, 1995	Multiple sites	5/10 years	83%/67%
Bickels, 2000	Proximal/Total femur	6.5 years	95%
Menendez, 2006	Proximal Femur	5/10 years	82%
Finstein, 2007	Proximal Femur	5 years	79%
Jeys, 2008	Multiple sites	10 years	75%
Bernthal, 2010	Proximal Femur	10/20 years	84%/56%
Shehadeh, 2010	Multiple sites	10 years	72%
Henderson, 2011	Multiple sites	Variable 10 years	Variable 80%
Pala, 2013	Multiple sites	4.2 years (2-8 years)	82%

He reported mechanical failure as the most prevalent at an average follow up of 15 years. [85] Most recent investigations, determine infection as the most prevalent reason for failure overall. A landmark study by Henderson et al. [81], reported the experience of 5 institutions from 3 different countries. [81] A total of 534 failures were analyzed and a new classification system for failures derived from this analysis. Henderson found infection to be the most common cause of failure overall but perhaps the most significant point of this investigation is that failure mechanism vary according to the type of prosthesis and anatomic location. It is clear that distal humeral replacements, despite being semiconstrained, experience higher stress forces at the cement bone interface when compared to proximal femoral replacements. As expected, distal humerus replacements fail more commoly due to mechanical reasons than infections. Time for failures to occur depends also on the cause. Infection can occur early or in a delayed fashion, whereas loosening tends to occur after two years of implantation. [81]

New technologies such as biologic fixation of stems such as the compress system by Biomet [86-89] or the press-fit cement-less stems from Stryker are part of the new technologies that are being used in the younger patient (Figure 9). Other prostheses with expandable capabilities have been developed to treat pediatric patients in which limb discrepancy secondary to resection of the growth plates at the distal femur or proximal tibia is a very challenging problem (Figure 10). Some promising results have been seen with these designs. [90, 91] However, complication rates are high and the number of surgeries multiple despite some of these prostheses being able to be lengthened through not invasive procedures. [90, 91] Many argue that options such as rotationplasty or amputation offer a better functional outcome with less complications and number of procedures. However, literature comparing both modalities of treatment is necessary before drawing any recommendations.

Allograft Reconstruction

The first of use of osseous allograft dates from 1881 when MacEwen replaced two-thrids of a humeral shaft with an interhuman transplantation, performing the first interacallary allograft.

In the 1940s and 1950s Perrish extended the use of bone transplants to reconstruct skeletal defects. [92] Since the late 1960 to nowdays the development and improvement of harvesting, processing and storage of bone allograft has developed inmensely.

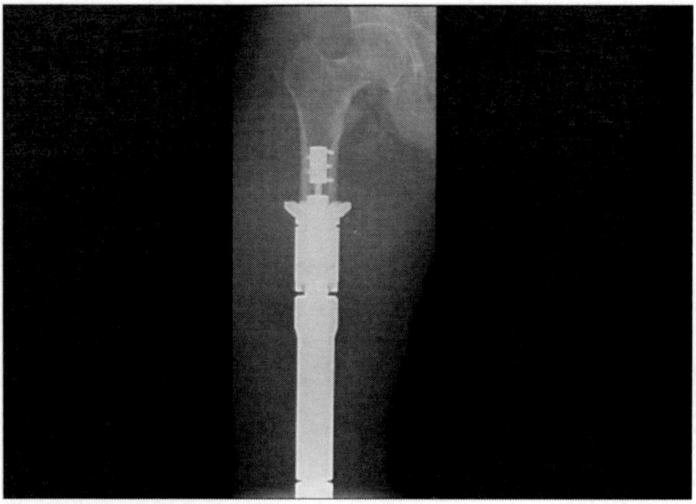

Courtesy of Megan Anderson, MD.

Figure 9. AP views of an expandible prosthesis for reconstruction of the distal femur.

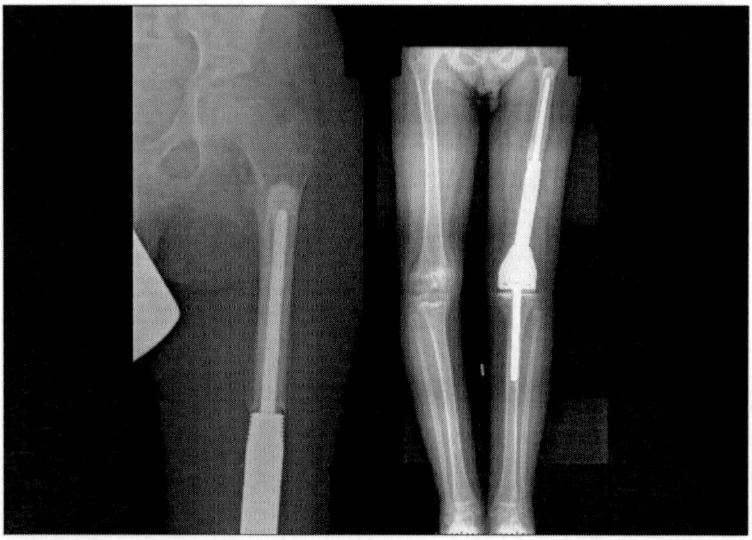

Courtesy of Megan Anderson, MD.

Figure 10. AP radiographic view of a prosthetic reconstruction with the compress mechanism.

The creation of bone banks with infection screening protocols have made safer the use of bone allografts, increasing as well the indications and options of use for surgeons as a reconstruction method; especially in the last 25 years of rapid development of limb reconstruction.

Allograft reconstruction emerged in the oncology world as a technique of reconstruction of preferable use in young or pediatric patients for whom endoprosthetic metallic reconstruction was not considered first line of treatment because of the need of subsequent surgical revision and the bone sacrificing nature of this procedure. [93] In addition, prosthesis use was also in development and complication rates were also high making this option of reconstruction (Allografts) appealing to surgeons and patients. [37, 93-98]

As mentioned in the endoprosthetic reconstruction section, oncologic outcomes are comparable between amputation and limb-sparing surgery. Published literature documenting this fact has triggered new research and techniques for limb-sparing surgery. The development of new fixation hardware devices such as locking plates and new surgical techniques have made this modality of treatment more popular.

Allografts can be classified as structural and non-structural. The former is subdivided in two main subtypes: osteoarticular and intercalary allografts. Ostearticular allografts contain the articular surface and soft-tissue attachments and structures of the closest involved joint. Intercalary allografts do not contain the articular portion and may or may not include soft-tissue attachments or structures.

A new subcategory for both groups is hemicondylar and hemi-intercalary allografts. The only difference is that these involve a portion of the osteoarticular or the intercalary graft. Figure 11 demonstrates different types of structural allografts.

Non-structural allografts and autografts are used in oncology and in other fields of orthopaedics. These are subdivided as cortical, cortico-cancellous and cancellous allografts. These are beyond the scope of this chapter but have an important role in the treatment of delayed union, non-union and revision of structural allografts. Lastly, autografts, structural and non-structural can be used to supplement allografts or treat complications related to allograft non-union or fracture.

Despite their bone preserving nature and the better soft tissue reconstruction achieved when compared to endoprosthetic reconstruction, allograft use is associated to complications as well. Major complications include fracture, non-union and infection, which often require removal or revision of the allograft. [37, 95, 99].

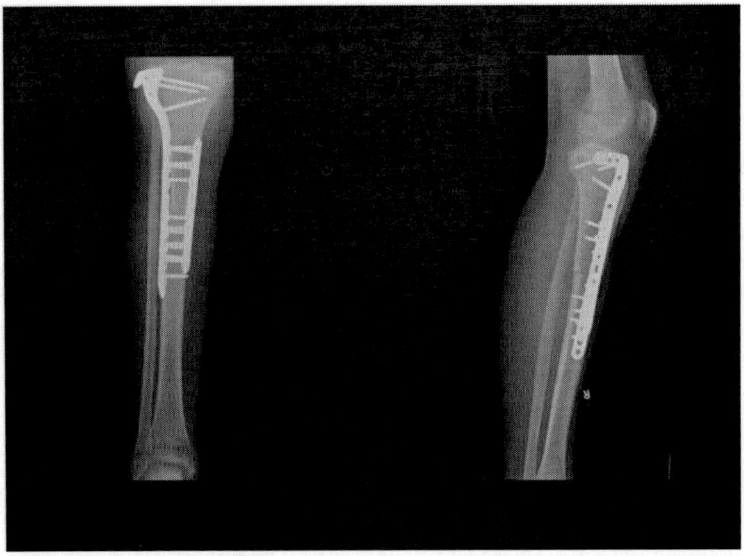

Courtesy of Mark Gebhardt, MD.

Figure 11A. AP and lateral views of an osteoarticular allograft for reconstruction of the proximal tibia.

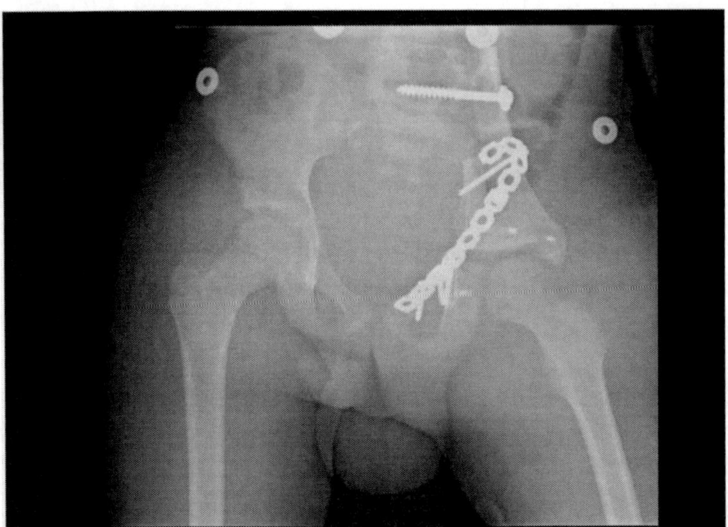

Courtesy of Mark Gebhardt, MD.

Figure 11B. AP view of the pelvis in a patient with Ewing's sarcoma of the ileum that after wide resection received reconstruction with osteoarticular allograft (Distal Tibia).

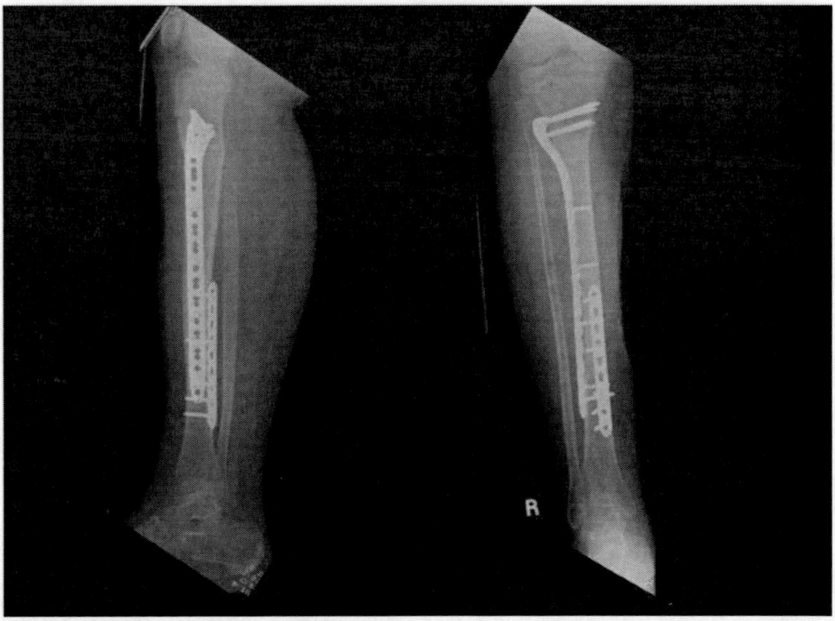

Courtesy of Megan Anderson, MD.

Figure 11C. AP and lateral radiographic views of an intercalary allograft reconstruction for a diaphyseal Ewing's Sarcoma of the Tibia.

The largest series of allografts demonstrated that most failures occur between the first and third years after surgery. Once the allograft passes this period, usually good function and survival can be expected. [37, 95, 99]

Intercalary allografts present traditionally better function and less complications than osteoarticular allografts. The largest series for intercalary femoral allografts from Aponte-Tinao and his group in Argentina reports on 83 patients with a survival rate of 85% at 5 years and 76% at 10. [100] The most common cause of revision was fracture followed by non-union (19%). Table 4 is a summary of the most relevant literature in terms of complications for allograft reconstructions.

As discussed earlier, this type of reconstruction is more commonly used in the pediatric population. Results are comparable with those in adults. Campanacci et al. [101] reported their experience with 25 pediatric patients with high-grade sarcomas of the distal femur or proximal tibia treated with allograft reconstruction and a minimal follow-up of at least 7 years. The overall survival rate was 70% at 5 years and 58% at 10 years for the distal femur and 45% at 5 years and 20% at 10 years in the proximal tibia.

Table 4. Survival rates and complications in allograft Reconstructions

Group	Allograft Type/Patient Number	Follow up	Survival rate	Complication
Lord et al, 1988	Variable (283)	10 years	59%	Infection 11.7%
Berrey et al, 1990	Variable (43)	7 years	64%	Fracture 16%
Mankin et al, 1996	Variable (873) Osteoarticular (53%) Intercallary (24%) Allograft/prosthesis (14%) Arthrodesis (9%)	5.6 years	76% at 5 years	Infection 11% Non-union 17% Fracture 19% Unstable joint 6%
Ortiz-Cruz et al, 1997	Interacallary (104)	5.6 years	92% at 5 years	Non-union 31% Infection 12% Fracture 18%
Hornicek et al, 2001	Multiple (945) Non-union (163)	6 years +/- 4 years	66%	Non-union 17%
Mankin et al, 2004	Multiple (648) Distal femur (222) Proximal tibia (109)	6 years +/- 4 years	68%	Infection 10% Fracture 16% Non-union 21%
Musculo et al., 2006	Review	Review	Review	Revision 25-30%
Campanacci et al, 2010	Osteoarticular Distal Femur (13) Osteoarticular Proximal Tibia (12) Pediatric Patients	10 years	70% at 5 years 58% at 10 years	Fracture 46% Infection 0%
Aponte-Tinao et al, 2012	Intercallary Allograft Femur (83)	10 years	85% at 5 years 76% at 10 years	Delayed union 13% Non-union 19% (Diaphyseal) Non-union 3% (Met) Fracture 17%

Function was determined to be good or acceptable in patients that retained the allograft. [101]

Lastly, the literature reporting on hemi-intercalary and hemicondylar allograft is limited and it is basically composed by small case series of patients treated mainly for pathology of low or intermediate grade. Concerns of this technique in terms of local control and recurrence exist. However, early results demonstrate comparable results to the other techniques discussed in this chapter with better functional outcome, better union rates and lower risk of fracture. Follow-up in the longer term still is pending for this technique. (Figure 12)

Allograft-Prosthesis Composite Reconstruction

Another alternative reconstruction technique is the combination of allograft and metallic prosthesis, known as allograft-prosthesis composites or APCs.

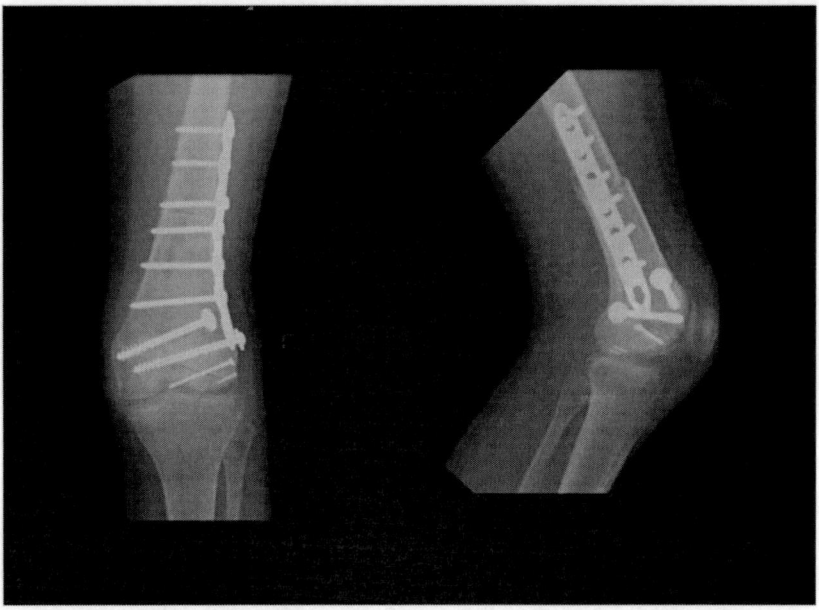

Courtesy of Mark Gebhardt, MD.

Figure 12. **A.** AP and lateral radiographic views of a hemi-Intercallary allograft reconstruction for a distal metaphyseal conventional osteosarcoma of the distal femur. **B.** AP and lateral radiographic views of a hemi-condylar allograft reconstruction.

This technique has been more commonly described in joints were the soft tissue reconstruction is key but where results with allograft or prosthetic reconstruction are not satisfactory such as the shoulder and proximal tibia. Most of this investigations are case series, being the most notorious the report of Abdeen and Healy in 2010 [102, 103] for proximal humeral reconstruction and the study from Lin et al. in 2009 [104] of 12 patients treated with APCs of the proximal tibia with a mean follow up of 40 months. Functional results were satisfactory with patients achieving in average 103° of knee flexion with 9 patients not presenting extensor lag. Functional outcome was 24.3 points out of 30 using the MSTS score or 81%. [104] Long-term follow-up with these techniques in under evaluation and publications in the near future will be available for evaluation and discussion. (Figure 13)

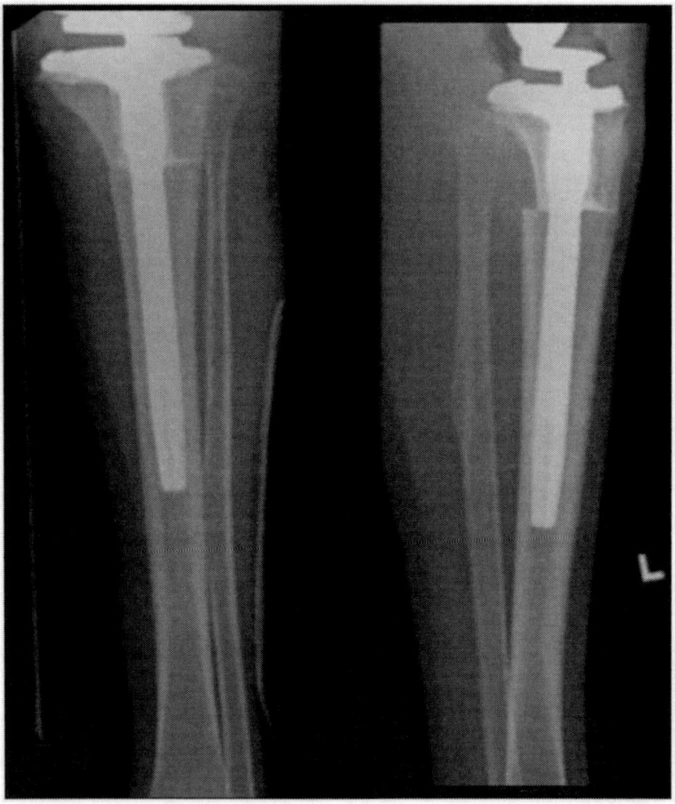

Figure 13. AP and lateral radiographic views of an allorgraft-prosthesis composite reconstruction of the proximal tibia for reconstruction after wide resection for an osteosarcoma of the proximal tibia.

Other Techniques

Other modalities of treatment that are usually reserved as salvage procedures after complications with the traditional techniques include arthrodesis of joints with allograft or autograft with plating or intramedullar fixation. This technique allows preservation of the extremity despite the lack of mobility. Even though function is not optimal, in the case of the shoulder it allows preservation of the hand with a stable post in the upper extremity and in the knee or ankle allows for a stable post for ambulation.

Other alternatives include resection arthroplasty in which a joint is left flail with no reconstruction. This is one of the oldest modalities of treatment for tumors and offers an acceptable but not optimal result. Patients can be functional despite limping and probably consuming less oxygen when ambulating when compared to patients with very high amputations or disarticulations.

Conclusion

Surgical treatment of ostosarcoma in the extremities is a key component of local control. Combination with adjuvant and neoadjuvant chemotherapy is crucial in improving patient survival and functional outcomes. There is a large number of techniques that have proved to be advantageous at some extend but not optimal to be recognized as the gold standard. Multiple techniques are available; most of them have been discussed and reviewed in this chapter. Literature comparing these modalities is scarce and future prospective and comparative studies are needed. However, the low prevalence of malignant primary bone tumors makes this task difficult. Multicenter investigations and combinations of registries are necessary to obtain the answers needed in this field.

The few available investigations, demonstrate comparable results in terms of function in patients treated with allograft or endoprosthesis. Differences are seen in the type and profile of complications experienced with each technique. The risk of fracture or non-union seen in allografts is not seen with prosthesis. Conversely, the mechanical failures and bone loss seen with prosthesis is not seen in allografts.

In conclusion, surgical treatment of primary malignant bone tumors is challenging and requires meticulous planning no matter what technique is chosen by the surgeon. Each modality has advantages and disadvantages and therefore, there is not a single best option for all patients. However, there is most of the time, a best option for each individual patient. It is the duty of the surgeon, to select the technique or modality of treatment that is going to satisfy the patient's functional demands with the lowest complication profile. This should be done always maintaining the oncologic principle of adequate radical resection and considering multiple factors such as the patient's age, tumor localization and grade, soft tissue involvement, life expectancy, level of activity, co-morbidities, anthropometric parameters, and social support among others. Making decisions taking into account all these aspects will guarantee a decision based in the holistic principle of treatment, which ultimately is going to benefit the patient the most.

REFERENCES

[1] Peltier L. F. Historical note on bone and soft tissue sarcoma. *J. Surg. Oncol.*, 1985, Dec.; 30(4):201-5. PubMed PMID: 3908827.
[2] Peltier L. Tumors of Bone and Soft Tissue. In: Peltier L, editor. Orthopaedics -A History and Iconography-. San Francisco: Norman; 1993. p. 264-91.
[3] Gross S. Sarcoma of the long bones. *Am. J. Med. Sci.*, 1879; 78(15-57): 338-77.
[4] Ferguson A. Treatment of osteogenic sarcoma. *J. Bone Joint Surg.*, 1940; 22:92-100.
[5] Lichtenstein L. Osteogenic Sarcoma in Bone. In: Lichtenstein L, editor. Bone Tumours. 2nd ed. St Louis: C.V. Mosby; 1959. p. 191-214.
[6] MacDonald I. B., J. W. Osteogenic Sarcoma. A modified nomenclature and review of 118 five-year cures. *Surg. Gynecol. Obst.*, 1943; 77: 413-21.
[7] Coley B. H., C. C. Jr. An analysis of fifty-nine cases of osteogenic sarcoma with survival for five years or more. *J. Bone Joint Surg.*, 1950; 32A:307-10.
[8] Thompson A. T.-W., R. T. Skeletal Sarcomata and Giant Cell Tumour. *J. Bone Joint Surg.*, 1955; 37B:266-303.
[9] Coventry M. D., D. C. Osteogenic Sarcoma: A critical analysis of 430 cases. *J. Bone Joint Surg.*, 1957; 39A:741-57.
[10] Marcove R. M., V.; Hajek, J. V.; Levin, A. G.; Hutter, R. V. P. Osteogenic Sarcoma under the age of twenty-one. A Review of one-

hundred and forty-five operative cases. *J. Bone Joint Surg*., 1970; 52A: 411-23.

[11] O'Hara J. M., Hutter R. V., Foote F. W., Jr., Miller T., Woodard H. Q. An analysis of thirty patients surviving longer than ten years after treatment for osteogenic sarcoma. *The Journal of bone and joint surgery American volume,* 1968, Mar.;50 (2):335-54. PubMed PMID: 5238720.

[12] Sweetnam R., Knowelden J., Seddon H. Bone sarcoma: treatment by irradiation, amputation, or a combination of the two. *British medical journal,* 1971, May 15;2 (5758):363-7. PubMed PMID: 4995895. Pubmed Central PMCID: 1795781.

[13] Sherman M., Irani R. N. Osteogenic sarcoma. Two cases of unexpectedly long survival. *The Journal of bone and joint surgery American volume,* 1962, Apr.;44-A:561-6. PubMed PMID: 14039203.

[14] Jaffe H. Tumours and Tumorous Conditions of the Bones and Joints. 1st Ed. ed. Philadelphia: Lea and Febiger; 1958.

[15] Lockshin M. H., I. Prognosis in Osteogenic Sarcoma. *Clin. Orthop.,* 1968;58:85-101.

[16] Dahlin D. C., Coventry M. B. Osteogenic sarcoma. A study of six hundred cases. *The Journal of bone and joint surgery American volume,* 1967, Jan.;49 (1):101-10. PubMed PMID: 5225072.

[17] Troup J. B., W. H. Malignant disease of the extremities treated by exarticulation. Analysis of two-hundred and sixty-four consecutive cases with survival rates. *J. Bone Joint Surg*., 1960; 42A:1041-50.

[18] Pack G. T. Major exarticulations for malignant neoplasms of the extremities: interscapulothoracic amputation, hip-joint disarticulation, and interilio-abdominal amputation; a report of end results in 228 cases. *The Journal of bone and joint surgery American volume*, 1956, Apr.;38-A(2):249-62. PubMed PMID: 13319386.

[19] Weinfeld M. S., Dudley H. R., Jr. Osteogenic sarcoma. A follow-up study of the ninety-four cases observed at the Massachusetts General Hospital from 1920 to 1960. *The Journal of bone and joint surgery American volume,* 1962, Mar.; 44-A:269-76. PubMed PMID: 14040209.

[20] Cade S. Osteogenic sarcoma; a study based on 133 patients. *Journal of the Royal College of Surgeons of Edinburgh,* 1955, Dec.;1(2):79-111. PubMed PMID: 13307660.

[21] Tudway R. C. Radiotherapy for Osteogenic Sarcoma. *J. Bone Joint Surg.,* 1961; 43B:61-7. PubMed PMID: 13923021.

[22] Tudway R. C. The place of external irradiation in the treatment of osteogenic sarcoma. *The Journal of bone and joint surgery British volume,* 1953, Feb.;35-B(1):9-21. PubMed PMID: 13034866.

[23] Lee E. S., Mackenzie D. H. Osteosarcoma. A Study of the Value of Preoperative Megavoltage Radiotherapy. *The British journal of surgery,* 1964, Apr.;51:252-74. PubMed PMID: 14138245.

[24] Allen C. V., Stevens K. R. Preoperative irradiation for osteogenic sarcoma. *Cancer*, 1973, Jun.;31(6):1364-6. PubMed PMID: 4196898.

[25] Sweetnam R. The surgical management of primary osteosarcoma. *Clinical orthopaedics and related research*, 1975, Sep. (111):57-64. PubMed PMID: 1057465.

[26] Suit H. D. Role of therapeutic radiology in cancer of bone. *Cancer*, 1975, Mar.;35 (3 suppl.):930-5. PubMed PMID: 1089475.

[27] Jenkin R. D., Allt W. E., Fitzpatrick P. J. Osteosarcoma. An assessment of management with particular reference to primary irradiation and selective delayed amputation. *Cancer,* 1972, Aug.;30 (2):393-400. PubMed PMID: 4506001.

[28] Cohen P. Osteosarcoma of the long bones. Clinical observations and experiences in the Netherlands. *European journal of cancer*, 1978, Sep.;14 (9): 995-1004. PubMed PMID: 280459.

[29] McKenna R. S., C. D.; Song, K. Y.; Higginbotham, N. L. Sarcomata of the osteogenic series (osteosarcoma, fibrosarcoma, chondrosarcoma, parosteal osteogenic saracoma and sarcoma arising in abonormal bone): An analysis of 552 cases. *J. Bone Joint Surg*., 1966;48A:1-26.

[30] Price C. H., Zhuber K., Salzer-Kuntschik M., Salzer M., Willert H. G., Immenkamp M., et al. Osteosarcoma in children. A study of 125 cases. *The Journal of bone and joint surgery British volume,* 1975, Aug.; 57(3): 341-5. PubMed PMID: 1057546.

[31] Friedman M. A., Carter S. K. The therapy of osteogenic sarcoma: current status and thoughts for the future. *J. Surg. Oncol.,* 1972; 4(5): 482- 510. PubMed PMID: 4566220.

[32] Peltier L. Historical note on bone and soft-tissue sarcoma. *J. Surg. Oncol.,* 1985;30:201-5.

[33] Dahlin D. General Aspects and an Analysis of 2276 cases. In: Dahlin D, editor. Bone Tumours. Springfield, Illinois: Charles C, Thomas; 1957.

[34] Jaffe N., Watts H. G. Multidrug chemotherapy in primary treatment of osteosarcoma. An editorial commentary. *The Journal of bone and joint surgery American volume,* 1976, Jul.;58 (5):634-5. PubMed PMID: 777004.

[35] Cores E. P., Holland J. F., Wang J. J., Sinks L. F. Doxorubicin in disseminated osteosarcoma. *JAMA: the journal of the American Medical Association,* 1972, Sep. 4;221 (10):1132-8. PubMed PMID: 4512088.

[36] Jaffe N. Recent advances in the chemotherapy of metastatic osteogenic sarcoma. *Cancer*, 1972, Dec.;30(6): 1627-31. PubMed PMID: 4539306.

[37] Mankin H. J., Hornicek F. J., Rosenberg A. E., Harmon D. C., Gebhardt M. C. Survival data for 648 patients with osteosarcoma treated at one institution. *Clinical orthopaedics and related research*, 2004, Dec. (429):286-91. PubMed PMID: 15577500.

[38] Goorin A. M., Andersen J. W. Experience with multiagent chemotherapy for osteosarcoma. Improved outcome. *Clinical orthopaedics and related research,* 1991 Sep(270):22-8. PubMed PMID: 1884543.

[39] Goorin A. M., Shuster J. J., Baker A., Horowitz M. E., Meyer W. H., Link M. P. Changing pattern of pulmonary metastases with adjuvant chemotherapy in patients with osteosarcoma: results from the multiinstitutional osteosarcoma study. *Journal of clinical oncology: official journal of the American Society of Clinical Oncology*, 1991, Apr.;9(4): 600-5. PubMed PMID: 2066757.

[40] Provisor A. J., Ettinger L. J., Nachman J. B., Krailo M. D., Makley J. T., Yunis E. J., et al. Treatment of nonmetastatic osteosarcoma of the extremity with preoperative and postoperative chemotherapy: a report from the Children's Cancer Group. *Journal of clinical oncology: official journal of the American Society of Clinical Oncology*, 1997, Jan.;15 (1): 76-84. PubMed PMID: 8996127.

[41] Picci P., Sangiorgi L., Rougraff B. T., Neff J. R., Casadei R., Campanacci M. Relationship of chemotherapy-induced necrosis and surgical margins to local recurrence in osteosarcoma. *Journal of clinical oncology: official journal of the American Society of Clinical Oncology,* 1994, Dec.;12 (12):2699-705. PubMed PMID: 7989947.

[42] Rougraff B. T., Simon M. A., Kneisl J. S., Greenberg D. B., Mankin H. J. Limb salvage compared with amputation for osteosarcoma of the distal end of the femur. A long-term oncological, functional, and quality-of-life study. *The Journal of bone and joint surgery American volume,* 1994, May;76 (5):649-56. PubMed PMID: 8175811.

[43] Eilber F. R., Morton D. L., Eckardt J., Grant T., Weisenburger T. Limb salvage for skeletal and soft tissue sarcomas. Multidisciplinary preoperative therapy. *Cancer,* 1984, Jun. 15;53 (12):2579-84. PubMed PMID: 6372980.

[44] Hudson M., Jaffe M. R., Jaffe N., Ayala A., Raymond A. K., Carrasco H., et al. Pediatric osteosarcoma: therapeutic strategies, results, and prognostic factors derived from a 10-year experience. *Journal of clinical oncology: official journal of the American Society of Clinical Oncology,* 1990 Dec.;8 (12):1988-97. PubMed PMID: 2230890.

[45] Jaffe N., Smith D., Jaffe M. R., Hudson M., Carrasco H., Wallace S., et al. Intraarterial cisplatin in the management of stage IIB osteosarcoma in the pediatric and adolescent age group. *Clinical orthopaedics and related research,* 1991, Sep. (270):15-21. PubMed PMID: 1884535.

[46] Petrilli A. S., Gentil F. C., Epelman S., Lopes L. F., Bianchi A., Lopes A., et al. Increased survival, limb preservation, and prognostic factors for osteosarcoma. *Cancer*, 1991, Aug. 15; 68(4):733-7. PubMed PMID: 1855172.

[47] Ruggieri P., De Cristofaro R., Picci P., Bacci G., Biagini R., Casadei R., et al. Complications and surgical indications in 144 cases of nonmetastatic osteosarcoma of the extremities treated with neoadjuvant chemotherapy. *Clinical orthopaedics and related research*, 1993, Oct. (295): 226-38. PubMed PMID: 8403653.

[48] Simon M. A. Limb salvage for osteosarcoma. *The Journal of bone and joint surgery American volume,* 1988, Feb.;70 (2):307-10. PubMed PMID: 3277972.

[49] Simon M. A., Aschliman M. A., Thomas N., Mankin H. J. Limb-salvage treatment versus amputation for osteosarcoma of the distal end of the femur. *The Journal of bone and joint surgery American volume,* 1986, Dec.;68(9):1331-7. PubMed PMID: 3465732.

[50] Springfield D. S., Schmidt R., Graham-Pole J., Marcus R. B., Jr., Spanier S. S., Enneking W. F. Surgical treatment for osteosarcoma. The *Journal of bone and joint surgery American volume*, 1988, Sep.;70 (8): 1124-30. PubMed PMID: 3166461.

[51] Ayerza M. A., Farfalli G. L., Aponte-Tinao L., Muscolo D. L. Does increased rate of limb-sparing surgery affect survival in osteosarcoma? *Clinical orthopaedics and related research,* 2010, Nov.;468(11):2854-9. PubMed PMID: 20559766. Pubmed Central PMCID: 2947695.

[52] Pardasaney P. K., Sullivan P. E., Portney L. G., Mankin H. J. Advantage of limb salvage over amputation for proximal lower extremity tumors. *Clinical orthopaedics and related research*, 2006, Mar.; 444: 201-8. PubMed PMID: 16449916.

[53] Malone J. M., Fleming L. L., Roberson J., Whitesides T. E., Jr., Leal J. M., Poole J. U., et al. Immediate, early, and late postsurgical

management of upper-limb amputation. *Journal of rehabilitation research and development*, 1984, May; 21 (1):33-41. PubMed PMID: 6527288.

[54] Thompson R. G. Amputation in the Lower Extremity. *The Journal of bone and joint surgery American volume,* 1963. Dec.;45: 1723- 34. PubMed PMID: 14083153.

[55] Van Ness C. Rotation-plasty for congenital defects of the femur. Making use of the ankle of the shortened limb to control the knee joint of a prosthesis. *J. Bone and Joint Surg*., 1950;32B:12-6.

[56] CP V. N. Rotation-plasty for congential defects of the femur. Making use of the ankle of teh shortened limb to control the knee joint of a prosthesis. *J. Bone Joint Surg*., 1950;32B:12-6.

[57] Agarwal M., Puri A., Anchan C., Shah M., Jambhekar N. Rotationplasty for bone tumors: is there still a role? *Clinical orthopaedics and related research,* 2007, Jun.;459:76-81. PubMed PMID: 17414168.

[58] Puri A., Agarwal M. Facilitating rotationplasty. *J. Surg. Oncol*., 2007, Mar. 15; 95(4):351-4. PubMed PMID: 17326128.

[59] Fuchs B., Kotajarvi B. R., Kaufman K. R., Sim F. H. Functional outcome of patients with rotationplasty about the knee. *Clinical orthopaedics and related research,* 2003, Oct. (415):52-8. PubMed PMID: 14612629.

[60] Mavrogenis A. F., Abati C. N., Romagnoli C., Ruggieri P. Similar survival but better function for patients after limb salvage versus amputation for distal tibia osteosarcoma. *Clinical orthopaedics and related research,* 2012, Jun.;470(6):1735-48. PubMed PMID: 22270466. Pubmed Central PMCID: 3348295.

[61] Hagberg E., Berlin O. K., Renstrom P. Function after through-knee compared with below-knee and above-knee amputation. *Prosthetics and orthotics international,* 1992, Dec.;16(3): 168-73. PubMed PMID: 1491950.

[62] Traugh G. H., Corcoran P. J., Reyes R. L. Energy expenditure of ambulation in patients with above-knee amputations. *Archives of physical medicine and rehabilitation,* 1975, Feb.;56(2): 67-71. PubMed PMID: 1124978.

[63] Waters R. L., Perry J., Antonelli D., Hislop H. Energy cost of walking of amputees: the influence of level of amputation. *The Journal of bone and joint surgery American volume,* 1976, Jan.;58 (1):42-6. PubMed PMID: 1249111.

[64] Ferguson P. C., McLaughlin C. E., Griffin A. M., Bell R. S., Deheshi B. M., Wunder J. S. Clinical and functional outcomes of patients with a pathologic fracture in high-grade osteosarcoma. *J. Surg. Oncol.*, 2010, Aug. 1;102(2):120-4. PubMed PMID: 20648581.

[65] Tan P. X., Yong B. C., Wang J., Huang G., Yin J. Q., Zou C. Y., et al. Analysis of the efficacy and prognosis of limb-salvage surgery for osteosarcoma around the knee. *European journal of surgical oncology: the journal of the European Society of Surgical Oncology and the British Association of Surgical Oncology*, 2012, Dec.;38 (12):1171-7. PubMed PMID: 22809860.

[66] Xie L., Guo W., Li Y., Ji T., Sun X. Pathologic fracture does not influence local recurrence and survival in high-grade extremity osteosarcoma with adequate surgical margins. *J. Surg. Oncol.*, 2012, Dec.;106 (7):820-5. PubMed PMID: 22740310.

[67] Scully S. P., Ghert M. A., Zurakowski D., Thompson R. C., Gebhardt M. C. Pathologic fracture in osteosarcoma: prognostic importance and treatment implications. *The Journal of bone and joint surgery American volume,* 2002, Jan.;84-A(1):49-57. PubMed PMID: 11792779.

[68] Moore A. T. B. H. Metal Hip Joint: A Case Report. *J. Bone and Joint Surg.,* 1943;25A:688-92.

[69] Marcove R. C., Lewis M. M., Rosen G., Huvos A. G. Total femur and total knee replacement. A preliminary report. *Clinical orthopaedics and related research*, 1977, Jul.-Aug. (126):147-52. PubMed PMID: 271530.

[70] Ward W. G., Johnston K. S., Dorey F. J., Eckardt J. J. Extramedullary porous coating to prevent diaphyseal osteolysis and radiolucent lines around proximal tibial replacements. A preliminary report. *The Journal of bone and joint surgery American volume,* 1993, Jul.;75(7):976-87. PubMed PMID: 8335673.

[71] Roberts P., Chan D., Grimer R. J., Sneath R. S., Scales J. T. Prosthetic replacement of the distal femur for primary bone tumours. *The Journal of bone and joint surgery British volume,* 1991, Sep.;73(5): 762-9. PubMed PMID: 1894662.

[72] Horowitz S. M., Glasser D. B., Lane J. M., Healey J. H. Prosthetic and extremity survivorship after limb salvage for sarcoma. How long do the reconstructions last? *Clinical orthopaedics and related research*, 1993, Aug. (293):280-6. PubMed PMID: 8339494.

[73] Capanna R., Morris H. G., Campanacci D., Del Ben M., Campanacci M. Modular uncemented prosthetic reconstruction after resection of tumours

of the distal femur. *The Journal of bone and joint surgery British volume,* 1994, Mar.;76(2):178-86. PubMed PMID: 8113272.

[74] Malawer M. M., Chou L. B. Prosthetic survival and clinical results with use of large-segment replacements in the treatment of high-grade bone sarcomas. *The Journal of bone and joint surgery American volume*, 1995, Aug.;77(8):1154-65. PubMed PMID: 7642659.

[75] Morris H. G., Capanna R., Campanacci D., Del Ben M., Gasbarrini A. Modular endoprosthetic replacement after total resection of the femur for malignant tumour. *International orthopaedics*, 1994, Apr.;18(2):90-5. PubMed PMID: 8039964.

[76] Bernthal N. M., Schwartz A. J., Oakes D. A., Kabo J. M., Eckardt J. J. How long do endoprosthetic reconstructions for proximal femoral tumors last? *Clinical orthopaedics and related research*, 2010, Nov.;468(11):2867-74. PubMed PMID: 20440661. Pubmed Central PMCID: 2947672.

[77] Menendez L. R., Ahlmann E. R., Kermani C., Gotha H. Endoprosthetic reconstruction for neoplasms of the proximal femur. *Clinical orthopaedics and related research*, 2006, Sep.;450:46-51. PubMed PMID: 16906093.

[78] Bickels J., Meller I., Henshaw R. M., Malawer M. M. Reconstruction of hip stability after proximal and total femur resections. *Clinical orthopaedics and related research,* 2000, Jun. (375):218-30. PubMed PMID: 10853173.

[79] Lackman R. D., Torbert J. T., Finstein J. L., Ogilvie C. M., Fox E. J. Inaccuracies in the assessment of femoral anteversion in proximal femoral replacement prostheses. *The Journal of arthroplasty*, 2008, Jan.;23(1):97-101. PubMed PMID: 18165037.

[80] Finstein J. L., King J. J., Fox E. J., Ogilvie C. M., Lackman R. D. Bipolar proximal femoral replacement prostheses for musculoskeletal neoplasms. *Clinical orthopaedics and related research,* 2007, Jun.;459:66-75. PubMed PMID: 17545760.

[81] Henderson E. R., Groundland J. S., Pala E., Dennis J. A., Wooten R., Cheong D., et al. Failure mode classification for tumor endoprostheses: retrospective review of five institutions and a literature review. The *Journal of bone and joint surgery American volume*, 2011, Mar. 2;93(5):418-29. PubMed PMID: 21368074.

[82] Pala E., Henderson E. R., Calabro T., Angelini A., Abati C. N., Trovarelli G., et al. Survival of current production tumor endoprostheses: complications, functional results, and a comparative

statistical analysis. *J. Surg. Oncol.*, 2013, Nov.;108(6):403-8. PubMed PMID: 24006247.

[83] Pala E., Mavrogenis A. F., Angelini A., Henderson E. R., Douglas Letson G., Ruggieri P. Cemented versus cementless endoprostheses for lower limb salvage surgery. *Journal of BUON: official journal of the Balkan Union of Oncology,* 2013, Apr.-Jun.; 18(2):496-503. PubMed PMID: 23818368.

[84] Shehadeh A., Noveau J., Malawer M., Henshaw R. Late complications and survival of endoprosthetic reconstruction after resection of bone tumors. *Clinical orthopaedics and related research*, 2010, Nov.; 468(11):2885-95. PubMed PMID: 20625951. Pubmed Central PMCID: 2947697.

[85] Jeys L. M., Kulkarni A., Grimer R. J., Carter S. R., Tillman R. M., Abudu A. Endoprosthetic reconstruction for the treatment of musculoskeletal tumors of the appendicular skeleton and pelvis. *The Journal of bone and joint surgery American volume,* 2008, Jun.; 90(6):1265-71. PubMed PMID: 18519320.

[86] Pedtke A. C., Wustrack R. L., Fang A. S., Grimer R. J., O'Donnell R. J. Aseptic failure: how does the Compress((R)) implant compare to cemented stems? *Clinical orthopaedics and related research*, 2012, Mar.; 470(3):735-42. PubMed PMID: 22045069. Pubmed Central PMCID: 3270164.

[87] Bhangu A. A., Kramer M. J., Grimer R. J., O'Donnell R. J. Early distal femoral endoprosthetic survival: cemented stems versus the Compress implant. *International orthopaedics*, 2006, Dec.; 30(6):465-72. PubMed PMID: 16983554. Pubmed Central PMCID: 3172732.

[88] O'Donnell R. J. Compressive osseointegration of tibial implants in primary cancer reconstruction. *Clinical orthopaedics and related research,* 2009, Nov.; 467(11):2807-12. PubMed PMID: 19653050. Pubmed Central PMCID: 2758992.

[89] Farfalli G. L., Boland P. J., Morris C. D., Athanasian E. A., Healey J. H. Early equivalence of uncemented press-fit and Compress femoral fixation. *Clinical orthopaedics and related research*, 2009, Nov.; 467(11):2792-9. PubMed PMID: 19513799. Pubmed Central PMCID: 2758982.

[90] Henderson E. R., Pepper A. M., Marulanda G., Binitie O. T., Cheong D., Letson G. D. Outcome of lower-limb preservation with an expandable endoprosthesis after bone tumor resection in children. *The Journal of*

bone and joint surgery American volume, 2012, Mar. 21;94(6):537-47. PubMed PMID: 22438003.

[91] Henderson E. R., Pepper A. M., Marulanda G. A., Millard J. D., Letson G. D. What is the emotional acceptance after limb salvage with an expandable prosthesis? *Clinical orthopaedics and related research*, 2010, Nov.; 468(11):2933-8. PubMed PMID: 20632139. Pubmed Central PMCID: 2947674.

[92] Parrish F. F. Allograft replacement of all or part of the end of a long bone following excision of a tumor. *The Journal of bone and joint surgery American volume,* 1973, Jan.; 55 (1): 1-22. PubMed PMID: 4570894.

[93] Clohisy D. R., Mankin H. J. Osteoarticular allografts for reconstruction after resection of a musculoskeletal tumor in the proximal end of the tibia. *The Journal of bone and joint surgery American volume*, 1994, Apr.; 76(4):549-54. PubMed PMID: 8150822.

[94] Mankin H. J., Doppelt S. H., Sullivan T. R., Tomford W. W. Osteoarticular and intercalary allograft transplantation in the management of malignant tumors of bone. *Cancer,* 1982, Aug. 15; 50 (4): 613-30. PubMed PMID: 7046906.

[95] Mankin H. J., Gebhardt M. C., Jennings L. C., Springfield D. S., Tomford W. W. Long-term results of allograft replacement in the management of bone tumors. *Clinical orthopaedics and related research*, 1996, Mar. (324):86-97. PubMed PMID: 8595781.

[96] Muscolo D. L., Ayerza M. A., Aponte-Tinao L. A. Massive allograft use in orthopedic oncology. *The Orthopedic clinics of North America*, 2006, Jan.; 37(1):65-74. PubMed PMID: 16311112.

[97] Muscolo D. L., Ayerza M. A., Aponte-Tinao L. A., Ranalletta M. Use of distal femoral osteoarticular allografts in limb salvage surgery. Surgical technique. *The Journal of bone and joint surgery American volume*, 2006, Sep.; 88 Suppl. 1 Pt 2:305-21. PubMed PMID: 16951102.

[98] Ortiz-Cruz E., Gebhardt M. C., Jennings L. C., Springfield D. S., Mankin H. J. The results of transplantation of intercalary allografts after resection of tumors. A long-term follow-up study. *The Journal of bone and joint surgery American volume,* 1997, Jan.; 79(1):97-106. PubMed PMID: 9010190.

[99] Hornicek F. J., Gebhardt M. C., Tomford W. W., Sorger J. I., Zavatta M., Menzner J. P., et al. Factors affecting nonunion of the allograft-host junction. *Clinical orthopaedics and related research*, 2001, Jan, (382): 87-98. PubMed PMID: 11154010.

[100] Aponte-Tinao L., Farfalli G. L., Ritacco L. E., Ayerza M. A., Muscolo D. L. Intercalary femur allografts are an acceptable alternative after tumor resection. *Clinical orthopaedics and related research*, 2012, Mar.; 470(3): 728-34. PubMed PMID: 21691906. Pubmed Central PMCID: 3270162.

[101] Campanacci L., Manfrini M., Colangeli M., Ali N., Mercuri M. Long-term results in children with massive bone osteoarticular allografts of the knee for high-grade osteosarcoma. *Journal of pediatric orthopedics*, 2010, Dec.; 30(8):919-27. PubMed PMID: 21102223.

[102] Abdeen A., Healey J. H. Allograft-prosthesis composite reconstruction of the proximal part of the humerus: surgical technique. *The Journal of bone and joint surgery American volume,* 2010, Sep.; 92 Suppl. 1 Pt 2:188-96. PubMed PMID: 20844174.

[103] Abdeen A., Hoang B. H., Athanasian E. A., Morris C. D., Boland P. J., Healey J. H. Allograft-prosthesis composite reconstruction of the proximal part of the humerus: functional outcome and survivorship. The *Journal of bone and joint surgery American volume*, 2009, Oct.; 91(10):2406-15. PubMed PMID: 19797576.

[104] Gilbert N. F., Yasko A. W., Oates S. D., Lewis V. O., Cannon C. P., Lin P. P. Allograft-prosthetic composite reconstruction of the proximal part of the tibia. An analysis of the early results. *The Journal of bone and joint surgery American volume*, 2009, Jul.;91 (7):1646-56. PubMed PMID: 19571087.

In: Osteosarcoma
Editors: Edwin Choy
ISBN: 978-1-63321-052-3

Chapter 3

RECENT DEVELOPMENTS IN THE IMAGING OF OSTEOSARCOMA

Timothy M. Meehan, MD. and Daniel I. Rosenthal, MD.
Department of Radiology, Massachusetts General Hospital, Harvard Medical School, Boston, MA, US

ABSTRACT

This chapter summarizes the advances in imaging of osteosarcoma that have occurred during last few decades. We consider that the recent past begins with the widespread adoption of MRI in the mid 1990s. It begins with a consideration of the more traditional role of imaging in diagnosis and staging of tumors. The next section deals with what has been learned about the implications of imaging findings on tumor prognosis, followed immediately with a description of the qualitative and quantitative features that may be user to evaluate the effects of treatment. Special attention is paid to the use of PET imaging and MRI for this purpose. The chapter concludes with a brief description of image-guided intervention, and post-treatment imaging.

INTRODUCTION

Osteosarcoma (OSA) is by definition a malignant neoplasm in which the tumor cells produce bone. The World Health Organization (WHO) recognizes eight types: conventional, telangiectatic, small cell, low grade central, secondary, parosteal, periosteal and high grade surface tumors. The "conventional" category is subdivided into osteoblastic, chondroblastic and fibroblastic types.

Although there are group differences in the imaging appearances of the categories of the WHO classification, with the possible exception of the parosteal tumors, there is substantial overlap. (Figures 1-5). This classification scheme is somewhat arbitrary and inconsistent, as two of the categories represent histological features (telangiectatic, small cell, Figures 6 and 7), four represent a combination of histological features and location (low grade central, parosteal, periosteal and high grade surface) and one considers only etiology (secondary).

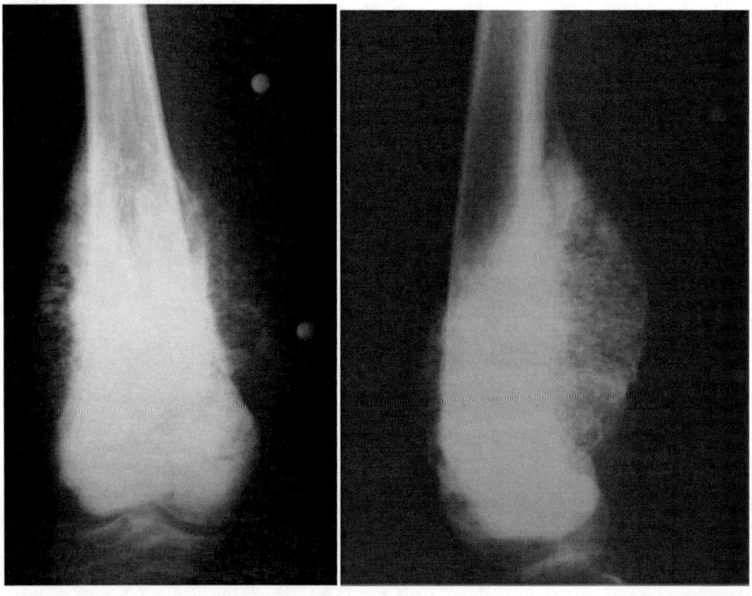

Figure 1. Classic osteoblastic osteosarcoma. The lateral and frontal radiographs demonstrate an osteosarcoma of the distal femur metaphysis with osteoid matrix and a classic "sunburst" periosteal reaction.

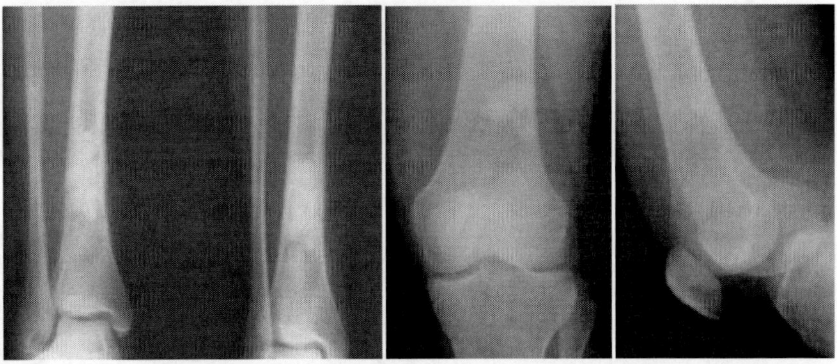

Figure 2. Two examples of well differentiated intramedullary osteosarcoma. Frontal and oblique radiographs demonstrate amorphous or "cloud-like bone formation in the medullary cavity of the metaphysis of the distal tibia(left) and feumur(right). Despite the innocent appearance, bone-forming lesions must always be regarded with suspicion. High-grade lesions are much more frequent than low grade. Note the lack of periosteal reaction due to the fact that the lesions have not yet extended beyond the marrow.

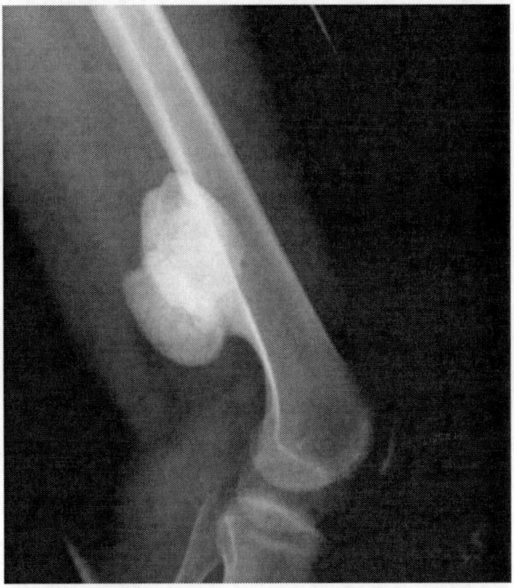

Figure 3. Parosteal osteosarcoma. Lateral radiograph shows a lobulated ossified exophytic tumor arising from the posterior distal femur. Anatomically, parosteal sarcomas originate from the outer fibrous later of the periosteum.

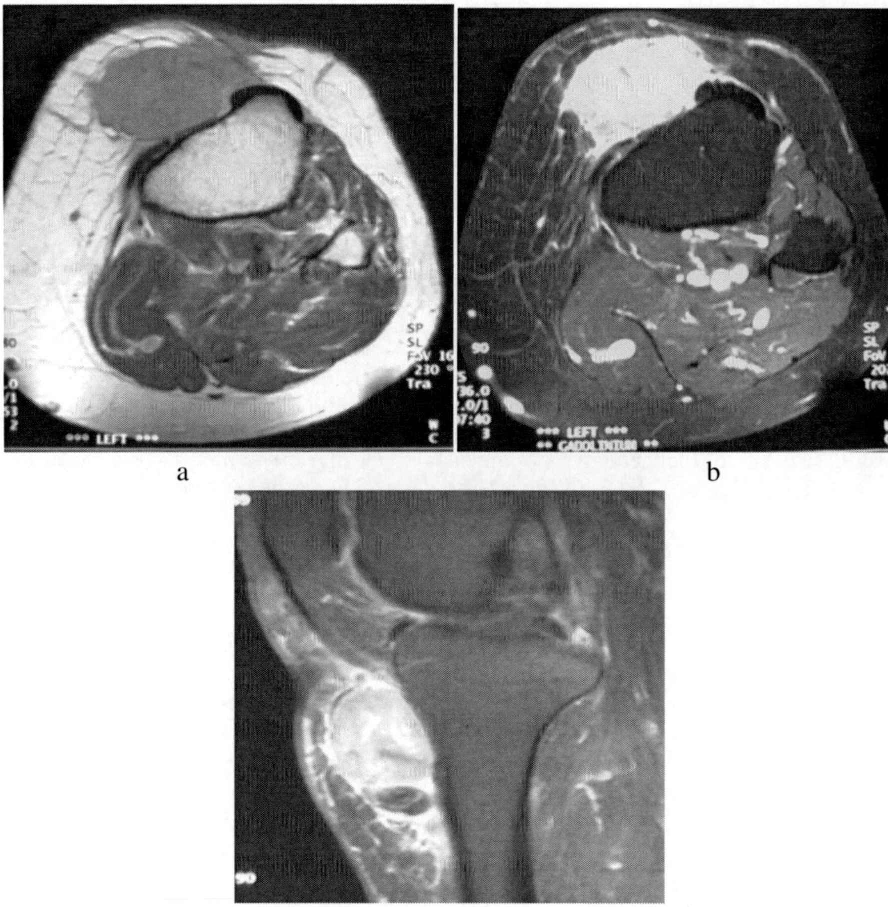

Figure 4. Surface osteosarcoma. Axial T1 pre-contrast (a) and axial (b) and sagittal (c) T1 post contrast images demonstrate an avidly enhancing high grade surface osteosarcoma adjacent to the proximal tibia. There is periosteal reaction but no marrow involvement.

DIAGNOSIS

The role of anatomical imaging in the diagnosis of osteosarcoma has been well documented over many years and has not undergone substantial change recently. Osteosarcoma can be identified on imaging when there is a destructive mass containing immature tumoral ossification. This can be difficult because lesions may show a variety of appearances. Each tumor may contain a mixture of cell types, and the imaging reflects the mixture of tissues. For example, a largely chondroblastic osteosarcoma may be difficult to distinguish from a chondrosarcoma (Figure 8). Accumulated experience has shown that some features previously thought to characterize benign conditions, such as fluid-fluid levels, are non-specific and may occur in both benign and malignant conditions, including osteosarcoma [1, 2] (Figure 9).

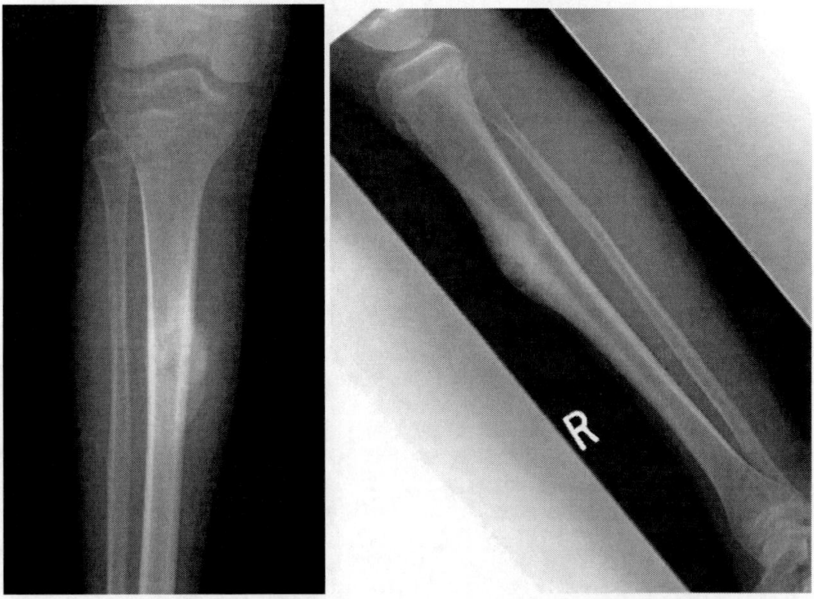

Figure 5. Intracortical osteosarcoma. Frontal and lateral radiographs of this rare low grade osteosarcoma demonstrate a broad-based area of eccentric cortical thickening with a small central luceny in the mid-shaft of the tibia. Note the coarse lamellar periosteal new bone formation.

In general, for tumors that produce an extra-cellular matrix such as osteosarcoma, the higher the grade of the lesion, the less the matrix resembles normal tissue. Four of the WHO categories of osteosarcoma tend to be low or intermediate grade (low grade central, parosteal, periosteal and intracortical) and therefore are likely to demonstrate recognizable bone on imaging studies.

The most common aggressive types (conventional, small cell, telangiectatic) usually arise from the endosteum (central), and may be so poorly differentiated that no macroscopic bone is recognizable, and therefore the diagnosis on imaging can be difficult or impossible.

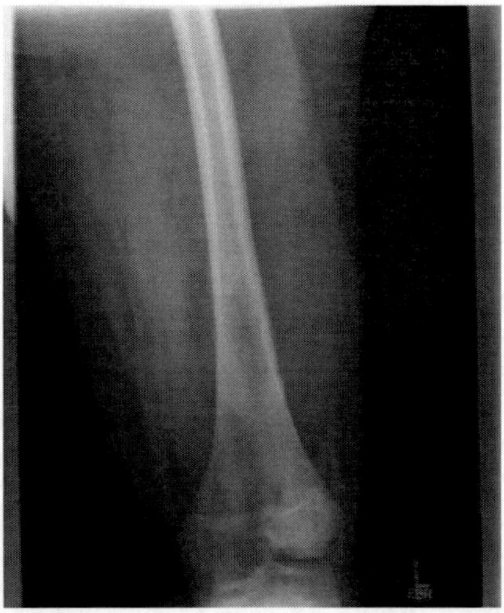

Figure 6. Small cell osteosarcoma. Frontal radiograph of the right femur demonstrates a mixed lytic and blastic tumor in the metaphysis with a pattern of permeative destruction. Small cell osteosarcoma is an exceedingly rare tumor, estimated to account for less than 1% of all cases of osteosarcoma.

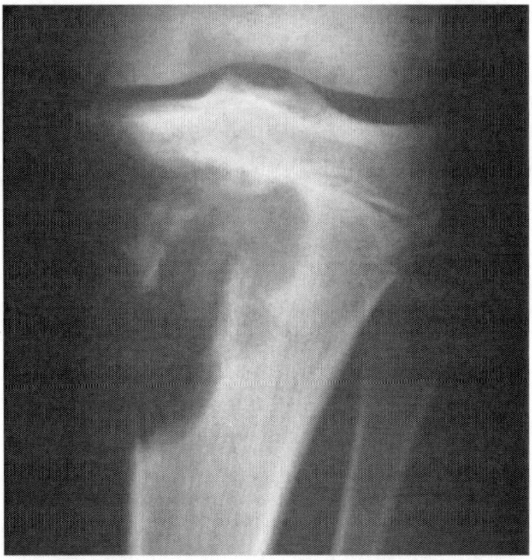

Figure 7. Telangectatic osteosarcoma. Frontal radiograph of the proximal tibia demonstrates a lytic lesion arising from the proximal metaphysis. There is aggressive destruction of the cortex and invasion of the joint space. There is no macroscopic bone recognizable on radiograph.

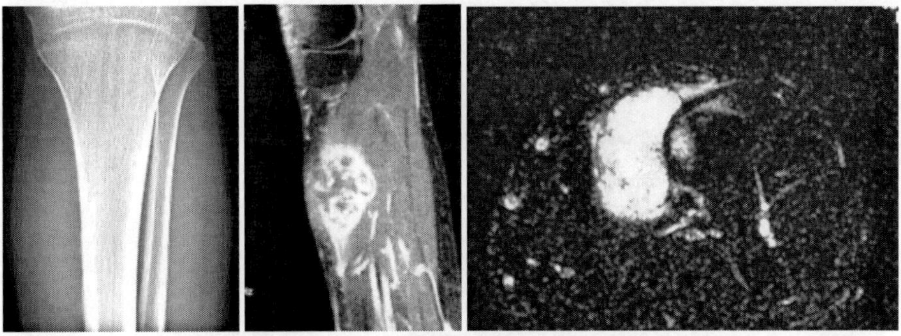

Figure 8. Periosteal chondroblastic osteosarcoma: Radiograph of the proximal tibia demonstrates subtle increased soft tissue attenuation. Sagittal T1 gadolinium enhanced images demonstrate an avidly enhancing lesion with peripheral and septal enhancement. There is lobular high intensity signal on T2 weighed imaging and lack of osseous formation on radiograph, making distinction from chondrosarcoma difficult.

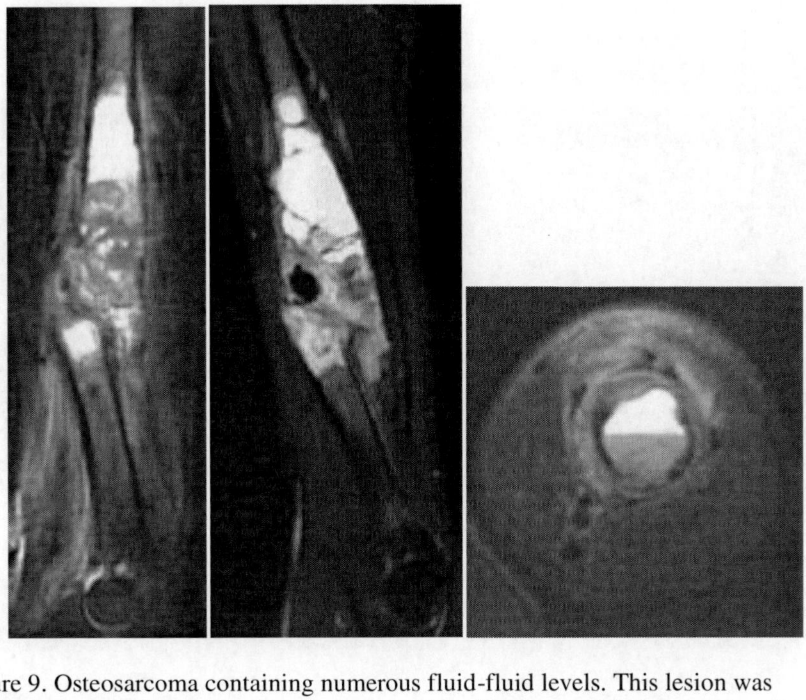

Figure 9. Osteosarcoma containing numerous fluid-fluid levels. This lesion was originally biopsied and thought to be an aneurismal bone cyst. Notice that there is a solid portion adjacent to the cystic component. A second biopsy directed at the solid portion seen on T1 sagittal contrast enhanced images demonstrated osteosarcoma.

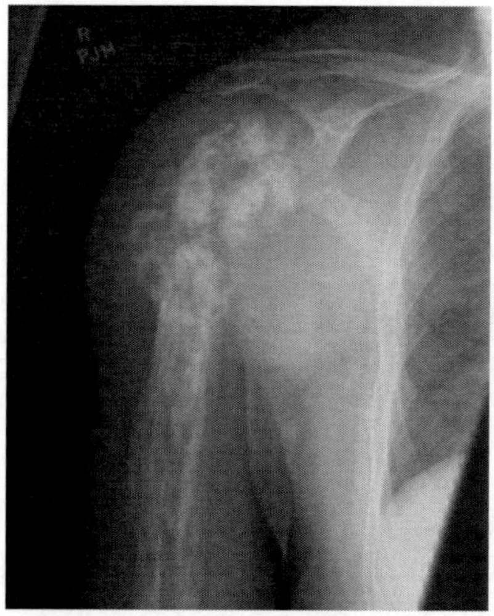

Figure 10. Osteosarcoma arising within Paget bone. The entire humerus is affected by Paget Disease, seen as disorganized thickening of the cortex and widening of the bone. A destructive lesion with amorphous bone formation is visible within the proximal end of the humerus.

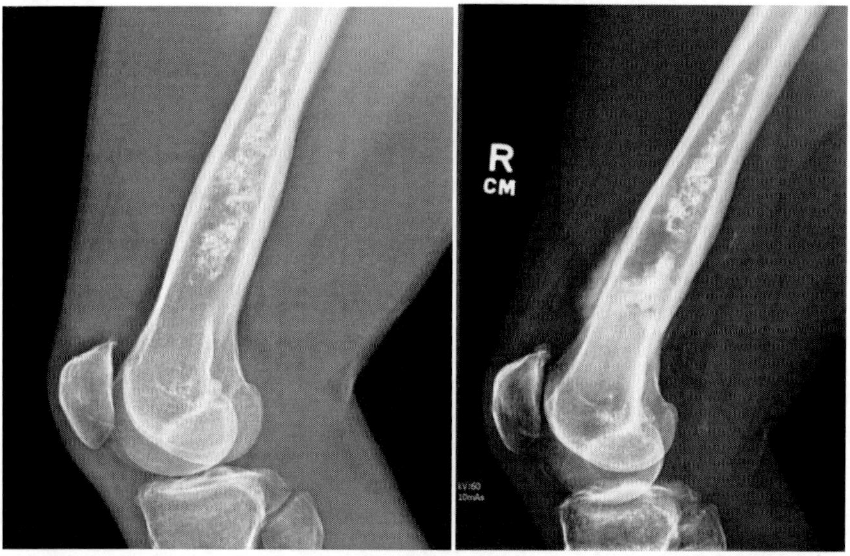

A B

Figure 11. Osteosarcoma arising from dedifferentiation. (A). A radiograph shows stippled calcifications in the medulla of the distal femur consistent with an enchondroma. (B) 10 years later, lateral radiographs demonstrate the development of an aggressive osteoblastic lesion in the distal femur.

Osteosarcoma may be secondary to a variety of pre-existing lesions and genetic syndromes. Perhaps the best known of these is Paget disease, (Figure 10) but a large number of precursor lesions have been identified. Tumors consisting of other cell lines (not bone) may transform into osteosarcoma through the mechanism of "dedifferentiation". (Figure 11) The list of lesions that may give rise to osteosarcoma keeps growing as rare transformations are encountered (such as from liposclerosing myxofibrous tumor [3]. Osteosarcoma has even been reported to arise from heterotopic ossification due to an electrical burn. [4] Hyperparathyroidism-induced osteosarcoma has been shown in a rat model using synthetic PTH, and the association has been reported in human case reports. [5]

It appears as though any lesion that causes chronic increases in bone turnover may predispose to osteosarcoma. The chance of degeneration of a benign condition to osteosarcoma may be increased following radiation treatment. There are several reports of radiation therapy of aneurysmal bone cyst provoking the occurrence of osteosarcoma. [6] Osteosarcoma that arises in pre-existing disease or after radiation generally has a poor prognosis. [7]

Some genetic syndromes of which osteosarcoma may be a feature include: Li Fraumeni syndrome, Familial retinoblastoma, and Werners syndrome. [8]

A few new diagnostic methods have been introduced in recent years. The use of labeled monoclonal antibody 791T/36 (anti-osteosarcoma) appears to detect OSA with high sensitivity (5/5), but specificity is poor, as 4/5 other primary sarcomas (of which only 2 were bone sarcomas) and two cases of infection also were positive. [9]

The use of MR spectroscopy to distinguish benign from malignant tumors has been somewhat disappointing. Single voxel spectroscopy can identify a clearly defined choline peak at 3.2 ppm in a large majority of malignant tumors, but false positive results are fairly frequent and false negative results may occur in low grade parosteal OSA. [10]

STAGING

Surgical planning decisions have become strongly influenced by imaging. A great deal of research was devoted to anatomical correlation of images during the 1980s and 1990s. Over the past several decades, limb-sparing surgery has become the norm, and amputation the exception, in large measure owing to the huge advances in cross-sectional imaging that have made pre-operative planning much more reliable and effective. Preoperative evaluation of tumor extent using magnetic resonance imaging is the best available method to ensure adequate margins. (Figure 12) [11]

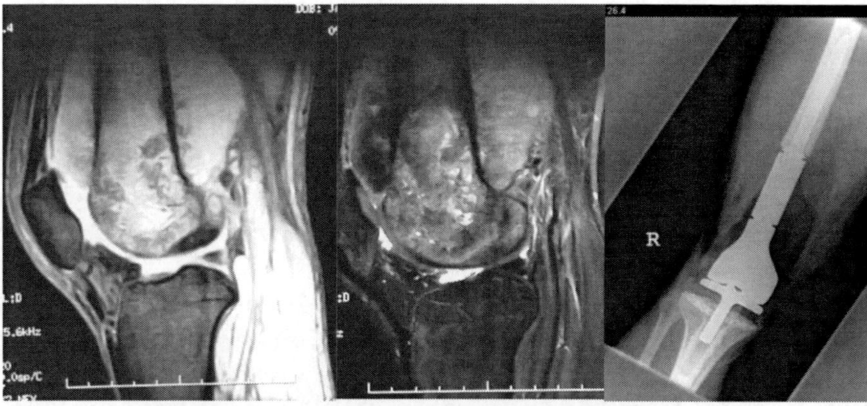

A

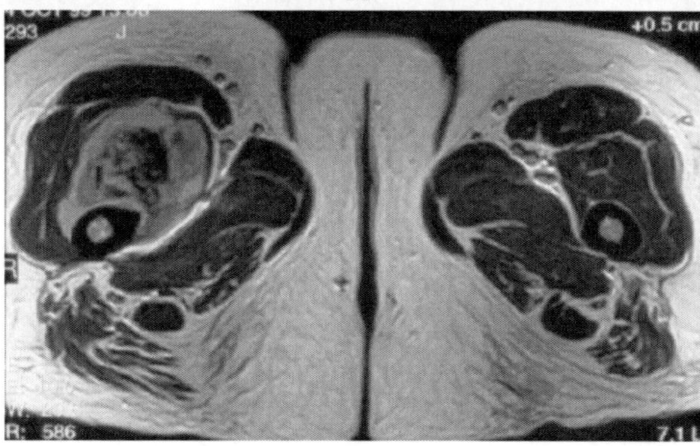

B

Figure 12. Osteosarcoma staging. A. Joint invasion. Sagittal T2 and T1 post contrast images demonstrate an osteosarcoma arising from the distal femur with concentric growth and joint invasion, necessitating total joint excision. Frontal radiograph showing reconstruction following resection of the distal femur and the knee joint. B. Vascular displacement: T1 weighted images demonstrate an osteosarcoma of the proximal right femur displacing but not invading the femoral vessels, an important distinction for surgical planning.

MR imaging is useful for estimating intraosseous extent of osteosarcoma prior to surgery. Tumor length can be most accurately measured using T1 weighted images, relying upon the natural contrast of fat within bone marrow. Heavily T2 weighted images (such as STIR) are more sensitive to the presence of tumor, due to their ability to detected increases in water content. However, these sequences also detect edema and reactive tissue and can lead to overestimation of tumor extent [12]. T2 weighted images are better for assessing soft tissue extent, although in this area too they may lead to overestimation due to peritumoral edema. For these reasons, the typical MR examination will include longitudinal (such as coronal) T1 or proton density-weighted images and axial T2 weighted images. Recently, it has been suggested that diffusion-weighted imaging is a good method to distinguish between tumor and peritumoral reactive edema.

Fat-suppressed gadolinium-enhanced T1 weighted images can be helpful if it is necessary to identify areas of cyst or cystic necrosis. This is of particular importance if planning a needle biopsy, since a necrotic area may yield non-diagnostic tissue, and vascular areas usually contain the highest grade tumor. However, these sequences are not usually essential for diagnosis or staging.
Although attention has largely shifted to other areas of research, investigations of gross morphology continue. For example, the fact that cartilage is only a relative barrier to tumor spread has been recognized only with the widespread adoption of pre-operative MRI. Contrary to older opinions, extension across joints (especially joints with little or no motion such as the sacroiliac joint), and open growth plates is relatively common. (Figure 13) [13]

Some of the pitfalls associated with modern and highly sensitive imaging methods are still being discovered. It may be more difficult to identify tumor limits precisely than it was initially thought. For example, an extended uptake pattern may be seen on bone scintigraphy due to regional hyperemia. This may cause overestimation of the size of the tumor. The extended uptake pattern is most often seen in bones across the joint but may occur anywhere in the same extremity. It has also been noted that decreased uptake or "cold" lesions may occur in osteosarcoma. [14]

In addition, many patients demonstrate increased radio-isotope uptake on bone scan at sites remote from the primary lesion that do not represent metastases. Frequent sites of "false positive" scans include ipsilateral weight-bearing joints. This phenomenon may affect joints that are proximal to the tumor, but is especially frequent at joints distal to the tumor. [15] Bone infarction may occur following chemotherapy for osteosarcoma (especially after intra-arterial chemotherapy) and may be mistaken for a new lesion. A useful distinguishing feature is the absence of gadolinium enhancement in an infarct. [16]

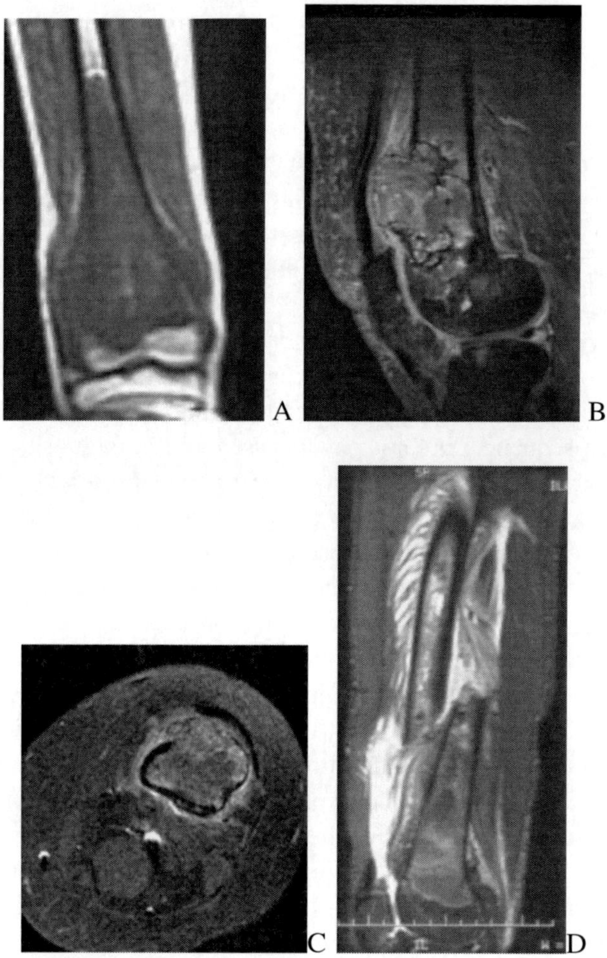

Figure 13. Osteosarcoma, tumor extent. A. Coronal T1 weighted imaging showing the extent of the tumor in the marrow. Tumor has violated the open growth plate. The normal fat content of the marrow serves as a clear boundary. B&C. Sagittal and axial T2 weighted images demonstrates cortical destruction with intramedullary as well as soft tissue tumor extension. Notice that abnormal signal extends well beyond the obvious mass. It can be difficult to distinguish tumor from edema using conventional T2 weighted imaging or contrast-enhanced imaging. D: Peritumoral Edema. T2 sagittal image demonstrates a pathologic fracture in the setting of osteosarcoma of the femur. Notice the feathery T2 hyperintensity involving the soft tissues related to pathologic fracture and edema, probably not macroscopic tumor extension, although the presence of microscopic disease is likely.

Peritumoral soft tissue edema can be observed adjacent to the tumor, even overlying intact periosteum. This may lead to difficulty in determining tumor margins on MRI [17]. A recent paper attempted to clarify the peritumoral signal abnormalities, in an effort to obtain better size estimates, and therefore facilitate more accurate surgical planning. The authors studied 27 osteosarcoma and 3 Ewing's sarcoma, attempting to distinguish between tumor margins and "peritumoral edema" Of the studied areas, 17.4% were positive for tumor (viable or necrotic). A feathery appearance on MRI correlated with tumor-negative areas whereas a bulky appearance correlated with tumor-positive regions. [18]

PROGNOSIS

Many factors have been identified that may influence the prognosis of osteosarcoma. These include size at the time of presentation, tumor subtype and grade, anatomical location of the tumor, whether it is primary or secondary to a pre-existing condition, and whether metastases are present at the time of presentation. While important, each of these is beyond the control of the physician. Adequacy of surgical treatment and effectiveness of chemotherapy are the only two that can be influenced (at least theoretically) by treatment decisions.

A recent paper re-examined some old ideas about tumor growth and prognosis using modern imaging. A large number of patients with osteosarcoma were divided into those with a concentric (225 tumors or 64.8% of the total), eccentric (71 or 20.5%), or longitudinal (51 or 14.7%). patterns of tumor growth (Figure 14). The type of tumor growth was found to be an independent prognostic factor. Eccentric tumors were usually small and responded well to chemotherapy, whereas concentric tumors were large and responded poorly. Moreover, longitudinally growing tumors were associated with better survival in AJCC stage IIB patients. [19] This study seems to reiterate older ideas derived from the tumor margin analysis in which concentric growth on cross-sectional imaging serves as a proxy for "permeated margins" as seen on radiography. [20]

Venous invasion is also increasingly recognized as a relatively common and ominous feature of osteosarcoma. MRI and/or CT with contrast or even venography can help to identify this occurrence. [13]

An additional imaging abnormality, pathologic fracture, has prognostic and treatment implications in the setting of osteosarcoma, either on presentation or during the course of chemotherapy. A study identified 52 patients with osteosarcoma and pathological fracture, matched to 55 patients without fracture but otherwise matched for age and tumor location.

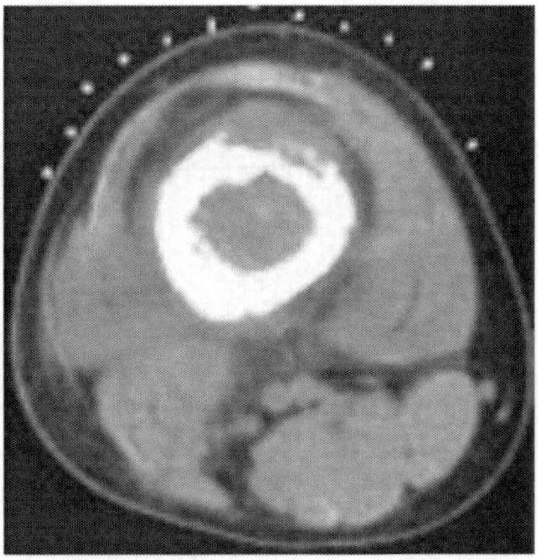

Figure 14. Osteosarcoma, concentric growth. CT of an osteosarcoma showing tumor from the medullary cavity of the femur permeating through the cortex to surround the femur circumferentially.

The presentation with fracture had poor implications for survival (55% at 5 years c/w 77% among the controls), with an increased risk of local recurrence. However, the performance of limb-salvage surgery, as compared to amputation, does not appear to worsen prognosis in eligible patients with a pathologic fracture. [21]

Conflicting evidence exists in regards to the presence of pulmonary metastasis at the time of diagnosis. Some reports in the literature deem it unimportant [22], while others recognize pulmonary metastatic disease as an indicator of poor prognosis [7].

Response to Treatment: Qualitative

Chemotherapeutic and surgical advances have improved current survival rates. Before 1970, 20% of patients treated with surgery alone survived 5 years. Current expectations are 60-80% survival and beyond. Patients surviving at least three years without recurrence are presumed to be cured. [3]

There are a number of qualitative findings that may be observed on various imaging studies in response to treatment (Figure 15). At one time, therapeutic response was judged solely on size, with response considered to be a 50% reduction in the product of the two largest diameters [24]. However, successfully treated osteosarcomas do not necessarily decrease in size (although they should not increase in size) and a number of other features may be recognized.

On plain films a dense rim of calcification and/or central calcification may be seen following chemotherapy. (Figure 16) The moth-eaten or permeated pattern of bone destruction on radiographs may transform to confluent areas of osteolysis. This may give the impression that bone destruction is worsening, when in fact the tumor is responding to treatment. [25]

Qualitative EVIDENCE OF
THERAPEUTIC EFFECT

1. ↓ SIZE
2. ↑ MARGINS
3. ↓ BRIGHTNESS
4. ↑CALCIFICATIONS
5. ↓ STRUCTURE
6. ↓ VASCULARITY
7. ↓ METABOLIC ACTIVITY

Figure 15. The qualitative changes associated with therapeutic osteosarcoma therapy.

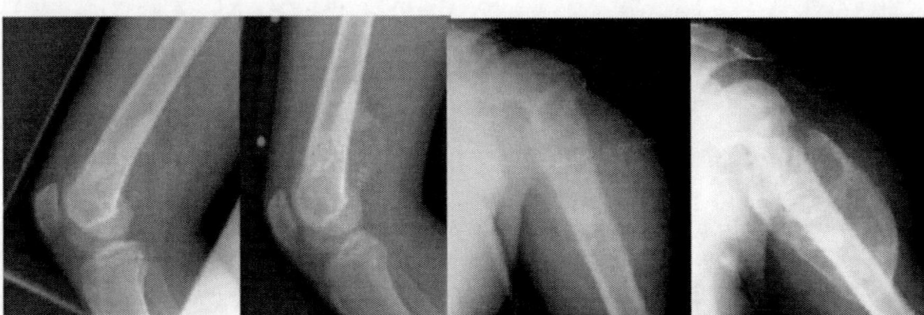

Figure 16. Qualitative changes due to treatment: Lateral radiographs of the femur and humerus before and after chemotherapy show increased ossification in the periphery of the treated tumor, a common finding after chemotherapy.

CT signs that the tumor is responding to chemotherapy include increasing peripheral and central ossification, decreased tumor mass, and return of identifiable fat planes adjacent to the tumor, possibly due to decreasing edema. [26]

A good scintigraphic response is considered to have occurred when there is more than a 20% decrease in the blood pool and clearance values compared to baseline. The blood pool values are slightly more meaningful than clearance. This observation does not apply to isotope uptake as seen on the usual static delayed images. This may actually increase in effectively treated tumors due to progressive ossification (Figure 17). Resolution of the gamma camera used for scintigraphy is limited to one cm making this technique less useful for very small tumors [27]. CT findings indicative of poor response include increasing bone destruction, marrow extension and increasing tumor size. [28]

Unfortunately, although these features may be seen in response to chemotherapy, they do not necessarily indicate that the response is adequate to affect outcomes. For that purpose, much more quantitative tools are required. [29, 22]

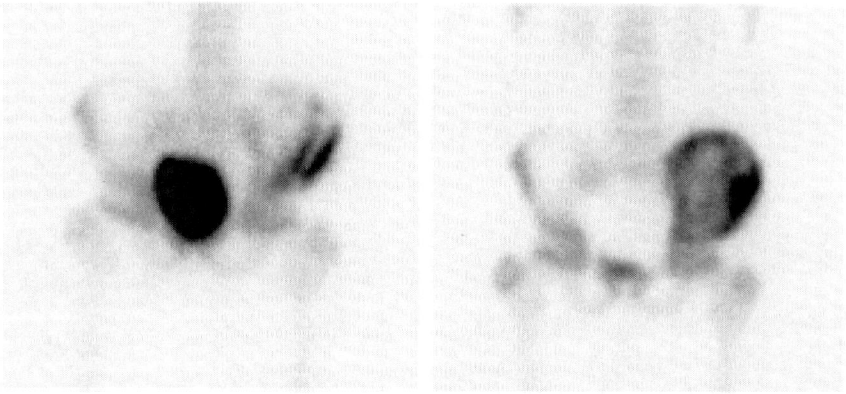

Figure 17. Ossification on Bone Scintigraphy. Frontal projections of two technetium MDP bone scans demonstrate increased tracer uptake before and shortly after chemotherapy. This finding is related to increased bone turnover and subsequent ossification and does not indicate tumor progression.

QUANTITATIVE APPROACHES TO EVALUATING TUMOR RESPONSE

Chemotherapeutic treatments have become more effective and more complex, with multiple agents that might or might not be effective in a particular case (for example, high dose methotrexate, vincristine, doxorubicin, cisplatin, bleomycin, actinomycin D, cyclophosphamide) replacing and producing better results than single agent (methotrexate) therapy. Since there is now a choice among effective therapeutic agents, it is no longer sufficient to note that the tumor either is or is not "responding". Reproducible quantitative measures of therapeutic response are needed to monitor how well the tumor is responding and, if necessary, guide changes in therapeutic direction. [30]

The "gold standard" for this purpose is 90% necrosis on histological evaluation after chemotherapy. Complete necrosis or scattered foci of viable tumor (90-99% necrosis) have equivalent good prognosis. Over the years a great many imaging features have been examined in an effort to find which (if any) can be used to predict response either as measured by disease-free survival or (more frequently) by correlating closely with >90% histological necrosis.

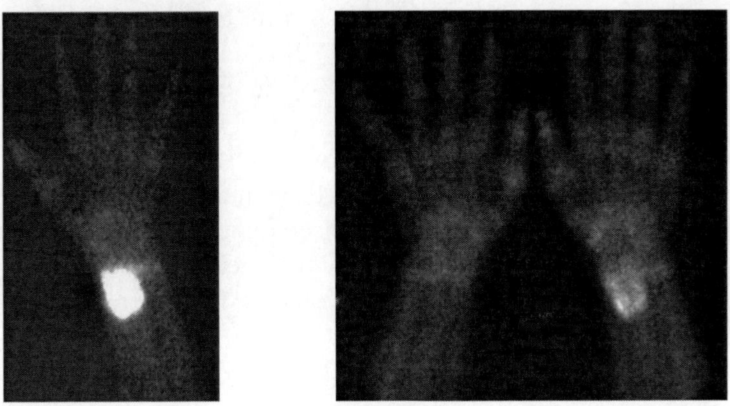

Figure 18. FDG PET Response. Frontal projections of an FDG PET exam demonstrate a high grade surface osteosarcoma of the right distal radius pretreatment and 2 months after therapy. Notice the qualitative change in metabolic tumor volume and intensity, which can be confirmed with SUV measurement.

PET AND PET CT

As mentioned, changes in tumor size do not correlate closely with histologic response. This observation has been made many times and appears to be related to the unchanging nature of the extracellular matrix of these tumors. PET imaging evaluates the metabolic activity of the tumor, and would therefore be expected to bear a relationship to prognosis and treatment response. Post-treatment standard uptake values (SUV) are usually found to be significantly lower in patients with a good response than in those with poor response as judged by histological criteria (>90% necrosis). (Figure 18) In some studies, the positive and negative predictive values of the post-treatment SUV (SUV2) or the ratio of SUV(2) to SUV(1) is very high, even approaching 100%. [31]

In most other studies the relationship between findings on PET imaging and chemotherapy response is not so conclusive. In one study of 40 patients with extremity OSA, a good FDG-PET response was defined as an SUV2<2.5 or a ratio of post treatment to pretreatment SUV less than 0.5. Using such measures FDG-PET imaging correlated only partially with a histologic response to neoadjuvant chemotherapy, being concordant with histologic response in 58% and 68% of patients, respectively. Interestingly, SUV2 was more strongly associated with outcome than with histological response, with 4-year disease free survival of 73% for SUV2<2.5 vs. 39% for SUV2>or=2.5; (P=.021) an observation that may suggest the limitations of histological necrosis as a parameter. [32]

Several measures have been derived from PET imaging to further refine its ability to predict outcome. The metabolic tumor volume (MTV) is a summation of all tumor-containing voxels (volume elements) that meet a specific activity threshold. In a recent study, when a specific uptake value (SUV) threshold of 2 was used to measure MTV before treatment, the metabolic volume appeared to correlate with metastasis-free survival independent of histological response. A MTV > 105 mL was a poor predictive value [33].

Since a single SUV threshold often fails to predict the percentage of histological necrosis perfectly, another approach is to identify definite responders, definite non-responders, and a "grey zone" requiring additional clarification. In a study of 70 consecutive patients with a high-grade osteosarcoma, five parameters were used in an effort to discriminate responders from nonresponders:

1. maximum standardized uptake values before chemotherapy (SUV1)
2. maximum standardized uptake values after chemotherapy(SUV2)
3. SUV change ratio
4. tumor volume change ratio
5. metabolic tumor volume change ratio (MTVCR)

Patients with an SUV2 of less than or equal to 2 showed a good histologic response, and patients with an SUV2 of greater than 5 showed a poor histologic response. The histologic response of a patient with an intermediate SUV2 (2 < SUV2 </= 5) was found to be predictable using the change in metabolic tumor volume. A patient with a ratio less than 0.65 is likely to be a good responder, whereas a patient with a ratio of post to pretreatment metabolic tumor volume greater than or equal to 0.65 is likely to be a poor responder. Using this combined predictor model, the predictive value for good responders was 97% (31/32) and for poor responders it was 95% (36/38) [34].

Another study looked at maximum SUV in 26 patients, 13 of whom were classified as good responders histologically, and 13 as poor responders. There was a significant correlation between SUVmax after chemotherapy and histological response. An SUV max >5 after chemotherapy identified the majority of histologic nonresponders (sensitivity 61%) with a positive predictive value of 89%. While interesting, it is doubtful whether this level of sensitivity is sufficient for clinical applications [35].

Contradictory results were found in another study. Change in the maximum standardized uptake value (SUVmax) between baseline and post-treatment scanning was not significantly associated with histologic response for either Ewing Sarcoma or osteogenic sarcoma. Interestingly, metabolic tumor volume (MTV) was predictive of response for osteosarcoma, but not for Ewing sarcoma. A 50% reduction in MTV (MTV2:1 < 0.5) was found to be significantly associated with favorable histologic response in osteosarcoma. Increasing the cut-off values for Ewing Sarcoma to a 90% reduction in MTV (MTV2:1 < 0.1) resulted in association with favorable histologic response. Perhaps response to neoadjuvant chemotherapy as reflected by changes in PET characteristics should be interpreted differently for Ewing Sarcoma and osteosarcoma. [36]

From the results reported above, it is clear that there is not yet uniform consensus on which PET parameter(s) to evaluate. In summary, at the present time it appears that parameters derived from PET imaging (SUV after treatment, the ratio of post treatment SUV to pretreatment SUV, average SUV, maximum SUV, and the Metabolic tumor volume) are significantly correlated with adequacy of treatment, but the ability to discriminate responders from non-responders is not yet adequate to allow decision making in an individual patient. Part of the difficulty is that most studies use histological necrosis as a proxy for response, and this measure can be difficult, complicated by the presence of necrosis in the pre-treatment sample, and an imperfect predictor of outcome.

Novel Isotope Imaging

Standard PET imaging is performed using FDG, and measures glycolytic activity. However, PET imaging can be performed with agents other than FDG.

Recent experimental work has shown that whereas PET imaging done with FDG is most intense in osteolytic lesions (mouse LM* osteosarcoma), PET imaging done with F18 (a pure bone agent) was most intense in osteoblastic tumors (human 143B cell line), and a novel agent (18)F-fluoromisonidazole [(18)F-FMISO] uptake correlated with hypoxic tumors (Caprin-1 stably overexpressing SaOS-2 cells). [37]

Another interesting technique that may have a clinical role in the future is the use of isotopes to scan for vascular endothelial growth factor (VEGF), an important angiogenic factor, whose receptors have been shown to be over expressed in various human carcinomas. In a small pilot study, two patients (a 15-year-old female and a 14-year-old male) with osteosarcoma were injected with 140 MBq (<130 pmol (<5 g) VEGF(165) per patient] of (123)I-VEGF(165). Dynamic acquisition SPECT imaging was initiated immediately after administration and carried out until 30 min after injection. Sequential images clearly showed increased (123)I-VEGF(165) activity in osteosarcoma lesions, suggesting that VEGF receptor scintigraphy may be useful for the visualization of highly malignant osteosarcoma. [38]

MRI Techniques

Conventional morphological MRI parameters (including volume change) do not significantly discriminate responders from non-responders (39) Tumors may shrink following effective chemotherapy (Figure 19) but they also may not (presumably due to the large quantity of extracellular matrix). It is generally agreed that an INCREASE in size after chemotherapy is a poor prognostic finding. Areas of T2 hyperintensity seen on post-treatment MRI may represent areas of residual viable tumor but can also be due to a host of other etiologies including tumor necrosis, edema, fibrosis and hemorrhage. (40) The same can be said for areas of gadolinium enhancement as seen on conventional post-contrast imaging. Large areas of necrosis may be seen before any treatment, and although they may increase after chemotherapy, it is not possible to distinguish adequate from inadequate treatment by this method (Figure 20). Delayed imaging after contrast injection may show increased uptake in necrotic tumor and granulation tissue. (This statement does not apply to dynamic contrast enhanced MRI –DCEMRI). Although decreased tumor volume is a weak predictor of treatment response and decreased peritumoral edema is also a weak predictor of response, neither can be relied upon for sufficient discrimination to guide the choice of therapy. (41) For this reason, efforts have been spent trying to identify special pulse sequences or techniques that could be helpful.

Magnetic resonance spectroscopy using Phosphorous-31 can be performed at baseline before standard chemotherapy as a metabolic evaluation. Osteosarcomas contain excess ATP and inorganic phosphate. In principle, metabolic tumor response can be monitored during chemotherapy by evaluating for increased Pi and loss of ATP, metabolic changes that indicate response. [42] This interesting technique is difficult and has not found its way into routine practice, nor has it been subjected to the sort of evaluation needed to establish clinical relevance.

Diffusion-weighted MRI is under active investigation for evaluation of prognosis and response to treatment. Diffusion-weighted MRI derives its signal using pulse sequences that are sensitive to inter-cellular diffusion and the movement of water molecules. Highly cellular tissues tend to show restricted diffusion, and therefore appear "bright" as diffusion results in a loss of signal due to incomplete rephasing. This phenomenon can be quantified using the Apparent Diffusion Coefficient (ADC). Decreased ADC correlates with low diffusion rates and therefore areas of restricted diffusion will appear "dark" on ADC maps.

Diffusion weighted MRI and PET imaging have been compared in their ability to evaluate the effects of treatment (as judged by >90% necrosis). A low SUVmax after therapy and/or a high ADC have both been shown to be good (but not excellent) predictors of successful treatment. [43]

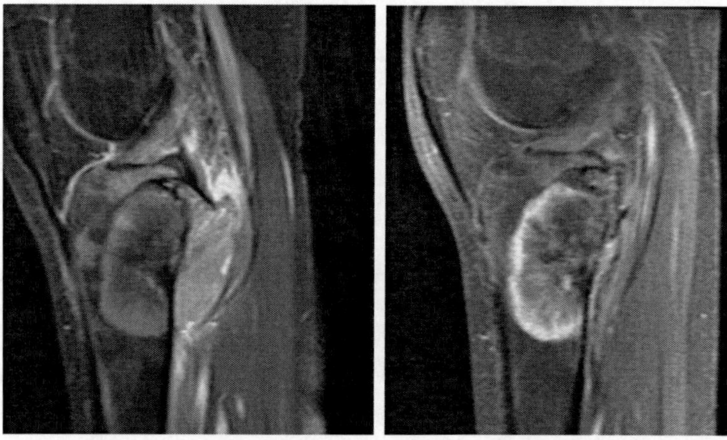

Figure 19. MRI Sagittal T1 post contrast images before and after chemotherapy. There is a marked decrease in tumor size. This observation, while encouraging, does not allow one to predict whether 90% of the remaining tumor is necrotic.

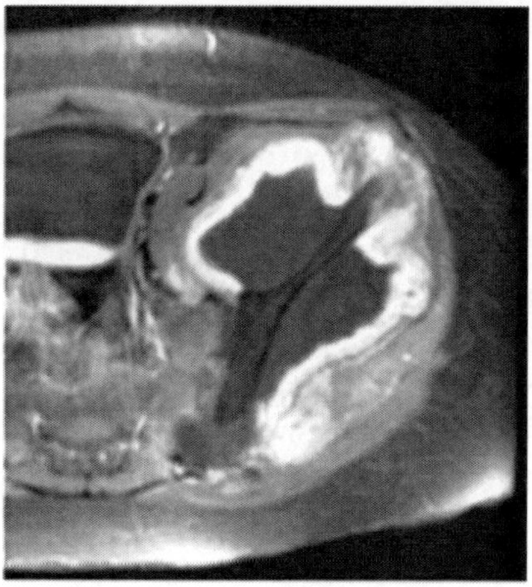

Figure 20. Tumor Necrosis. T1 axial post contrast image demonstrates a large volume of non-vascularized necrotic tumor with surrounding vascularized pseudocapsule. Although regions of non-enhancing tumor may increase after treatment this observation cannot be used to assess the adequacy of treatment because necrotic tumor and granulation tissue may enhance in a delayed fashion.

Other studies have found that an increase in ADC after chemotherapy is a good prognostic finding. In a prospective series of 7 adolescents treated for long-bone osteosarcoma, diffusion-weighted MR examinations were performed at diagnosis, at mid-course of chemotherapy, and immediately before surgery and compared to histological evaluation of tumor response. Patients with no increase in ADC showed a poor response to chemotherapy on their histological results. At mid-course, the change in ADC was significantly different among the 4 good responders compared to the 3 poor responders. The difference in ADC enabled complete separation (100% specificity) of the groups, suggesting that diffusion-weighted imaging might be able to indicate response fairly early during treatment. [44]

Despite these encouraging results, in another indication of the complexity of identifying predictor variables, it appears that perhaps the size of the lesion must be taken into account in evaluating the ADC. In one study, apparent diffusion coefficient did not correlate with necrosis; however, on adjusting for volume, significant correlation was found, leading to a new parameter: diffusion per unit volume.(45) This observation bears a certain similarity to the finding that SUV on PET imaging might have to be adjusted for metabolic tumor volume in predicting responsiveness (see above).

In yet another similarity to PET imaging, some authorities believe that the average ADC conveys different information from the minimum ADC (analogous to SUV vs. SUVmax). In a study of 22 patients with osteosarcoma both the average ADC and the minimum ADC, were significantly higher post-chemotherapy than pre-chemotherapy values ($P < 0.05$). However, the patients with a good histological response had a significantly higher minimum ADC ratio than those with a poor response (1.01 + or - 0.22 and 0.55 + or - 0.29 respectively, $P < 0.05$) but no difference in the average ADC. [46]

As it can with PET imaging, tumoral hypoxia can also be evaluated using MRI. Blood oxygen-dependent (BOLD) sequences have been shown to correlate with both (18)F-misonidazole PET/CT and histological findings of hypoxia, although not with diffusion weighted imaging. [47]

BLOOD FLOW

It has been known for many decades that there is a relationship between blood flow, prognosis, and response to chemotherapy. It is important to distinguish between vascularity and blood flow. Highly vascular lesions may or may not show high levels of blood flow. For example, typical hemangiomas are highly vascular, but have little blood flow. A critical distinction is the rate at which tumors enhance with contrast or show uptake of isotope. Tumors with residual areas of high blood flow after treatment carry a poor prognosis. This phenomenon was initially observed with angiography [25, 48].

Slightly more recently, nuclear bone scans have been used to demonstrate that early uptake of Technetium (Tc) 99m in the tumor correlates with viability. After chemotherapy, there is decreased early uptake in all tumors responding to therapy. Differences in early uptake are related to blood flow, not to incorporation of isotope by the tumor, which is delayed. [49]

Similarly, decreased thallium uptake scores appear to predict effective chemotherapy. It is likely that this is due to the blood pool effect of thallium (TI), but it is also possible that thallium uptake is due to active intracellular transport and measures more than simply blood flow. [50, 51]

A recent study investigated the use of the blood pool scanning agent (99m)Tc-hexakis-2-methoxyisobutyl-isonitrile ((99m)Tc-MIBI) scintigraphy in evaluating the response to chemotherapy of patients with osteosarcoma in comparison with (201)TI scintigraphy and angiography. The therapeutic effect was assessed by histopathological examination of the resected specimens. The tumors of poor responders showed less than 90% necrosis, whereas the tumors of good responders showed 90% or more necrosis. The scanning agents were compared to each other and to angiography based upon the ability to identify a "cut-off" levels which would predict therapeutic success with the greatest degree of accuracy. (Table 1) Tc-MIBI scintigraphy performed slightly better than the other two methods. If scanning is to be used to determine that a particular therapeutic approach is not working, then specificity becomes more important than sensitivity in prediction, and in this regard Tc-MIBI scintigraphy was definitely preferred.

Although predictive of chemotherapy response at some level of certainty, scanning methods based upon blood flow may still be inadequate to predict event-free survival. [53] This may be partly due to inherent limitations of the technique. Isotope scanning also lacks the spatial resolution to constitute a complete evaluation of response as small residual foci of tumor can be overlooked.

Table 1. comparing the sensitivity and specificity in predicting histologically adequate (>90%) necrosis of ((99m)Tc-MIBI) scintigraphy, thallium scintigraphy, and conventional angiography [52]

	Sensitivity	Specificity	Accuracy
MIBI	74	84	79
TI	80	61	72
Angiography	92	35	66

Contrast-enhanced CT has also been used to evaluate tumor blood flow, as has ultrasound with color Doppler. After one cycle of chemotherapy, Doppler ultrasound demonstrated no change in the quotient of resistive indexes (QRI) of the tumor in responders to treatment when compared to non-responders. After two cycles, there was a statistically significant (p=0.03) increase in the QRI of the tumor in responders to treatment when compared to non-responders. Decreases in qualitative blood flow and Doppler shift was also observed but was not statistically significant. After completion of chemotherapy, these changes were even more marked, becoming significant for all measures. Due to inherent limitations in the ultrasound technique, these findings could only be seen in the extra-osseous parts of tumors, rendering this modality unsuitable for purely intra-osseous tumor. [54]

DYNAMIC CONTRAST ENHANCED MRI (DCE-MRI)

Recently, however, most attention has been focused on dynamic contrast-enhanced MRI (DCE-MRI) as the preferred method to evaluate response. Dynamic contrast-enhanced MRI evaluates response as indicated by blood flow changes. It has rather stringent technical requirements, and is distinctly different than the post-contrast images that are usually obtained.

DCE-MRI should include fast T1-weighted sequences with a temporal resolution of at least 3 seconds. Section thickness of at least 10mm is preferred to minimize sampling error. Intra-venous gadolinium can be administered using a bolus technique of 0.1 mmol/kg at rate of 2 ml/s, beginning 5 seconds after the start of data acquisition or using bolus triggering settings. Scanning should be in a plane that best shows the tumor and an artery. DCE-MRI methods have advanced from single-slice acquisitions to sequences that enable image acquisition to be performed volumetrically, such that the pharmacodynamic properties of a large tumor may be analyzed in its entirety as opposed to just representative slices. [55]

Computer algorithms that subtract enhanced imaging sequences from precontrast acquisition are becoming the norm and can be used to evaluate enhancement at various points in time. Changes in signal intensity can be plotted to create time-intensitycurves. Early enhancement is defined as enhancement that occurs during the arterial phase of imaging, generally identified by observing contrast enhancement in an adjacent artery.

The pattern of enhancement can be classified into one of four categories: 1) none 2) gradual increase 3) Rapid initial increase followed by plateau,

4) rapid initial increase followed by washout. Viable tumor is generally characterized by rapid initial and sustained early enhancement (category 3). Total viable tumor volume can be measured using computer programs or by summating manual traces made on multiple images if necessary.

When early and sustained or progressive enhancement is identified, it corresponds to viable tumor, although tumor nodules measuring less than 3-5 mm may be overlooked. [56, 57, 58]

Rapid uptake is defined by the slope of the time intensity curve, where slope is defined as (%/min) = (SI max – SI base)x 100/[SIbase X (tmax-Tbase)] Using this definition, there has been shown to be a good correlation with viable tumor when the slope is at least 45%. However, there were some false positives due to intensely vascular proliferating fibroblasts – presumably a response to chemotherapy. [59]

If the slope of the time intensity curve decreases by 50 or 60 percent, this indicates an excellent response to chemotherapy (P<.01) [60]. In principle, this result could be achieved using the less complex methods of isotope scanning, but the results with DCEMRI are better than those obtained using three phase scintigraphy to measure blood flow. [61] Following chemotherapy, persistent regions of fast and sustained uptake indicate residual tumor, which should disappear if treatment has been efficacious. [57] Conversely, unchanged perfusion on dynamic MRI is a good predictor of a non-responder. [60]

Sophisticated methods for modeling dynamic enhancement have been developed. Because of the irregular size and shape of many sarcomas, conventional circular or square regions of interest may fail to include some areas of tumor, or may include non-tumorous tissue. To address this, "FAMIS" or factor analysis medical imaging sequences, was used to identify pixel-by-pixel changes in signal intensity. Using this method, it was shown that early uptake disappeared in five patients who responded to chemotherapy, whereas it persisted in four of five nonresponders. However, small foci of tumor measuring less than 5mm still could not be detected in 3 patients. [61]

Despite the occurrence of some false negative and positive examinations, [62] dynamic contrast-enhanced MRI has been shown to predict event-free survival [63] (Figure 21).

An open question is how early during the course of treatment can success or failure be predicted using these methods based upon blood flow. In one study to look at this problem, dynamic MRI and skeletal angioscintigraphy both predict response with reasonable accuracy at the conclusion of chemotherapy, but neither was accurate at the midpoint (after 2 cycles), limiting utility to assess for mid-cycle treatment response as a means to potentially alter chemotherapy in non-responders. [64]

Although the analysis is straightforward, and the results are highly promising, the use of signal intensity changes on DCE- MRI to assess tumor responsiveness is subject to a number of limitations. For example, signal intensity change may not accurately reflect tumor contrast concentration due to the non-linear nature of gadolinium enhancement and variation in cardiac output. The appearance of enhancement is also influenced by scanner settings, limiting comparisons between patients and systems. Thus, it is still unclear exactly which parameters to measure and how.

One possible way around this problem is to use contrast agent concentration rather than signal intensity. This can be done by using pharmacokinetic modeling techniques.

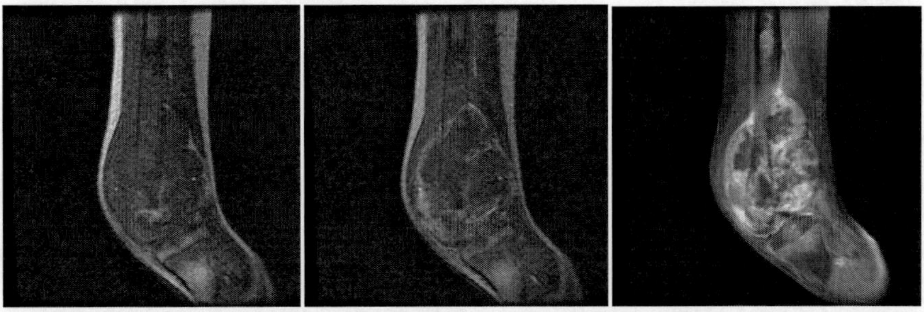

Figure 21. DCE- MRI after chemotherapy. Sagittal T1 post contrast images were performed every 3 seconds for 150 seconds with subsequent delayed imaging. The first image shows lack of early enhancement. There is minimal peripheral enhancement at 150 seconds (image 2) with no visible nodules of residual tumor. Delayed sagittal image demonstrates progressive peripheral enhancement in the necrotic tumor and reactive zone.

Using a recognized pharmacokinetic model, concentration-time curves are mathematically fitted to signal intensity changes during dynamic enhancement acquisitions and quantitative modeling parameters are derived. At the present time, there is considerable interest in evaluating the following quantitative parameters that are calculated in this fashion:

K(trans) (the influx volume transfer constant, a marker for transendothelial contrast permeability)
v(p) (the relative vascular plasma space)
k(ep) (efflux rate constant) indicative of histologic response

v(e) (the relative extravascular extracellular space, or leakage space per unit volume of tissue)

The three major factors that determine contrast media behavior in tissues are blood perfusion, transport of contrast across vessel walls and diffusion of contrast medium in the interstitial space. These parameters are based on the observation that gadolinium-based contrast agents are able to traverse the vascular endothelium and leak into the interstitial space but cannot enter the intracellular space. In flow-limiting situations or where vascular permeability is greater than inflow, blood perfusion will be the dominant factor determining contrast kinetics. In this circumstance K(trans) approximates tissue blood flow. This situation is commonly observed in tumors. In addition, tumors (including osteosarcoma) exhibit a more permeable vasculature and have a different composition of extracellular and extravascular space compared to normal tissues. Distinct contrast enhancement and concentration patterns can thus be identified and quantified when compared to normal tissue. Necrotic regions with poor blood supply may have a low K(trans) despite high intrinsic permeability.

Experimental validation of these parameters has been obtained in mice by comparison with laser microscopy. It is known that the abnormal blood vessel organization, structure, and function found in solid tumors can give rise to enhanced vascular permeability and changes in these abnormalities may predict therapeutic responses. The permeability and architecture of the microvasculature in human osteosarcoma tumors growing in dorsal window chambers in athymic mice were measured by confocal laser scanning microscopy (CLSM) and dynamic contrast enhanced magnetic resonance imaging (DCE-MRI). A significant correlation was found between permeability indicators. The extravasation rate K(i) as measured by CLSM correlated positively with DCE-MRI parameters, such as the volume transfer constant K(trans) and the initial slope of the contrast agent concentration-time curve. [65]

In pediatric patients undergoing chemotherapy for osteosarcoma, all permeability parameters decreased significantly from week 0 to week 9 and week 12. The parameters K(trans), v(p) and k(ep) were significantly different after 9 weeks of treatment between responders and nonresponders (P = .046, P = .021, and P = .008, respectively), and are therefore considered to be indicative of histologic response. The parameter v(e) did not correlate with histological response but was a significant prognostic factor for both event free survival (P = .02) and overall survival (P = .03) at baseline. [66]

A baseline native tissue T1 relaxation time value is typically needed for dynamic contrast-enhanced DCE-MRI studies to quantify enhancement. This can be difficult to calculate. An assumed baseline value has to be used when real measurements are not available. A systematic investigation of the dependence on baseline relaxation times of the commonly used DCE-MRI parameters (K(trans), k(ep), v(e) and initial area under the curve, IAUC) as well as several newly defined parameters (the normalized ratios (NRs) of k(ep), K(trans) and v(e), which are measures of relative changes in these parameters between two time points) was performed for a spoiled gradient-echo pulse sequence. Both simulations and in vivo studies were done. Effects of various scanning factors on the baseline dependence were also assessed using simulations. The DCE-MRI parameters k(ep) and the NR of k(ep) appear to be largely independent of baseline T1 relaxation, especially when larger flip angles are used (e.g., 30-40 degrees). Their estimations therefore do not require any knowledge of baseline values. The normalized ratios of K(trans), v(e) and IAUC also exhibit independence of baseline values, but only when there is no change between pre- and post-treatment scans. The estimation of parameters themselves (K(trans), v(e) and IAUC) is highly dependent on the baseline value. [67]

Another attempt to get around the need for a baseline longitudinal relaxation rate compared the DCE-MRI parameters derived when the relaxation rate constant was measured individually using the two-point determination method compared to the same parameters derived from an average R(10). In 18 patients with lower extremity osteosarcomas, the authors found that the whole tumor and histogram median K(trans) and v(e) obtained with the individual relaxation measurement was not significantly different from that obtained with the average approach. The results suggest that it might be possible to substitute a population-based measurement for individual determination of baseline relaxation rates. [68]

Similar efforts are underway to characterize and quantify MRI data without any prerequisites by using a semi-quantitative analysis of the curve patterns (CPA) resulting from DCE-MRI. In a simulation study, parametric maps were generated using novel CPA methods and a pharmacokinetic model-based method for comparison. It was possible to identify CPA parameters that varied less than 2% when T(1) changed from 300 msec to 1500 msec, and less than 10% when the flip angle changed from 30 degrees to 40 degrees. These studies also showed that the CPA parameters had a strong correlation with k(ep), with correlation coefficients of 0.9983 in the simulation and 0.95 in the in vivo studies suggesting a possible alternative to quantifying DCE-MRI studies that minimizes variations potentially induced by arterial input function (AIF) and T(1) estimations and model dependence. However, CPA analysis can also be quite complex, and it is also influenced by pulse sequence selection. [69]

It is possible that DCE-MRI may shed some light on tumor angiogenesis. As was mentioned in the discussion of novel isotope imaging, levels of vascular endothelial growth factor (VEGF) have been shown to correlate with pulmonary metastases in addition to poor prognosis. Dynamic contrast enhanced MRI can be used to correlate histologically with VEGF positive and negative tumors. VEGF-positive tumors show higher mean vascular permeability when compared with VEGF-negative tumors. [70]

Time-intensity curves obtained using dynamic contrast-enhanced MRI have been characterized as either high (plateau and washout type) or low (persistent type) microvascular permeability. These patterns were correlated with VEGF expression as assessed in biopsy. [71]

The authors found that qualitative analysis of time intensity curves correctly identified all 28 VEGF positive samples at baseline and 24/25 (96%) of VEGF positive samples and 5/6 (83%) of VEGF negative samples after chemotherapy. None of the pre-treatment VEGF negative samples were correctly identified (0/3). The change in curve pattern from washout/plateau to persistent type was in agreement with corresponding decrease in VEGF expression, however the initial evaluation of pretreatment VEGF expression may be limited using this method. VEGF expression did not correlate with DW-MRI and PET-CT parameters. The authors contend that their qualitative analysis of VEGF may add an additional independent tool for risk stratification.

IMAGE-GUIDED INTERVENTION

Image-guided interventions have been useful in treatment of small primary bone tumors (generally not osteosarcoma) and metastatic bone disease. [72] Little attention has been given to their application to primary sarcomas. This is partly a technical limitation due to the inability to treat large volumes of tumor. However, some success has been claimed for the use of high-energy focused ultrasound (HIFU). High-intensity focused ultrasound (HIFU) is a technique to destroy tissue at depth within the body. In theory, structures along the path of the beam are not affected because the ultrasonic intensity at the beam focus is much higher than that outside of the focus.

Although successful treatment of osteosarcoma using high intensity focused ultrasound has been reported, these results have not been validated in clinical trials. [73] In a small safety and efficacy study, one patient with osteosarcoma was said to achieve a "complete response" using this method. [74]

By far the largest experience with this technique comes from China. In 1997, a patient with osteosarcoma was first successfully treated with ultrasound imaging-guided HIFU in Chongqing, China. Since then it has been used many times, and great success has been reported. [75] However, documentation of the results has been scant, and given the improbable nature of using this therapeutic tool for osteosarcoma, a great deal more evidence is required before accepting it as a therapeutic alternative.

POST-TREATMENT IMAGING: TREATMENT RELATED FINDINGS

Long term survival of osteosarcoma can lead to various unfamiliar findings and co-morbidities that can be confusing on post-treatment imaging. For example in a retrospective study of 48 patients with a minimum of 10 year survival, there was significantly reduced bone mass. Given this finding it may be prudent to assess for early osteoporosis in long term survivals with DEXA analysis. [76]

Benign enlargement of the sciatic nerve after amputation for osteosarcoma is innocuous. It is proportional to the length of time after amputation. [77]

A curiosity not related to the effectiveness of chemotherapy is the observation of dense metaphyseal bands at the growth plates in long bones, sclerosis of epiphyseal ossification centers, anterior rib ends, sternum and spine that were observed following Pamidronate therapy of children with osteosarcoma. These changes were seen quite frequently, with osseous change being visible on CT in more than half of patients. A bone-within-bone appearance in the spine and ossification centers was identified on radiography in 36%. [78]

Marrow suppression by chemotherapy results in fatty conversion of the marrow, a condition that is not likely to be mistaken for anything else. However treatment of marrow suppression with granulocyte colony-stimulating factor (GCSF) may lead to marked reconversion of marrow treatment possibly causing confusion with metastatic disease. The effect is dose-dependent and marrow findings can often be identified in tandem with evaluation of the primary tumor. [79]

Surveillance for Recurrence

Early results are promising for FDG PET as a surveillance method for tumor recurrence and metastasis (Figure 22). In one study comparing FDG PET CT to conventional imaging (MRI of the tumor site, chest CT and bone scan) the sensitivity, specificity and accuracy of PET was similar to the combined methods.(Figure 23) In addition FDG PET CT was slightly better at detecting osseous and soft tissue local recurrence. [80]

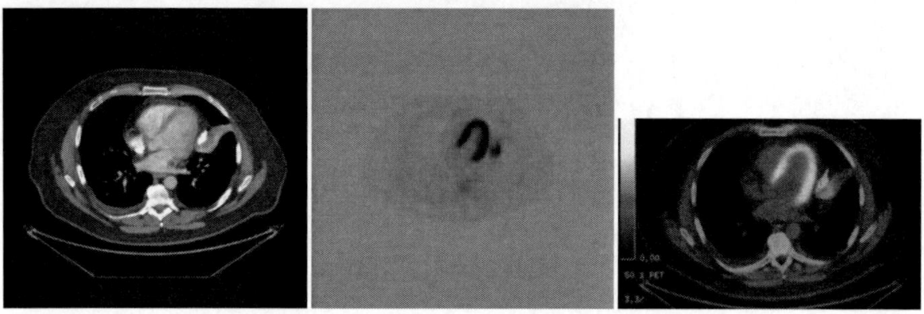

Figure 22. Osteoblastic pulmonary metastatic disease. CT with contrast and PET with and without fusion demonstrate a partially calified metastic lesion in the left lung with intense FDG avidity. Fusion images and SUV analysis are helpful for anatomic localization and characterization.

Whole-body MR imaging has also been advocated for post-surgical surveillance for the detection of local recurrence and distant metastatic disease. In one study a total of 39 patients were evaluated using PET CT, MRI and isotope bone scan. 18 patients were negative for metastatic disease as judged by clinical follow up. All 18 were negative with whole MRI and bone scan, but two had false positive on FDG PET. FDG PET had the highest overall sensitivity. Of note most false negative involving whole body MRI studies were located in the ribs, skull and small bones of the hand. The majority of false negative scintigraphy was located in the spine. [81]

The tremendous successes of imaging in evaluation of the patient with sarcoma may have led to some over-enthusiastic use. Recent work suggests that perhaps some bone scans can be omitted. In a retrospective review of 85 patients, no patient with localized disease developed metastatic disease to the skeletal system before local treatment; those with localized disease who developed metastases did so some time after completion of the treatment plan. As the probability of developing bone metastatic disease while receiving therapy is very low, routine bone scan in asymptomatic patients before local treatment may safely be omitted. [82]

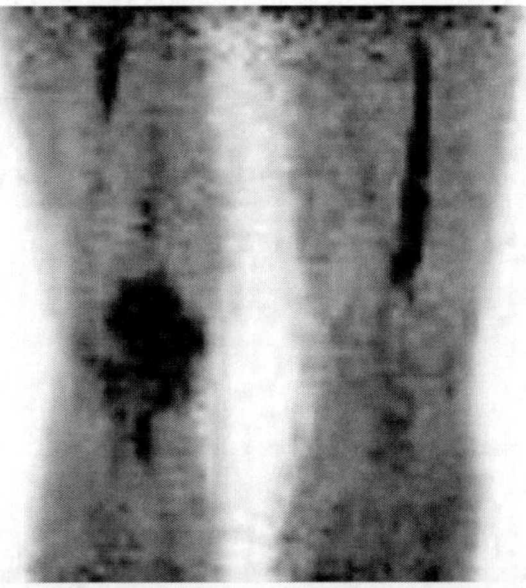

Figure 23. Tumor Surveillance. Frontal FDG PET MIP image demonstrating intense tracer uptake in the right distal femur associated with osteosarcoma recurrence.

Our own work suggests that despite the relative accuracy of imaging to detect local recurrence, it may be unnecessary to perform surveillance scans, as very few asymptomatic recurrences are discovered. [83]

CONCLUSION

Recent developments in the imaging of osteosarcoma have been due to the gradual accumulation of experience as well as incremental refinements in existing tools. Although a future state in which imaging can serve as a substitute for biopsy in determining tumor viability is within sight, it is not yet within grasp. Progress in imaging of osteosarcoma has been subject to the same limitations as progress in therapy: rarity of the lesions, and variability in histology and anatomy. Although it is not possible at this time to give definitive answers to any fundamental questions about how to diagnose, treat or follow the lesions, sustained slow progress continues to be made.

REFERENCES

[1] Tsai JC, Dalinka MK, Fallon M, Zlatkin MB, Kressel HY. Fluid-fluid level: a nonspecific finding in tumors of bone and soft tissue. *Radiology* 1990;175(3):779-782.

[2] Grey AC, Mangham DC, Davies AM, Grimer RJ. Fluid-fluid level in an intraosseous ganglion. *Skeletal Radiol*. 1997;26(11):667–670.

[3] Kransdorf MJ, Murphey MD, Sweet DE. Liposclerosing myxofibrous tumor: a radiologic-pathologic-distinct fibro-osseous lesion of bone with a marked predilection for the intertrochanteric region of the femur. *Radiology* 1999;212(3):693-698.

[4] Aboulafia AJ, Brooks F, Piratzky J, Weiss S. Osteosarcoma arising from heterotopic ossification after an electrical burn. A Case Report. *J. Bone Joint Surg. Am*. 1999;81(4):564-570.

[5] Jutte PC, Rosso R, De Paolis M, Errani C, Pasini E, Campanacci L. Osteosarcoma associated with hyperparathyroidism. *Skeletal Radiol.* 2004;33(8):473–476.

[6] Hsu CC, Wang JW, Huang CH, Chen WJ. Osteosarcoma at the Site of a Previously Treated Aneurysmal Bone Cyst, A Case Report. *J. Bone Joint Surg. Am.* 2005;87(2):395-398.

[7] Grimer RJ, Carter SR, Tillman RM, Spooner D, Mangham DC, Kabukcuoglu Y. Osteosarcoma of the pelvis. *J. Bone Joint Surg. Br.* 1999;81(5):796-802.

[8] Tsuji Y, Kusuzaki K, Kanemitsu K, Matsumoto T, Ishikawa Y, Hirasawa Y. Calcaneal osteosarcoma associated with werner syndrome A case report with mutation analysis. *J. Bone Joint Surg. Am.* 2000;82(9):1308-1308.

[9] Armitage NC, Perkins AC, Pimm MV, Wastie M, Hopkins JS, Dowling F, et al. Imaging of bone tumors using a monoclonal antibody raised against human osteosarcoma. *Cancer* 1986;58(1):37-42.

[10] Wang CK, Li CW, Hsieh TJ, Chien SH, Liu GC, Tsai KB. Characterization of Bone and Soft-Tissue Tumors with in Vivo 1H MR Spectroscopy: Initial Results1. *Radiology* 2004;232(2):599-605.

[11] Meyer MS, Spanier SS, Moser M, Scarborough MT. Evaluating marrow margins for resection of osteosarcoma: a modern approach. *Clin. Orthop. Relat. Res*. 1999;363:170-175.

[12] Onikul E, Fletcher BD, Parham DM, Chen G. Accuracy of MR imaging for estimating intraosseous extent of osteosarcoma. *AJR Am. J. Roentgenol.* 1996;167(5):1211-1215.

[13] Fahey M, Spanier SS, Vander Griend RA. Osteosarcoma of the pelvis. *J. Bone Joint Surg. Am.* 1992;74(3):321-330.

[14] McLean RG, Murray IP. Scintigraphic patterns in certain primary malignant bone tumours. *Clin. Radiol*. 1984;35(5):379-383.

[15] Keller SM, Rosenbaum RC, Rosenberg SA. The significance of bone scan abnormalities in patients with primary osteogenic sarcoma. *J. Surg. Oncol*. 1984;26(2):122-129.

[16] Ollivier L, Leclere J, Vanel D, Forest M, Pouillart P, Riche MC, et al. Femoral infarction following intraarterial chemotherapy for osteosarcoma of the leg: a possible pitfall in magnetic resonance imaging. *Skeletal Radiol.* 1991;20(5):329–332.

[17] Golfieri R, Baddeley H, Pringle JS, Leung AW, Greco A, Souhami R, et al. Primary bone tumors: MR morphologic appearance correlated with pathologic examinations. *Acta Radiol*. 1991;32(4):290-298.

[18] Masrouha KZ, Musallam KM, Samra AB, Tawil A, Haidar R, Chakhachiro Z, et al. Correlation of non-mass-like abnormal MR signal intensity with pathological findings surrounding pediatric osteosarcoma and Ewing's sarcoma. *Skeletal Radiol*. 2012;41(11):1453-1461.

[19] Kim MS, Lee SY, Cho WH, Song WS, Koh JS, Lee JA, et al. Growth patterns of osteosarcoma predict patient survival. *Archives of orthopaedic and trauma surgery* 2009;129(9):1189-1196.

[20] Brown KT, Kattapuram SV, Rosenthal DI. Computed tomography analysis of bone tumors: patters of cortical destruction and soft tissue extension. *Skeletal Radiol*. 1986;15(6):448–451.

[21] Scully SP, Ghert MA, Zurakowski D, Thompson RC, Gebhardt MC. Pathologic Fracture in Osteosarcoma Prognostic Importance and Treatment Implications. *J. Bone Joint Surg. Am*. 2002;84(1):49-57.

[22] Wunder JS, Paulian G, Huvos AG, Heller G, Meyers PA, Healey JH. The histological response to chemotherapy as a predictor of the oncological outcome of operative treatment of Ewing sarcoma. *J. Bone Joint Surg. Am*. 1998;80(7):1020-1033.

[23] Link MP, Goorin AM, Horowitz M, Meyer WH, Belasco J, Baker A, et al. Adjuvant chemotherapy of high-grade osteosarcoma of the extremity. *Clinical Orthop. Relat. Res*. 1991;(270):8-14.

[24] Miller AB, Hoogstraten B, Staquet M, Winkler A. Reporting results of cancer treatment. *Cancer* 1981;47(1):207–214.

[25] Chuang VP, Benjamin R, Jaffe N, Wallace S, Ayala AG, Murray J, et al. Radiographic and angiographic changes in osteosarcoma after

intraarterial chemotherapy. *AJR Am. J. Roentgenol.* 1982;139(6):1065-1069.

[26] Shirkhoda A, Jaffe N, Wallace S, Ayala A, Lindell MM, Zornoza J. Computed tomography of osteosarcoma after intraarterial chemotherapy. *AJR Am. J. Roentgenol.* 1985;144(1):95-99.

[27] Knop J, Delling G, Heise U, Winkler K. Scintigraphic evaluation of tumor regression during preoperative chemotherapy of osteosarcoma. Correlation of 99mTc-methylene diphosphonate parametric imaging with surgical histopathology. *Skeletal Radiol.* 1990;19(3):165-172.

[28] Mail JT, Cohen MD, Mirkin LD, Provisor AJ. Response of osteosarcoma to preoperative intravenous high-dose methotrexate chemotherapy: CT evaluation. *AJR Am. J. Roentgenol.* 1985;144(1):89-93.

[29] Lawrence JA, Babyn PS, Chan HS, Thorner PS, Pron GE, Krajbich IJ. Extremity osteosarcoma in childhood: prognostic value of radiologic imaging. *Radiology* 1993;189(1):43-47.

[30] Goorin AM, Andersen JW. Experience with multiagent chemotherapy for osteosarcoma. *Clin. Orthop. Relat. Res.* 1991;(270):22-28.

[31] Hamada K, Tomita Y, Inoue A, Fujimoto T, Hashimoto N, Myoui A, et al. Evaluation of chemotherapy response in osteosarcoma with FDG-PET. *Ann. Nucl. Med.* 2009;23(1):89–95.

[32] Hawkins DS, Rajendran JG, Conrad EU 3rd, Bruckner JD, Eary JF. Evaluation of chemotherapy response in pediatric bone sarcomas by [F-18]-fluorodeoxy-D-glucose positron emission tomography. *Cancer* 2002;94(12):3277–3284.

[33] Byun BH, Kong CB, Park J, Seo Y, Lim I, Choi CW, et al. Initial Metabolic Tumor Volume Measured by 18F-FDG PET/CT Can Predict the Outcome of Osteosarcoma of the Extremities. *J. Nucl. Med.* 2013;54(10):1725-1732.

[34] Cheon GJ, Kim MS, Lee JA, Lee SY, Cho WH, Song WS, et al. Prediction model of chemotherapy response in osteosarcoma by 18F-FDG PET and MRI. *J. Nucl. Med.* 2009;50(9):1435-1440.

[35] Kong CB, Byun BH, Lim I, Choi CW, Lim SM, Song WS, et al. 18F-FDG PET SUVmax as an indicator of histopathologic response after neoadjuvant chemotherapy in extremity osteosarcoma. *Eur. J. Nucl. Med. Mol. Imaging* 2013;40(5):728-736.

[36] Gaston LL, Di Bella C, Slavin J, Hicks RJ, Choong PF. 18F-FDG PET response to neoadjuvant chemotherapy for Ewing sarcoma and osteosarcoma are different. *Skeletal Radiol.* 2011;40(8):1007-1015.

[37] Campanile C, Arlt MJ, Kramer SD, Honer M, Gvozdenovic A, Brennecke P, et al. Characterization of different osteosarcoma phenotypes by PET imaging in preclinical animal models. *J. Nucl. Med.* 2013;54(8):1362-1368.

[38] Holzer G, Hamilton G, Angelberger P, Lai D, Ubl P, Dudczak R, et al. Imaging of highly malignant osteosarcoma with iodine-123-vascular endothelial growth factor. *Oncology* 2012;83(1):45-49.

[39] Denecke T, Hundsdörfer P, Misch D, Steffen I, Schönberger S, Furth C, et al. Assessment of histological response of paediatric bone sarcomas using FDG PET in comparison to morphological volume measurement and standardized MRI parameters. *Eur. J. Nucl. Med. Mol. Imaging* 2010;37:1842–1853.

[40] Sanchez RB, Quinn SF, Walling A, Estrada J, Greenberg H. Musculoskeletal neoplasms after intraarterial chemotherapy: correlation of MR images with pathologic specimens. *Radiology* 1990;174(1):237-240.

[41] Holscher HC, Bloem JL, Vanel D, Hermans J, Nooy MA, Taminiau AH, et al. Osteosarcoma: chemotherapy-induced changes at MR imaging. *Radiology* 1992;182(3):839-844.

[42] Ross B, Helsper JT, Cox IJ, Young IR, Kempf R, Makepeace A, et al. Osteosarcoma and other neoplasms of bone. Magnetic resonance spectroscopy to monitor therapy. *Arch. Surg.* 1987;122(12):1464-1469.

[43] Byun BH, Kong CB, Lim I, Choi CW, Song WS, Cho WH, et al. Combination of 18F-FDG PET/CT and diffusion-weighted MR imaging as a predictor of histologic response to neoadjuvant chemotherapy: preliminary results in osteosarcoma. *J. Nucl. Med.* 2013;54(7):1053-1059.

[44] Baunin C, Schmidt G, Baumstarck K, Bouvier C, Gentet JC, Aschero A, et al. Value of diffusion-weighted images in differentiating mid-course responders to chemotherapy for osteosarcoma compared to the histological response: preliminary results. *Skeletal Radiol.* 2012; 41(9):1141-1149.

[45] Bajpai J, Gamnagatti S, Kumar R, Sreenivas V, Sharma MC, Khan SA, et al. Role of MRI in osteosarcoma for evaluation and prediction of chemotherapy response: correlation with histological necrosis. *Pediatr. Radiol.* 2011;41(4):441-450.

[46] Oka K, Yakushiji T, Sato H, Hirai T, Yamashita Y, Mizuta H. The value of diffusion-weighted imaging for monitoring the chemotherapeutic response of osteosarcoma: a comparison between average apparent

diffusion coefficient and minimum apparent diffusion coefficient. *Skeletal Radiol.* 2010;39(2):141-146.

[47] Dallaudiere B, Hummel V, Hess A, Lincot J, Preux PM, Maubon A, et al. Hypoxia in osteosarcoma in rats: preliminary study of blood oxygenation level-dependent functional MRI and 18F-misonidazole PET/CT with diffusion-weighted MRI correlation. *AJR Am. J. Roentgenol.* 2013; 200(2):W187-192.

[48] Kumpan W, Lechner G, Wittich GR, Salzer-Kuntschik M, Delling G, Kotz R, et al. The angiographic response of osteosarcoma following pre-operative chemotherapy. *Skeletal Radiol*. 1986;15(2):96-102.

[49] Sommer HJ, Knop J, Heise U, Winkler K, Delling G. Histomorphometric changes of osteosarcoma after chemotherapy. Correlation with 99mTc methylene diphosphonate functional imaging. *Cancer* 1987;59(2):252-258.

[50] Menendez LR, Fideler BM, Mirra J. Thallium-201 scanning for the evaluation of osteosarcoma and soft-tissue sarcoma. A study of the evaluation and predictability of the histological response to chemotherapy. *J. Bone Joint Surg. Am*. 1993;75(4):526–531.

[51] Kunisada T, Ozaki T, Kawai A, Sugihara S, Taguchi K, Inoue H. Imaging assessment of the responses of osteosarcoma patients to preoperative chemotherapy. *Cancer* 1999;86(6):949-956.

[52] Miwa S, Shirai T, Taki J, Sumiya H, Nishida H, Hayashi K, et al. Use of 99mTc-MIBI scintigraphy in the evaluation of the response to chemotherapy for osteosarcoma: comparison with 201Tl scintigraphy and angiography. *Int. J. Clin. Oncol*. 2011;16(4):373-378.

[53] Magnan H, Chou AJ, Chou JF, Yeung HW, Healey JH, Meyers PA. Noninvasive imaging with thallium-201 scintigraphy may not correlate with survival in patients with osteosarcoma. *Cancer* 2010;116(17):4147-4151.

[54] Van der Woude HJ, Bloem JL, Van Oostayen JA, Nooy MA, Taminiau AH, Hermans J, et al. Treatment of high-grade bone sarcomas with neoadjuvant chemotherapy: the utility of sequential color Doppler sonography in predicting histopathologic response. *AJR Am. J. Roentgenol.* 1995;165(1):125-133.

[55] Seng K, Maderwald S, De Greiff A, Quick HH, Laub G, Schmitt P, et al. Dynamic contrast-enhanced magnetic resonance angiography of the thoracic vessels: an intraindividual comparison of different kspace acquisition strategies. *Invest. Radiol*. 2010;45(11):708–714.

[56] Van der Woude HJ, Bloem JL, Verstraete KL, Taminiau AH, Nooy MA, Hogendoorn PC. Osteosarcoma and Ewing's sarcoma after neoadjuvant chemotherapy: value of dynamic MR imaging in detecting viable tumor before surgery. *AJR Am. J. Roentgenol*. 1995;165(3):593-598.
[57] van Rijswijk CS, Geirnaerdt MJ, Hogendoorn PC, Peterse JL,. Van Coevorder F, Taminiau A, et al. Dynamic contrast-enhanced MR imaging in monitoring response to isolated limb perfusion in high-grade soft tissue sarcoma: Initial results. *Eur. Radiol*. 2003;13(8):1849-1858.
[58] Hanna S, Parham D, Fairclough D, Meyer W, Le A, Fletch D. Assessment of osteosarcoma reponse to preoperative chemotherapy ysing dynamic FLASH gadolinium-DTPA-enhanced magnetic resonance mapping. *Invest. Radiol*. 1992;27(5):367-373.
[59] Shapeero LG, Henry-Amar M, Vanel D. Response of osteosarcoma and Ewing sarcoma to preoperative chemotherapy: assessment with dynamic and static MR imaging and skeletal scintigraphy. *Invest. Radiol.* 1992;27(11):989-991.
[60] Maas R, Winkler K, Delling G, Heise U. The potential of MRI in preoperative evaluation of chemotherapy-induced necrosis in osteosarcoma and Ewing's sarcoma. *Chir. Organi. Mov.* 1990;75(1 Suppl):41-44.
[61] Charpentier E, Bonnerot V, Frouin F, Vanel D, Charlotte F, Kalifa C, et al. Factor analysis of dynamic magnetic resonance imaging in predicting the response of osteosarcoma to chemotherapy. *Invest. Radiol.* 1992;27(10):847-855.
[62] De Baere T, Vanel D, Shapeero LG, Charpentier A, Terrier P, Di Paola M. Osteosarcoma after chemotherapy: evaluation with contrast material-enhanced subtraction MR imaging. *Radiology* 1992;185(2):587-592.
[63] Schwab JH, Springfield DS, Raskin KA, Mankin HJ, Hornicek FJ. What's New in Primary Bone Tumors. *J. Bone Joint Surg. Am.* 2012;94(20):1913-1919.
[64] Ongolo-Zogo P, Thiesse P, Sau J, Desuzinges C, Blay JY, Bonmartin A, et al. Assessment of osteosarcoma response to neoadjuvant chemotherapy:comparative usefulness of dynamicgadolinium-enhanced spin-echo magneticresonance imaging and technetium-99m skeletal angioscintigraphy. *Eur. Radiol*. 1999;9(5):907–914.
[65] Reitan NK, Thuen M, Goa PE, de Lange Davies C. Institution characterization of tumor microvascular structure and permeability: comparison between magnetic resonance imaging and intravital confocal imaging. *J. Biomed. Opt*. 2010;15(3):1-11.

[66] Guo J, Reddick WE, Glass JO, Ji Q, Billups CA, Wu J, et al. Dynamic contrast-enhanced magnetic resonance imaging as a prognostic factor in predicting event-free and overall survival in pediatric patients with osteosarcoma. *Cancer* 2012;118(15):3776-3785.

[67] Guo JY, Reddick WE, Rosen MA, Song HK. Dynamic contrast-enhanced magnetic resonance imaging parameters independent of baseline T10 values. *Magn. Reson. Imaging* 2009;27(9):1208-1215.

[68] Huang W, Wang Y, Panicek DM, Schwartz LH, Koutcher JA. Feasibility of using limited-population-based average R10 for pharmacokinetic modeling of osteosarcoma dynamic contrast-enhanced magnetic resonance imaging data. *Magn. Reson. Imaging* 2009;27(6):852-858.

[69] Guo JY, Reddick WE. DCE-MRI pixel-by-pixel quantitative curve pattern analysis and its application to osteosarcoma. *J. Magn. Reson. Imaging* 2009;30(1):177-184.

[70] Hoang BH, Dyke JP, Koutcher JA, Huvos AG, Mizobuchi H, Maza BA, et al. VEGF expression in osteosarcoma correlates with vascular permeability by dynamic MRI. *Clin. Orthop. Relat. Res.* 2004;(426):32–38.

[71] Bajpai J, Gamanagatti S, Sharma MC, Kumar R, Vishnubhatla S, Khan SA, et al. Noninvasive imaging surrogate of angiogenesis in osteosarcoma. *Pediatr. Blood Cancer* 2010;54(4):526-531.

[72] Rosenthal D, Callstrom MR. Critical review and state of the art in interventional oncology: benign and metastatic disease involving bone. *Radiology* 2012;262(3):765–780.

[73] Gebauer B, Tunn PU. Thermal ablation in bone tumors. *Recent Results Cancer Res.* 2006;167:135-146.

[74] Orgera G, Monfardini L, DellaVigna P, Zhang L, Bonomo G, Arnone P, et al. High-intensity focused ultrasound (HIFU) in patients with solid malignancies: evaluation of feasibility local tumor response and clinical results. *Radiol. Med.* 2011;116(5):734-748

[75] Zhang L, Wang ZB. High-intensity focused ultrasound tumor ablation: Review of ten years of clinical experience. *Front Med. China* 2010;4(3):294-302.

[76] Holzer G, Krepler P, Koschat MA, Grampp S, Dominkus M, Kotz R. Bone mineral density in long-term survivors of highly malignant osteosarcoma. *J. Bone Joint Surg. Br.* 2003;85(2) 231-237.

[77] Hill SC, Baker AR, Barton NW, Wexler LH, Scott LJ. Sciatic nerve:paradoxic hypertrophy after amputation in young patients. *Radiology* 1997;205(2):559–562.

[78] Price AP, Abramson SJ, Hwang S, Chou A, Bartolotta R, Meyers P, et al. Skeletal imaging effects of pamidronate therapy in osteosarcoma patients. *Pediatr. Radiol.* 2011;41(4):451-458.

[79] Ryan SP, Weinberger E, White KS, Shaw DW, Patterson K, Nazar-Stewart V, et al. MR imaging of bone marrow in children with osteosarcoma: effect of granulocyte colony-stimulating factor. *AJR Am. J. Roentgenol.* 1995;165(4):915-920.

[80] Franzius C, Daldrup-Link HE, Wagner-Bohn A, Sciuk J, Heindel WL, Jürgens H, et al. FDG–PET for detection of recurrences from malignant primary bone tumors: comparison with conventional imaging. *Ann. Oncol.* 2002;13(1):157-160.

[81] Daldrup-Link HE, Franzius C, Link TM, Laukamp D, Sciuk J, Jürgens H, et al: Whole-body MR imaging for detection of bone metastases in children and young adults: Comparison with skeletal scintigraphy and FDG PET. *AJR Am. J. Roentgenol.* 2001;177(1):229-236.

[82] Bakri D, Bar-Shalom R, Ben Arush MW, Postovsky S. Value of routine bone scans in patients with bone sarcomas before local treatment. *J. Pediatr. Hematol. Oncol.* 2011;33(2):103-106.

[83] Cheney MD, Giraud C, Goldberg SI, Rosenthal DI, Hornicek FJ, Choy E, et al. MRI surveillance following treatment of extremity soft tissue sarcoma. *J. Surg. Onco.* 2013; [epub ahead of print].

In: Osteosarcoma
Editors: Edwin Choy

ISBN: 978-1-63321-052-3

Chapter 4

PROMISING THERAPEUTIC APPROACHES FOR OSTEOSARCOMA TARGETING MIDKINE

Mine Ergüven, M.D., Ph.D. [1,*]
[1]İstanbul Aydın University, Faculty of Engineering,
İstanbul, Turkey

ABSTRACT

A heparin binding small protein midkine (MK) with growth factor and cytokine actions comprises a family with pleiotrophin/heparin-binding growth-associated molecule. MK is highly expressed at mid-gestation period, however its' expression decreased and/or lost in adults. MK showed its activity through several receptors including anaplastic lenfoma kinase, proteine tyrosine phosphatase zeta, Notch 2, low density lipoprotein receptor-related protein, proteoglycans and integrins. MK has significant roles in *inflammation and immunity* (vascular stenosis, diabetic nephropathy, Crohn's Disease, haptotaxi, migration, wound healing, rheumatoid arthritis), *blood pressure* (chronic kidney diesease-related hypertansion, renin-angiotensin system), *development* (epithelial-mesenchymal interactions and transformations, mesoderm migration, neural tube development, mitogenesis, reproduction and aging), *tissue protection/renewal/repair* (myocardial and cerebral infarction, anti-apoptosis, stem cell, wound healing), *cancer* (tumour growth, chemoresistance, transformation, anti-apoptosis, epithelial-

* Phone: + 90 (535) 782 30 66; E-mail: mine.erguven@gmail.com; Work Phone: +90 (212) 4116100-57201.

mesenchymal interactions) and the *determination of cell fate* (from autophagy to cell resistance/survival or autophagic cell death/apoptosis). High MK expression is determined in several cancer types including osteosarcoma (OS) in preclinic and clinic studies. Knocking out or knocking down of MK gene using small interfering RNA or inhibition of MK signaling via anti-MK monoclonal antibody showed promising results in the treatment of primary OS and its' metastatic action. MK itself is widely expected as treatment for tissue repair/renewal/repair. MK provides innovative opportunity to compansate lost bone tissue. In this review, considering MKs' multiple adverse mechanisms of actions, this chapter focused to discuss promising therapeutic approaches for OS targeting MK.

Keywords: Osteosarcoma, Midkine, Biomarker, Therapeutic target

INTRODUCTION

OS is the most common primary malignant bone tumor in children and adolescents, comprising almost 60% of all bone sarcomas [1,2]. It is an osteoid producing solid tumor that occurs more often in larger bones close to epiphyseal areas of rapid growth. The incidence of OS is approximately 4–5 children per year per million in the US. It shows a bimodal age distribution with a peak incidence of OS in young adults. A second peak of incidence was identified in elderly adults where it is associated with defective bone remodeling [3, 4]. With the advent of chemotherapy, the long-term cure rate after surgery for non-metastatic OS has risen from 25% to 60% [5]. However, despite advances in chemotherapy and surgery, the survival rate for OS has reached a plateau and 40% of OS patients eventually died from the disease. The majority of OS are high grade and are often metastatic [6]. They are associated with poor prognosis and the overall survival rate for patients with advanced disease remains low at 20% [7, 8]. A high proportion of patients will have a relapse due to metastasis to the lung, the primary site of OS metastasis. Up to 20% of OS patients present with detectable lung metastasis at initial diagnosis, whereas 80% of patients with only primary tumors develop metastasis in the lung following surgical resection [6]. Metastases are often resistant to conventional chemotherapy and current aggressive treatments pose a significant challenge and do not guarantee long-term survival [9].

A better understanding of OS biology and pathogenesis is needed to advance the development of targeted therapies for both primary and metastatic OS. Understanding OS biology still remains a complex challenge that an unknown etiology, high genetic instability of OS cells, a wide histological heterogeneity, lack of biomarkers, high local aggressiveness, and a rapid metastasizing potential haven't solved yet. Recent progresses in identifying tumor associated pathways and specific mediators of OS pathogenesis, progression, and prognosis has led to novel targeted treatment approaches. Hence in this review, the contribution of old but newly pronounced biomarker named MK was discussed as one of the missing/neglected piece of OS treatment puzzle.

Search Strategy and Selection Criteria

We searched PubMed for the past 13 years (January 2001–March 2014) with the terms "Osteosarcoma" and "midkine". The abstracts were screened to identify those research studies and review articles we judged relevant to our objectives. This procedure identified only 8 publications.

Osteosarcoma

OS, although rare, is the most frequently occurring primary malignant bone tumor, affecting mainly the metaphysis of long bones in children and adolescents. The term "OS" as opposed to "osteogenic sarcoma" is preferred by the World Health Organization (WHO). WHO classification separates conventional OS into three major subtypes: osteoblastic, condroblastic and fibroblastic, reflecting the predominant type of matrix within the tumor. In addition to classical OS, the WHO classification recognizes additional histological variants, including telangiectatic OS, small cell OS, parosteal and periosteal OSs, as well as low grade central and high grade surface OSs. The classical central subtypes are nearly always WHO grade III high malignant tumors, whereas surface OSs are mostly low grade I or intermediate grade II tumors [10]. In the majority of primary OS, the etiology is unknown. Cytogenetic studies have shown various complex changes involving some chromosomes but without any specific pattern. Two genes – a hereditary mutation of retinoblastoma (Rb), and an autosomic recessive mutation of p53 in the Li-Fraumeni syndrome – localized in 13q14 and 17p13, respectively, are currently proposed to be involved in a stepwise accumulation of genomic defect [10, 11].

OS revealed several key signaling networks in which multiple genes were altered at the chromosomal level. These include the vascular endothelial growth factor (VEGF) and mammalian target of rapamycin (mTOR) signaling pathways, in which amplifications occur, and the wingless-type MMTV integration site family (Wnt), cellular adhesion molecules, and Hedgehog signaling pathways, in which deletions occur. Further investigation of the VEGF pathway revealed that VEGF-alpha (VEGFA) gene amplification is a poor prognostic factor for tumor-free survival of OS patients. VEGFA is abundantly expressed in 74.1% of OS cases, and patients with VEGFA-positive OSs had significantly worse tumor-free survival rates than patients with VEGFA-negative OSs [12].

A recent study identified syndecan-2 as a Wnt target and provided evidence supporting the pathologic role of Wnt signaling pathway in OS [13]. In contrast, Cai and coworkers showed that the Wnt pathway is inactivated in OS and therefore plays a potential tumor suppressor role, as stimulation of the pathway inhibits proliferation or promotes differentiation [14]. WNT5a and receptor tyrosine kinase-like orphan receptor (ROR)-2, which are highly expressed in OS, are both correlated with tumor metastasis and proliferation [15]. Similarly, the physiological interaction of WNT5b and ROR2 can also enhance cell migration [16]. Notably, Wnt5a/ROR2 signaling induces expression of matrix metalloproteinases (MMPs)-13, and this effect is abrogated by an inhibitor of the sarcoma (Src)-family protein tyrosine kinases (SFKs) [17].

The frequency of tumor supressor genes' proteins as RB-1 and tumor protein p53 (TP53) alterations in sporadic OS ranges from 30 to 40%, and patients with tumors harboring alterations in either gene seem to have poorer prognosis than those with tumors lacking such alterations. Other tumor supressor WW domain-containing oxidoreductase (WWOX) gene is deleted in 30% of human OSs, and the WWOX protein is undetectable in 61.8%, which indicates that loss of WWOX, whether by deletion of the gene or loss of protein expression, is likely anearly event in OS pathogenesis [18]. Another mechanism of OS pathogenesis is oncogene aberration. A multifunctional DNA repair enzyme APEX nuclease (APEX)-1 gene which increases the expression of VEGF is amplified in OSs. APEX1 protein expression independently predicts local recurrence and/or metastasis [19]. Myc amplification has been associated with OS pathogenesis and chemoresistance.

A recent study showed that alternate splicing of Murine Double Minute (MDM)-2 was superior to p53 mutation as a prognostic biomarker in OS.

Molecules involved in OS cell migration and invasion may be good therapeutic targets. Highly expressed integrin beta-4 (integrin b-4) promotes OS metastasis and interacts with ezrin which contains a binding site for p-glycoprotein (p-gp) [20]. The Notch pathway downregulates osteoclastogenesis/osteoblastogenesis and plays critical roles in OS. Targeting of Notch, induced G2/M arrest and MMPs inhibition in OS cells [21].

In OS, expression of aldolase A, fructosebisphosphate (ALDOA) and/or sulfotransferase family 3A, member 1 (SULT1A3) was significantly higher in patients with shorter survival time, suggesting these proteins are negative survival markers of OS [19]. In addition, B-cell lymphoma (BCL)-2-associated athanogene (BAG)-3 alters the interaction between heat shock protein (HSP)-70 and inhibitor of kappa B kinase gamma (IKK-g), increasing availability of IKK-g and protecting it from degradation in SAOS-2 OS cells. This, in turn, increases nuclear factor kappa-light-chain-enhancer of activated B cells (NF-kB) activity and promotes survival [20]. Myc inactivation caused proliferative arrest and promoted differentiation in OS [21].

The proapoptotic molecule Bcl-2-interacting mediator (BIM) also plays a role in apoptosis, autophagy, and anoikis in OS [22, 23]. Polo-like kinase (PLK)-1 increases mitotic cell cycle and shows anti-apoptotic effect in several OS cell lines and increased the growth in vivo [24]. High hypoxia inducible factor-1 alpha subunit (HIF-1a) expression is also frequently seen [25].

For OS patients, high levels of Bcl-xL are highly associated with poorer survival compared with low levels. Bcl-xL downregulation or upregulation significantly reduced or increased proliferation, respectively, in OS cells. Furthermore, B-cell lymphoma-extra large (Bcl-xL) downregulation significantly enhanced chemosensitivity or radiosensitivity of OS cells in vitro, and this might be associated with elevated caspase-3 activity [26].

The molecules of the coagulation cascade may play an important role in tumor growth and be pharmaceutical targets to disrupt OS growth. It's reported that venous thrombi adjacent to OS harbor tumor surrounded by fibrin-expressing coagulation cofactors, which is associated with poor prognosis. More aggressive OS cell lines had higher surface expression of procoagulant factors, generated more thrombin, and proliferated in response to thrombin compared with their less aggressive counterparts [27].

Cell surface receptor expression patterns in standard and patientderived OS cell lines. Insulin-like growth factor (IGF)-2R was consistently overexpressed on the cell surface across all tested cell lines. Substantial expression of met proto-oncogene (hepatocyte growth factor receptor), v-erb-b2 erythroblastic leukemia viral oncogene homolog 2 (HER-2), IGF-1R, fms-related tyrosine kinase 4, insulin receptor (IR), and platelet-derived growth factor receptor, beta polypeptide was also detected, suggesting that these receptors may contribute to the aggressiveness and biological heterogeneity of OS and may serve as potential targets for OS patients [28].

HSP90 is also a relevant target for therapeutic intervention in OS [29]. Rb gene mutations in OS result in increased activity of the elongation factor E2F1. In human primary OSs and E2F1- inducible OS cell lines, high E2F1 levels exerted a growth-suppressing effect (including p73 induction) that relied on the integrity of the DNA damage response network [30].

Signal Transducer and Activator of Transcription, or Signal Transduction and Transcription (STAT) 3 is also highly expressed in OS tissues and is associated with poor tumor differentiation, metastasis, and low 5-year overall and relapse-free survival rates. STAT3 inhibition resulted in proliferation and enhanced apoptosis in OS cells through the inhibition of antiapoptotic genes, including Myc and cyclin D1 [31, 32].

OS cells are osteoclastic lineage cells, which are characterized by cells secreting the osteoclast-inducing factor named receptor activator of NF-kB ligand. Receptor activator of NF-kB-Fc, osteoprotegerin, bisphosphonates, and sarcoma (Src) inhibitör control various aspects of osteoclast function [33]. In addition, BCL2-like 11 mediates the antitumor effects of several chemotherapeutic agents, whereas BIM suppression supports chemoresistance [34].

Autophagy, a catabolic process that is critical to maintaining cellular homeostasis and responding to cytotoxic insult, can either promote or inhibit anti-tumor drug resistance, depending on both the nature and duration of treatment-induced metabolic stress and the tumor type. In OS cells, high mobility group box (HMGB)-1 protein-mediated autophagy is a remarkable contributor to drug resistance. HMGB1 binds to the autophagy protein Beclin 1, regulating Beclin 1-Class III phosphatidylinositol 3-kinase (PI3KC3) complex formation and autophagic progression [35].

Cancer stem cells (CSCs) in OS was first determined by Gibbs and coworkers [36]. They showed that human OS samples and cell lines contain a subpopulation of cells that are capable of growing in spherical, clonal clusters in suspension under serum-free conditions and have the properties of self renewal and multipotency [36]. These cell clusters named as sarcospheres or osteospheres can be dissociated and form secondary spheres, and have the ability to undergo osteogenic and adipogenic differentiation. It's also proven that sphere-forming cells from OS lines can initiate tumors, and are more drug-resistant to chemotherapeutic agents [37]. Mesenchymal stem cell (MSC) cell surface glycoprotein markers CD133 (prominin), CD 117 (c-kit) and Stro-1 were detected in OS [38, 39].

OSs is generally characterized by increased proliferation and defective differentiation. Loss of differentiation is a prognostic feature of high grade OS while low grade disease is associated with more differentiated morphology. There is a clear link between tumorigenesis and defective differentiation in OS. As mentioned before, Rb and p53 are commonly inactivated in OS, are also required for controlled osteoblast differentiation. Rb and p53 deficient osteoblasts have an increased capacity to form multipotent spheres and show defective bone differentiation along with a high propensity for the development of OS [40]. It's proposed that Rb and p53 mutations change the bone differentiations program, thereby selecting for immature progenitors with defective DNA damage checkpoints and a propensity to accumulate further mutations. OSs and mesenchymal stem cells (MSCs) have other common characteristic as deubiquitination mechanism: Rb-inhibitors of DNA binding proteins (ID)-the deubiquitinating enzyme (USP1). High levels of ID promoted the stem cell features and blocked osteoblastic differentiation in MSCs, and USP1 knockdown in OS led to ID destabilization, growth arrest and differentiation [41]. MSCs could maintain OS cells in an undifferentiated state through secretion of cytokines such as interleukin-6 [42].

Hedgehog, Notch and mitogen activated protein kinase (MAPK) signaling pathways play a role in maintaining stem cells in the osteoblast lineage and maintaining OS CSCs. Bone morphogenetic proteins (BMPs) are members of the tumor growth factor-beta (TGF-β) superfamily and play a critical role in skeletal development, bone formation and stem cell differentiation. Disruptions in bone morphogenetic protein (BMP) signaling result in a variety of skeletal and extraskeletal anomalies. it was shown that BMPs with a pro-differentiation function decreases OS CSCs [40, 43]. BMP9 is a poorly characterized member of the BMP family and is among the most osteogenic BMPs, promoting osteoblastic differentiation of MSCs both in vitro and in vivo [44]. Wnt signaling is inactive in sphere forming stem cells [45].

MIDKINE

A 13 kDA protein MK is a heparin-binding growth factor with cytokine actions. MK was found as the product of a gene up-regulated at an early stage of retinoic acid-induced differentiation of teratocarcinoma stem cells and became the founding member of a small protein family, the other member of which is pleiotrophin (PTN), also called heparin-binding growth associated molecule (HBGAM). MK promotes proliferation, migration, anti-apoptotic manner, mitogenesis, transforming and angiogenesis various cells. MK showed its activity through several receptors including anaplastic lenfoma kinase (ALK), protein tyrosine phosphatase zeta (PTPζ), Notch 2, low density lipoprotein receptor-related protein (LRP), proteoglycans and integrins. MK has significant roles in inflammation and immunity [vascular stenosis, diabetic nephropathy, Crohn's Disease, haptotaxi, migration, wound healing, rheumatoid arthritis], blood pressure [chronic kidney diesease-related hypertansion, renin-angiotensin system], development [epithelial-mesenchymal interaction (EMT) and transformation, mesoderm migration, neural tube development, mitogenesis, reproduction and aging], tissue protection/renewal/repair (myocardial and cerebral infarction, anti-apoptosis, stem cell, wound healing), cancer [tumour growth, chemoresistance, transformation, anti-apoptosis, EMT] and determination of cell fate [from autophagy to cell resistance/survival or autophagic cell death/apoptosis] [46, 47].

PTPζ is a transmembrane protein with intracellular tyrosine phosphatase domain and extracellular chondroitin sulfate chain and also serves as a PTN receptor. Chondroitin sulfate portion of PTPζ is important for binding to MK [46, 48]. As an MK receptor, PTPζ has been shown to be involved in migration of embryonic neurons [48] and UMR106 osteoblast-like cells [49], survival of embryonic neurons [50] and B cells [51] and suppression of the proliferation of osteoblasts [52]. After MK or PTN binds to PTPζ, tyrosine phosphorylation is increased in cytoplasmic signaling molecules such as protein kinase B (Akt) [51] and β-catenin [52]. After binding PTPζ is dimerized, leading to inactivation of the intracellular phosphatase domain, and results in increased tyrosine phosphorylation. β-catenin is a critical step in canonical Wnt signalling. In osteoblasts, MK has been shown to inhibit osteoblast proliferation by interfering in Wnt signalling by inhibiting PTPζ-mediated dephosphorylation of β-catenin [52]. Multiple kinases as PI3K, MAPK, a Src family kinase and protein kinase C (PKC) appear to be involved in signaling downstream from PTPζ [49]. PTPζ inactivates Src through dephosphorylation. PI3K in the signalling involves in MK-induced phosphorylation of Akt [49].

LRP-1 is a member of the LRP family and binds to MK. LRP-1 serves as an MK receptor upon survival of embryonic neurons [53] and prevention of hypoxic injury in mouse embryonic stem cells [54]. It's shown that MK partially prevented hypoxic injury through activation of Akt, HIF-1a via LRP-1 [54]. The underlying mechanism of the anchorage-independent cell growth of cancer cells is also related to LRP [55, 56]. In addition to LRP-mediated signalling, a portion of MK has been shown to exert its effect directly in the nucleus. MK is internalized after binding to LRP-1 and is then transported to the nucleus by binding to nucleolin. MK can also be transferred to the nucleolus for the synthesis of ribosomal RNA [46].

The integrins are components of MK receptors to increase cell migration and function in a molecular complex. α4β1-integrin serves as an MK receptor upon migration of UMR-106 osteoblastic cells, and α6β1-integrin for neurite outgrowth of embryonic neurons. In addition MK promotes complex formation of integrins, LRP-6 ectodomain and PTPζ. MK increases the tyrosine phosphorylation of integrin-associated molecule paxillin in osteoblastic cells [57]. MK binds to tetraspanin and α6β1-integrin and enhances their association, leading to activation of focal adhesion kinase (FAK), paxillin and STAT1α pathway, resulting in enhanced migration and invasiveness in cancer cells [58].

ALK is involved in the tumourigenesis of at least several malignant tumours including anaplastic large cell lymphoma [59]. After stimulation by MK, ALK phosphorylates insülin receptor substrate-1, leading to activation of MAPK, PI3K and NF-κB [60]. However, it is not established whether ALK directly binds to MK with high affinity. Furthermore, ALK formed a complex with LRP-6 ectodomain and integrins [H. Muramatsu et al. unpublished results, 46] which means that ALK may work in the receptor complex for MK.

Notch-2, a transmembrane protein belonging to the Notch family, is an MK receptor inducing EMT. Direct binding of MK and Notch-2 has been shown. After MK stimulation, JAK2 and STAT3 signalling pathway is activated [60-62]. MK induces cleavage of the Notch-2 cytoplasmic domain and stimulates the expression of NF-κB. It's also shown that the Notch signalling system took part in chemokine production of MK [63]. The possibility that Notch-2 acts in the receptor complex which includes a Notch-related transmembrane protein DNER and PTPζ [63].

Most MK activities are inhibited by heparin or digestion with heparitinase or chondroitinase, indicating the importance of carbohydrate recognition in MK signalling. Two oligomeric carbohydrate structures, namely heparan sulfate trisulfated units and chondroitin sulfate E units, have been shown to bind to MK strongly [64]. Chondroitin sulfate chains are present in PTPζ and a chondroitin-sulfate binding partner of MK and pericellular protein named versican also binds to MK to deliver MK to the receptor [65].

Downstream targets as the PI3K/Akt system and MAPK play central roles that the PI3K/Akt system is involved in the survival of B cells [51], prevention of hypoxic injury in embryonic stem cells [54], and migration of osteoblast-like cells [49]. MK can suppress caspase and activate Bcl-2 [64]. Transcriptional factors, whose activities are regulated by signalling cascades activated/promoted by MK, can be listed as NF-κB [62], HIF-1a [54] and STATs [58, 63, 66, 67]. STATs have different roles as the MK-STAT3 pathway plays a necessary role in mitotic clonal expansion, differentiation, EMT and cytokine production [63], MK-STAT1 pathway involved in the migration [58], MK-STAT5 decreased the Treg cell population through decreasing the master transcriptional factor of Treg cell differentiation Foxp3 [66].

Midkine and Osteosarcoma

MK levels are high during embryogenesis especially in mid-gestation period. After that, it decreases and in adults, expression of the MK protein is only detected in the kidney at very low level [46, 69]. In contrast, its increased expression in tumors as glioblastoma, esophageal, gastric, pancreatic, colorectal, prostate, lung, cervical, brain, neuroblastoma, and Wilm's tumor including OS regardless of tissue type with high frequency was found [46]. In general, MK expression increases along with advancing tumor stage and closely correlates with poor prognosis that the blood MK level is frequently elevated with advance of human carcinomas, decreased after surgical removal of the tumors and/or other therapy applications [46]. Knock down or knock out of MK gene frequently resulted in response to treatment in cancer era, however MK itself is needed for recovery state of some disease state as wounds: Both cases are concluded as the result of high growth, proliferation and self-renewal capacity of MK. [46, 64, 68, 69]. MK has alsosignificant role in tumour recurrence and drug resistance, which is directly related to partial response/treatment failure with the lack of life quality [46, 64, 68, 69].

The study of Maehara and coworkers showed the relationship between MK and OC [71]. They showed that MK is overexpressed in OS and the level of MK expression is correlated with prognosis fate thus it can be evaluated as candidate therapeutic target for OCs. They investigated several factors like alkalen phosphotase (ALP), tumor size, intensity of bone scintigraphy in tumors including MK expression in seven patients with OS, and examined the effects of the anti-MK antibody against four cell lines of OS in vitro [71]. They found that only factor correlated with prognosis was MK. They used functional antibodies against MK which suppresses growth of OC cell lines, 9N2, 3N1, Saos-2, and NOS-1, to 25–65% of untreated controls. They also mentioned that the expression of truncated MK, which is pronounced as a tumor marker in progessed carcinomas [72, 73], was not detected in any of their OS cell lines and tumors, thus they conluded that the truncated form can not be used as a tumor marker in OS [71].

In the study of Sueyoshi and coworkers, they proceeded MK knockdown by small interfering RNA (siRNA) and used also recombinant MK in vitro and in vivo [74]. They significantly induced apoptosis in OC cells by siRNA, however they increased cell proliferation by recombinant MK application. Inhibition of MK signaling by anti-MK monoclonal antibody (anti-MK mAb) suppressed growth of OC cells both in vitro and in vivo. In addition, they found that inhibition of MK function significantly suppressed lung metastasis in xenograft transplantation model [74].

Mirkin and coworkers generated doxorubicin (DXR)-resistant OC cells (Saos-2/R) and found that they express higher amounts of MK than their drug-sensitive counterparts [75]. In addition, they also transfected Saos cells with MK, they found that these cells express MK in a manner that was almost equivalent to that of DXR-resistant cells. In their study, MK-transfected wild-type cells acquired a significant level of drug resistance as compared to their non-transfected parental cells [75]. They showed that MK can protect drug-sensitive cells from drug toxicity and induce drug resistance. The underlying mechanism of this cytoprotection explained by them as the activation of the Akt pathway and the inhibition of drug-induced proliferation arrest as well as apoptosis (the inhibition of caspase-3 activity) [75]. They concluded that there are intercellular cytoprotective signals which means the development of resistance to chemotherapy such as the one mediated by MK, originating from cells with acquired drug resistance to protect neighboring drug-sensitive cells [75].

Takagi-Kimura and co-workers proceeded oncolytic virotherapy for human OS using MK promoter-regulated adenoviruses in xenograft models and *in vitro* [76]. They developed a tumor-specific MK promoter-regulated oncolytic vectors based on two different human adenovirus serotypes named MOA5 and MOA35. They first checked MK mRNA expression and its promoter activity in OS cell lines, they detected that they were significantly high in five human OS cell lines, but was restricted in normal cells. In addition, they also evaluated the expressions of Ad5 receptor (coxsackievirus/adenovirus receptor; CAR) and Ad35 receptor (CD46) for each cell line. They found very low levels of Ad5 receptor expression were observed in only two human OS cell types as MNNG-HOS and MG-63 cells, whereas high levels of CAR expression were seen in the other human OS cell lines. Interesting results coming from their study that infectivity and in vitro cytocidal effect of MOA35 was significantly enhanced in MNNG-HOS and MG-63 cells compared with MOA5, although the cytocidal effects of MOA5 were sometimes higher in high CAR-expressing cell lines. In MG-63 xenograft models, MOA35 showed highest therapeutic efficacy compared with MOA5. They concluded that MOA5 and MOA35 allow tailored virotherapy and facilitate more effective treatments for OS [76].

In conlusion, anti-MK treatment modalities with various methods resulted in proliferation/growth inhibition in OS at pre-clinical and clinical studies, suggesting MK would be a promising biomarker for diagnosis and prognosis of OS. Few studies has been procedeed for defining MK role(s) in OS up-to now. MK and OC pathways have many common pathways as Notch, HIF-1, Wnt... etc. which are still waiting to be elucidated for OC etiology and new treatment modality.

Conflict of Interest

None declared.

References

[1] Cormier J. N., Pollock R. E. Soft tissue sarcomas. *CA Cancer J. Clin.*, 2004; 54:94-109.

[2] Heare T., Hensley M. A., Dell'Orfano S. Bone tumors: OS and Ewing's sarcoma. *Curr. Opin. Pediatr.*, 2009; 21:365-72.

[3] Hansen M. F., Seton M., Merchant A. OS in Paget's disease of bone. *J. Bone Miner Res.*, 2006; 21:P58-63.

[4] Ottaviani G., Jaffe N. The epidemiology of OS. *Cancer Treat. Res.*, 2009; 152:3-13.

[5] Caudill J. S., Arndt C. A. Diagnosis and management of bone malignancy in adolescence. *Adolesc. Med. State Art. Rev.*, 2007; 18:62-78.

[6] Marina N., Gebhardt M., Teot L., et al. Biology and therapeutic advances for pediatric OS. *Oncologist,* 2004; 9:422-41.
[7] Meyers P. A., Heller G., Healey J., et al. Chemotherapy for nonmetastatic osteogenic sarcoma: the Memorial Sloan-Kettering experience. *J. Clin. Oncol.*, 1992; 10:5-15.
[8] Meyers P. A., Schwartz C. L., Krailo M., et al. OS: a randomized, prospective trial of the addition of ifosfamide and/or muramyl tripeptide to cisplatin, doxorubicin, and high-dose methotrexate. *J. Clin. Oncol.,* 2005; 23:2004-11.
[9] Posthuma De Boer J., Witlox M. A., Kaspers G. J., et al. Molecular alterations as target for therapy in metastatic OS: a review of literature. *Clin. Exp. Metastasis*, 2011; 28:493-503.
[10] Ritter J., Bielack S. S. OS. *Ann. Oncol.*, 2010; 21:vii320-5.
[11] Yang J., Zhang W. New molecular insights into OS targeted therapy. *Curr. Opin. Oncol.,* 2013; 25:398-406.
[12] Yang J., Yang D., Sun Y., et al. Genetic amplification of the vascular endothelial growth factor (VEGF) pathway genes, including vegfa, in human OS. *Cancer,* 2011; 117:4925–4938.
[13] Dieudonne F. X., Marion A., Hay E., et al. High wnt signaling represses the proapoptotic proteoglycan syndecan-2 in OS cells. *Cancer Res.,* 2010; 70:5399–5408.
[14] Cai Y., Mohseny A. B., Karperien M., et al. Inactive wnt/beta-catenin pathway in conventional high-grade OS. *J. Pathol.*, 2010; 220:24–33.
[15] Ebb D., Meyers P., Grier H., et al. Phase ii trial of trastuzumab in combination with cytotoxic chemotherapy for treatment of metastatic OS with human epidermal growth factor receptor 2 overexpression: a report from the children's oncology group. *J. Clin. Oncol.,* 2012; 30: 2545–2551.
[16] Lu B. J., Wang Y. Q., Wei X. J., et al. Expression of WNT-5a and ROR2 correlates with disease severity in OS. *Mol. Med. Rep.,* 2012; 5:1033-6.
[17] Morioka K., Tanikawa C., Ochi K., et al. Orphan receptor tyrosine kinase ROR2 as a potential therapeutic target for OS. *Cancer Sci.,* 2009; 100:1227-33.
[18] Yang J., Cogdell D., Yang D., et al. Deletion of the wwox gene and frequent loss of its protein expression in human OS. *Cancer Lett.,* 2010; 291:31–38.

[19] Yang J., Yang D., Cogdell D., et al. Apex1 gene amplification and its protein overexpression in OS: correlation with recurrence, metastasis, and survival. *Technol. Cancer Res. Treat.*, 2010; 9:161–169.

[20] Brambilla D., Zamboni S., Federici C., et al. P-glycoprotein binds to ezrin at amino acid residues 149-242 in the ferm domain and plays a key role in the multidrug resistance of human OS. *Int. J. Cancer*, 2012; 130: 2824–2834.

[21] Li Y., Zhang J., Ma D., et al. Curcumin inhibits proliferation and invasion of OS cells through inactivation of notch-1 signaling. *FEBS J.,* 2012; 279:2247–2259.

[22] Akiyama T., Dass C. R., Choong P. F. Bim-targeted cancer therapy: a link between drug action and underlying molecular changes. *Mol. Cancer Ther.*, 2009; 8:3173–3180.

[23] Gillings A. S., Balmanno K., Wiggins C. M., et al. Apoptosis and autophagy: Bim as a mediator of tumour cell death in response to oncogene-targeted therapeutics. *FEBS J.,* 2009; 276:6050–6062.

[24] Yamaguchi U., Honda K., Satow R., et al. Functional genome screen for therapeutic targets of OS. *Cancer Sci*., 2009; 100:2268–2274.

[25] Liang D., Yang M., Guo B., et al. HIF-1 alpha induced by beta-elemene protects human OS cells from undergoing apoptosis. *J. Cancer Res. Clin. Oncol.,* 2012; 138:1865–1877.

[26] Wang Z. X., Yang J. S., Pan X., et al. Functional and biological analysis of bcl-xl expression in human OS. *Bone*, 2010; 47:445–454.

[27] Ichikawa J., Cole H. A., Magnussen R. A., et al. Thrombin induces OS growth, a function inhibited by low molecular weight heparin in vitro and in vivo: Procoagulant nature of OS. *Cancer*, 2012; 118:2494–2506.

[28] Hassan S. E., Bekarev M., Kim M. Y., et al. Cell surface receptor expression patterns in OS. *Cancer*, 2012; 118:740–749.

[29] Akiyama T., Dass C. R., Choong P. F. Novel therapeutic strategy for OS targeting osteoclast differentiation, bone-resorbing activity, and apoptosis pathway. *Mol. Cancer Ther.*, 2008; 7:3461–3469.

[30] McCleese J. K., Bear M. D., Fossey S. L., et al. The novel hsp90 inhibitor sta-1474 exhibits biologic activity against OS cell lines. *Int. J. Cancer*, 2009; 125:2792–2801.

[31] Liontos M., Niforou K., Velimezi G., et al. Modulation of the e2f1-driven cancer cell fate by the DNA damage response machinery and potential novel e2f1 targets in OSs. *Am. J. Pathol.*, 2009; 175:376–391.

[32] Wang Y. C., Zheng L. H., Ma B. A., et al. Clinical value of signal transducers and activators of transcription 3 (stat3) gene expression in human OS. *Acta. Histochemica*, 2011; 113:402–408.

[33] Enomoto M., Hayakawa S., Itsukushima S., et al. Autonomous regulation of OS cell invasiveness by wnt5a/ror2 signaling. *Oncogene,* 2009; 28:3197–3208.

[34] Akiyama T., Dass C. R., Choong P. F. Bim-targeted cancer therapy: a link between drug action and underlying molecular changes. *Mol. Cancer Ther.*, 2009; 8:3173–3180.

[35] Huang J., Liu K., Yu Y., et al. Targeting HMGB1-mediated autophagy as a novel therapeutic strategy for OS. *Autophagy*, 2012; 8:275-277.

[36] Gibbs C. P., Kukekov V. G., Reith J. D., et al. Stem-like cells in bone sarcomas: implications for tumorigenesis. *Neoplasia,* 2005; 7:967-76.

[37] Fujii H., Honoki K., Tsujiuchi T., et al. Sphere-forming stem-like cell populations with drug resistance in human sarcoma cell lines. *Int. J. Oncol.,* 2009; 34:1381-6.

[38] Adhikari A. S., Agarwal N., Wood B. M., et al. CD117 and Stro-1 identify OS tumor-initiating cells associated with metastasis and drug resistance. *Cancer Res.,* 2010; 70:4602-12.

[39] Li J., Zhong X. Y., Li Z. Y., et al. CD133 expression in OS and derivation of $CD133^+$ cells. *Mol. Med. Rep.*, 2013;7:577-84.

[40] Rubio R., Gutierrez-Aranda I., Sáez-Castillo A. I., et al. The differentiation stage of p53-Rb-deficient bone marrow mesenchymal stem cells imposes the phenotype of in vivo sarcoma development. *Oncogene*, 2013;32:4970-80.

[41] Williams S. A., Maecker H. L., French D. M., et al. USP1 deubiquitinates ID proteins to preserve a mesenchymal stem cell program in OS. *Cell,* 2011; 146:918-30.

[42] Bian Z. Y., Fan Q. M., Li G., et al. Human mesenchymal stem cells promote growth of OS: involvement of interleukin-6 in the interaction between human mesenchymal stem cells and Saos-2. *Cancer Sci.,* 2010; 101:2554-60.

[43] Wang L., Park P., Zhang H., et al. BMP-2 inhibits the tumorigenicity of cancer stem cells in human OS OS99-1 cell line. *Cancer Biol. Ther.*, 2011; 11:457-63.

[44] Lamplot J. D., Qin J., Nan G., et al. BMP9 signaling in stem cell differentiation and osteogenesis. *Am. J. Stem Cells*, 2013;2:1-21.

[45] Basu-Roy U., Seo E., Ramanathapuram L., et al. Sox2 maintains self renewal of tumor-initiating cells in OSs. *Oncogene*, 2012; 31:2270-82.

[46] Erguven M., Muramatsu T., Bilir A. (eds.). Midkine: From Embryogenesis to Pathogenesis and Therapy. Springer: Dordrecht,the Netherlands, 2012.

[47] Muramatsu T., Kadomatsu K. Midkine: an emerging target of drug development for treatment of multiple diseases. *Br. J. Pharmacol.,* 2014; 171:811-3.

[48] Maeda N., Ichihara-Tanaka K., Kimura T., et al. A receptor-like protein-tyrosine phosphatase PTPζ/RPTPβ binds a heparin-binding growth factor midkine. Involvement of arginine 78 of midkine in the high affinity binding to PTPζ. *J. Biol. Chem.*, 1999; 274: 12474–12479.

[49] Qi M., Ikematsu S., Maeda N., et al. Haptotactic migration induced by midkine. Involvement of protein-tyrosine phosphatase zeta. Mitogen-activated protein kinase, and phosphatidylinositol 3-kinase. *J. Biol. Chem.,* 2001; 276:15868-75.

[50] Sakaguchi N., Muramatsu H., Ichihara-Tanaka K., et al. Receptor-type protein tyrosine phosphatase zeta as a component of the signaling receptor complex for midkine-dependent survival of embryonic neurons. *Neurosci. Res.,* 2003; 45:219-24.

[51] Cohen S., Shoshana O. Y., Zelman-Toister E., et al. The cytokine midkine and its receptor RPTPζ regulate B cell survival in a pathway induced by CD74. *J. Immunol.*, 2012; 188:259-69.

[52] Liedert A., Mattausch L., Röntgen V., et al. Midkine-deficiency increases the anabolic response of cortical bone to mechanical loading. *Bone,* 2011; 48:945-51.

[53] Muramatsu H., Zou K., Sakaguchi N., et al. LDL receptor-related protein as a component of the midkine receptor. *Biochem. Biophys. Res. Commun.*, 2000; 270:936–941.

[54] Lee S. H., Suh H. N., Lee Y. J., et al. Midkine prevented hypoxic injury of mouse embryonic stem cells through activation of Akt and HIF-1α via low-density lipoprotein receptor-related protein-1. *J. Cell Physiol.,* 2012; 227:1731-9.

[55] Chen S., Bu G., Takei Y., et al. Midkine and LDL-receptor-related protein 1 contribute to the anchorage-independent cell growth of cancer cells. *J. Cell Sci.*, 2007;120:4009-15.

[56] Erguven M., Bilir A., Yazihan N., et al. Decreased therapeutic effects of noscapine combined with imatinib mesylate on human glioblastoma in vitro and the effect of midkine. *Cancer Cell Int.*, 2011; 11:18.

[57] Muramatsu H., Zou P., Suzuki H., et al. alpha4beta1- and alpha6beta1-integrins are functional receptors for midkine, a heparin-binding growth factor. *J. Cell Sci.*, 2004; 117:5405-15.

[58] Huang Y., Sook-Kim M., Ratovitski E. Midkine promotes tetraspanin-integrin interaction and induces FAK-Stat1α pathway contributing to migration/invasiveness of human head and neck squamous cell carcinoma cells. *Biochem. Biophys. Res. Commun.*, 2008; 377:474-478.

[59] Kadomatsu K., Kishida S., Tsubota S. The heparin-binding growth factor midkine: the biological activities and candidate receptors. *J. Biochem.*, 2013; 153: 511–521.

[60] Kuo A. H., Stoica G. E., Riegel A. T., et al. Recruitment of insulin receptor substrate-1 and activation of NF-kappaB essential for midkine growth signaling through anaplastic lymphoma kinase. *Oncogene,* 2007; 26:859-69.

[61] Kishida S., Mu P., Miyakawa S., et al. Midkine promotes neuroblastoma through Notch2 signaling. *Cancer Res.,* 2013; 73:1318-27.

[62] Güngör C., Zander H., Effenberger K. E., et al. Notch signaling activated by replication stress-induced expression of midkine drives epithelial-mesenchymal transition and chemoresistance in pancreatic cancer. *Cancer Res.,* 2011; 71:5009-19.

[63] Huang Y., Hoque M. O., Wu F., et al. Midkine induces epithelial-mesenchymal transition through Notch2/Jak2-Stat3 signaling in human keratinocytes. *Cell Cycle*, 2008; 7:1613-22.

[64] Muramatsu T. Midkine, a heparin-binding cytokine with multiple roles in development, repair and diseases. *Proc. Jpn. Acad. Ser. B. Phys. Biol. Sci.,* 2010; 86:410-25.

[65] Zou K., Muramatsu H., Ikematsu S., et al. A heparin-binding growth factor, midkine, binds to a chondroitin sulfate proteoglycan, PG-M/versican. *Eur. J. Biochem.*, 2000; 267:4046-53.

[66] Takeuchi H. Midkine and multiple sclerosis. *Br. J. Pharmacol.,* 2014; 171:931-5.

[67] Cernkovich E. R., Deng J., Hua K., et al. Midkine is an autocrine activator of signal transducer and activator of transcription 3 in 3T3-L1 cells. *Endocrinology,* 2007; 148:1598-604.

[68] Erguven M., Bilir A., Yazihan N., et al. Imatinib mesylate decreases the cytotoxic effect of roscovitine on human glioblastoma cells in vitro and the role of midkine. *Oncol. Lett.,* 2012; 3:200-208.

[69] Bilir A., Ergüven M.; Midkine Signaling in Glioblastoma: A Novel Developmental Drug Target?; In Management of CNS Tumors; Miklos Grami (ed.), 59-74. New York: Intech, 2011.

[70] Ergüven M.; Aquaporin, Midkine and Glioblastoma; In Evolution of the Molecular Biology of Brain Tumors and the Therapeutic Implications; Terry Lichtor (ed.), 355-376. New York: Intech, 2013.

[71] Maehara H., Kaname T., Yanagi K., et al. Midkine as a novel target for antibody therapy in OS. *Biochem. Biophys. Res. Commun.,* 2007; 358: 757-62.

[72] Kaname T., Kadomatsu K., Aridome K., et al. The expression of truncated MK in human tumors. *Biochem. Biophys. Res. Commun.,* 1996; 219: 256-60.

[73] Miyashiro I., Kaname T., Nakayama T., et al. Expression of truncated midkine in human colorectal cancers. *Cancer Lett.*, 1996; 106:287-91.

[74] Sueyoshi T., Jono H., Shinriki S., et al. Therapeutic approaches targeting midkine suppress tumor growth and lung metastasis in OS. *Cancer Lett.,* 2012; 316:23-30.

[75] Mirkin B. L., Clark S., Zheng X., et al. Identification of midkine as a mediator for intercellular transfer of drug resistance. *Oncogene,* 2005; 24:4965–4974.

[76] Takagi-Kimura M., Yamano T., Tagawa M., et al. Oncolytic virotherapy for osteosarcoma using midkine promoter-regulated adenoviruses. *Cancer Gene Ther.*, 2014; 21:126-32.

In: Osteosarcoma
Editors: Edwin Choy
ISBN: 978-1-63321-052-3

Chapter 5

INORGANIC PHOSPHATE AS A NOVEL SIGNALING MOLECULE: ITS POTENTIAL USE IN THE OSTEOSARCOMA THERAPY

Annamaria Spina, Luca Sorvillo, Francesca Di Maiolo, Luigi Sapio and Silvio Naviglio*
Department of Biochemistry, Biophysics and General Pathology, Second University of Naples, Medical School, Naples, Italy

ABSTRACT

There is a pressing need for the development of new and alternative approaches to the treatment of osteosarcoma. In this regard, naturally occurring molecules with antitumor activity and with the least toxicity to normal tissues are suggested as possible candidates to be investigated for their synergistic efficacy in combination with anticancer drugs.

Inorganic phosphate (Pi) is an essential nutrient to the living organisms. It is required as a component of energy metabolism, kinase/phosphatase signaling and in the formation and function of lipids, carbohydrates and nucleic acids and, at systemic level, it plays a key role for the normal skeletal and dentin mineralization. Pi represents an abundant dietary element and its intestinal absorption is efficient and minimally regulated. The kidney is a major regulator of the Pi

* Correspondence to: Silvio Naviglio, e-mail: silvio.naviglio@unina2.it.

homeostasis and can increase or decrease its Pi reabsorptive capacity to accommodate the Pi need.

Relevantly, Pi is emerging as an important signaling molecule capable of modulating multiple cellular functions by altering signal transduction pathways, gene expression and protein abundance in many cell types.

Recently, a series of articles directed at determining the consequences of elevated Pi on the behaviour of human osteosarcoma cells has been published. Overall, evidence has been accumulating that enhances the proposal of Pi as a signaling molecule and indicates that Pi may act as a potent antitumor agent in osteosarcoma cells.

The main results, the underlying molecular mechanisms, the potential clinical significance and therapeutic applications by these studies will be presented.

Osteosarcoma is the most common primary malignant tumor of bone, occurring most frequently in children and adolescents [1].

Surgery, radiotherapy and intensive chemotherapy are mainly effective in patients with localized disease and have improved overall survival over the last years [2].

However, clinically evident metastatic disease is present in 10-20% of patients at diagnosis. Despite aggressive treatment, more than one third of patients develop recurrent high-grade osteosarcomas, with metastatic disease typically affecting the lung, liver and bone itself, so that the 5-year survival rates are still not more than 60% [3]. The frequent acquisition of drug-resistant phenotypes and occurrence of second malignancies associated with chemotherapy remain serious problems. Moreover, toxic effects of the chemotherapy still remain a major drawback in the treatment of osteosarcoma patients [4].

In addition, since osteosarcomas have highly variable biological and genetic features and pursue different clinical courses, there is a concrete risk that osteosarcoma patients might be denied access to new "personalized treatments" due to difficulties to efficiently translate genetic and biological knowledge into clinical practice [5].

Thus, there is a pressing need for the development of new and alternative approaches to the treatment of osteosarcoma [6].

At this regard, dietary supplements, phytotherapeutic agents and naturally occurring molecules with antitumor activity and with the least toxicity to normal tissues are suggested as possible candidates to be investigated for their synergistic efficacy in combination with anticancer drugs [7].

Inorganic phosphate (Pi) is an essential nutrient to the living organisms. It is required as a component of energy metabolism, kinase/phosphatase signaling and in the formation and function of lipids, carbohydrates and nucleic acids and, at systemic level, it plays a key role for the normal skeletal and dentin mineralization [8].

Pi represents an abundant dietary element and its intestinal absorption is efficient and minimally regulated. The kidney is a major regulator of Pi homeostasis and can increase or decrease its Pi reabsorptive capacity to accommodate the Pi need.

The maintenance of proper Pi homeostasis is a critical event and the serum Pi level is maintained within a narrow range through an elaborate network of humoral interactions and feedback loops involving intestine, kidney, parathyroid gland, and bone and depends on the activity of a number of hormones, including parathyroid hormone, 1,25-dihydroxy vitamin D, and fibroblast growth factor 23 (FGF-23) as major regulators of the Pi homeostasis [9].

As a cell's interior is electronegative relative to the exterior, the movement of Pi into the cell does not occur by simple diffusion, but it is mediated by Na^+-coupled Pi cotransporters and is a regulated event [10].

Numerous recent data have strengthened a long-established hypothesis that a phosphate-sensing mechanism would detect changes in serum or local phosphate concentration and would inform the body, the local environment, or the individual cell [11, 12]. Relevantly, Pi is emerging as an important signaling molecule capable of modulating multiple cellular functions by altering signal transduction pathways, gene expression and protein abundance in many cell types [12-14].

In the last years, we have published a series of articles directed at determining the consequences of elevated Pi on the behaviour of human osteosarcoma cells, and on the underlying molecular mechanisms [15-18]. Throughout our studies, we have used a spectrum of final concentration of Pi [1-10 mM] to cover the physiologic range in humans and in agreement with most of the published studies on the Pi-triggered effects.

Overall, our data enrich the proposal of Pi as a signaling molecule and indicate that Pi may act as a potent antitumor agent in osteosarcoma cells. Here, our main findings are highlighted and summarized.

First, we found that the Pi treatment of human osteosarcoma U2OS cells resulted in the cell growth inhibition by slowing-down the cell division cycle, accompanied by a decrease of both intracellular cAMP levels and adenylate cyclase activity [15]. These effects were blunted by the inhibitor of Na-Pi transporters, phosphonoformic acid (PFA). In addition, cAMP elevating agents, such as forskolin, prevented the cell growth inhibition in response to Pi.

The human osteosarcoma U2OS cells grow as adherent cells and are easily detached from monolayers by brief exposure to the trypsin. However, when we started to perform experiments aimed to studying the effects of elevated Pi on the behaviour of osteosarcoma cells, we immediately noted that the U2OS cells became extremely hard to dislodge with the trypsin when cultured in presence of Pi supplementation, whereas other cells, including the human osteosarcoma Saos cells, did not.

Later on, we investigated such phenomenon and demonstrated that the U2OS cells became resistant to the trypsin action in response to the Pi treatment in a dose and time dependent manner [16]. The Pi-induced increase of the adherence capabilities of the U2OS cells was accompanied by an inhibition of the pro-proliferative and pro-metastatic ERK1/2 signaling pathway and a down-regulation of the pro-metastatic beta3 integrin subunit expression, and also by an upregulation of the Rap1 function [16].

To note, the ERK1/2 inhibition in response to Pi was preceded by a rapid and transient increase of ERK1/2 phosphorylation followed by a prolonged inhibition, in agreement with a biphasic effect of Pi on the ERK1/2 signaling pathway, reported previously [19].

Importantly, most of the effects elicited by Pi in U2OS cells (that contain wild p53) could not be seen in p53 null Saos cells, suggesting that Pi can produce discrete effects depending on the cell type and genetic background.

More recently, we have described that in wild p53 containing osteosarcoma U2OS cells, and not in p53 null Saos and p53 mutant MG63 osteosarcoma cells, Pi is capable of inducing sensitization to doxorubicin [17]. We provided evidence that the enhancement of doxorubicin-induced cytotoxicity by Pi occurs via p53-dependent apoptosis and through a mechanism involving ERK1/2 down-regulation [17].

Importantly, so far we are accumulating evidence that the ERK1/2 inhibition in response to Pi is accompanied by a consistent down-regulation of protein levels of the upstream B-Raf and Raf-1 kinases and these events are actually under our investigation to further explore and explain how Pi affects the ERK1/2 function to inhibit the cell viability and to enhance the doxorubicin-induced cytotoxicity in U2OS osteosarcoma cells.

Finally, we have analyzed the possible antitumor effects of combined treatments with Pi and other commonly used chemotherapeutic agents in osteosarcoma cells [18].

Interestingly, we found that Pi augmented the cytotoxic effect and showed a synergistic induction of apoptosis in osteosarcoma U2OS cells when combined with either doxorubicin or taxol "G2/M blocking" agents, whereas no additive antiproliferative effects could be seen in combined treatments with Pi and "G1/S blocking" 5-FU agent [18].

Notably, the fact that Pi enhances the antiproliferative effects of doxorubicin and taxol in U2OS cells, but not those of 5-fluorouracil suggests that Pi does not act in a widespread way, but can have discrete effects on the cell proliferation depending very likely on the cell cycle phase(s) in which they occur.

The molecular mechanisms underlying the Pi-mediated chemosensitivity of osteosarcoma cells to anticancer drugs are just starting to be understood. Similarly to doxorubicin case [14], a possible role of p53 and/or ERK1/2 in the enhancement of taxol-induced cytotoxicity by Pi in U2OS is actually under our investigation.

Importantly, in our studies Pi was found to have a positive pharmacological interaction even with a low dose (0.1 μM) doxorubicin and of taxol (0.05 μM) that are expected to be more tolerable and associated to minimal undesired side-effects in patients, thus increasing the potential clinical relevance of our data.

New drug delivery systems have been developed that incorporate anticancer drugs into phosphate containing nanoparticles to maintain high concentrations of anticancer drugs at bone local site [20, 21]. Very interestingly, the release of inorganic phosphate by phosphate containing nanoparticles and its retention in bone microenvironment is predicted to occur, thus affecting locally the Pi concentrations.

In addition, keeping in mind that phosphate is the most abundant anion in the cell with a high intracellular concentration (of about 100 mmol/L), it is easy to imagine that an increase of extracellular Pi can be found in the tumor microenvironment upon its release from death cells during the chemotherapy.

Relevantly, the combination chemotherapy is receiving particular attention in order to find compounds that could increase the therapeutic index of antineoplastic drugs while limiting their potential toxicity.

Notably, the burden of the cancer is growing and becoming a major financial issue. The number of cancer patients and the cost of their treatment are constantly increasing. Thus, the charge of anticancer therapies in the developed world is spiraling and its economic impact is increasingly becoming more relevant for National Health Services [22].

Efficacious and cheaper anticancer strategies compatible with a public National Health System are strongly warranted.

Our findings that the inorganic phosphate, very simple "naturally occurring molecule", can have antitumor effects on osteosarcoma cells and can achieve additive cytotoxic effects when combined with relevant chemotherapeutic agents illustrates its potential for clinical applications [23].

In this context, further positive results from in vivo studies could indicate that controlling the Pi levels at local sites might contribute to the development of novel and cheap modalities for therapeutic intervention in osteosarcoma.

REFERENCES

[1] Chou AJ, Geller DS and Gorlick R: Therapy for osteosarcoma: where do we go from here? *Paediatr. Drugs* 10, 315-327 (2008).

[2] Dai X, Ma W, He X and Jha RK: Review of therapeutic strategies for osteosarcoma, chondrosarcoma, and Ewing's sarcoma. *Med. Sci. Monit.*17, 177-190 (2011).

[3] Kim SY and Helman LJ: Strategies to explore new approaches in the investigation and treatment of osteosarcoma. *Cancer Treat. Res.*152, 517-528 (2009).

[4] Hattinger CM, Pasello M, Ferrari S, Picci P and Serra M: Emerging drugs for high-grade osteosarcoma. *Expert Opin. Emerg. Drugs.*15, 615-634 (2010).

[5] Gutierrez ME, Kummar S and Giaccone G: Next generation oncology drug development: opportunities and challenges. *Nat. Rev. Clin. Oncol.* 6, 259-265 (2009).

[6] Yang J, Zhang W. New molecular insights into osteosarcoma targeted therapy. *Curr. Opin. Oncol.* 25, 398-406 (2013).

[7] Naviglio S, Della Ragione F. Naturally occurring molecules and anticancer combination therapies in the era of personalized medicine and economic crisis. *Curr. Pharm. Des.* 19, 5325-6 (2013).

[8] Takeda E, Taketani Y, Sawada N, Sato T, Yamamoto H: The regulation and function of phosphate in the human body. *Biofactors* 21, 345-55 (2004).

[9] Bergwitz C, Jüppner H: Regulation of phosphate homeostasis by PTH, vitamin D, and FGF23. *Annu. Rev. Med.* 61, 91-104 (2010).

[10] Tenenhouse HS: Phosphate transport: Molecular basis, regulation, and pathophysiology. *J. Steroid Biochem. Mol. Biol.* 103, 572–577 (2007).

[11] Bergwitz C, Jüppner H: Phosphate sensing. *Adv. Chronic Kidney Dis.* 18, 132-44 (2011).
[12] Sabbagh Y: Phosphate as a sensor and signaling molecule. *Clin. Nephrol.* 79, 57-65 (2013).
[13] Khoshniat S, Bourgine A, Julien M, Weiss P, Guicheux J, Beck L: The emergence of phosphate as a specific signaling molecule in bone and other cell types in mammals. *Cell Mol. Life Sci.* 68, 205-18 (2011).
[14] Anderson JJ. Potential health concerns of dietary phosphorus: cancer, obesity, and hypertension. *Ann. N. Y. Acad. Sci.* Oct;1301:1-8 (2013).
[15] Naviglio S, Spina A, Chiosi E, Fusco A, Illiano F, Pagano M, Romano M, Senatore G, Sorrentino A, Sorvillo L, Illiano G: Inorganic phosphate inhibits growth of human osteosarcoma U2OS cells via adenylate cyclase/cAMP pathway. *J. Cell Biochem.* 98, 1584-96 (2006).
[16] Naviglio S, Di Gesto D, Borrelli V, Forni M, Illiano F, D'Auria R, Sorrentino A, Chiosi E, Illiano G, Spina A: Novel molecular mechanisms by inorganic phosphate in osteosarcoma U2OS cells. *Frontiers in Bioscience.* E3,1249-1258 (2011).
[17] Spina A, Sorvillo L, Di Maiolo F, Esposito A, D'Auria R, Di Gesto D, Chiosi E, Naviglio S: Inorganic phosphate enhances sensitivity of human osteosarcoma U2OS cells to doxorubicin via a p53-dependent pathway. *J. Cell Physiol.* 228,198-206 (2013).
[18] Spina A, Sorvillo L, Chiosi E, Esposito A, Di Maiolo F, Sapio L, Caraglia M and Naviglio S: Synergistic cytotoxic effects of inorganic phosphate and chemotherapeutic drugs on human osteosarcoma cells. *Oncol. Rep.* 29, 1689-96 (2013).
[19] Beck Jr GR, Knecht N: Osteopontin regulation by inorganic phosphate is ERK1/2-, protein kinase C-, and proteasome-dependent. *J. Biol. Chem.* 278, 41921–9 (2003).
[20] Qing F, Wang Z, Hong Y, Liu M, Guo B, Luo H, Zhang X. Selective effects of hydroxyapatite nanoparticles on osteosarcoma cells and osteoblasts. *J. Mater. Sci. Mater. Med.* 23, 2245-51 (2012).
[21] Min KH, Lee HJ, Kim K, Kwon IC, Jeong SY, Lee SC: The tumor accumulation and therapeutic efficacy of doxorubicin carried in calcium phosphate-reinforced polymer nanoparticles. *Biomaterials.* 33, 5788-97 (2012).
[22] Sullivan R, Peppercorn J, Sikora K, et al: Delivering affordable cancer care in high-income countries. *Lancet Oncol.*12, 933-80 (2011).

[23] Spina A, Sorvillo L, Esposito A, Borgia A, Sapio L, Naviglio S. Inorganic phosphate as a signaling molecule: a potential strategy in osteosarcoma treatment. *Curr. Pharm. Des.*19, 5394-403 (2013).

In: Osteosarcoma
Editors: Edwin Choy
ISBN: 978-1-63321-052-3

Chapter 6

MICRORNAS IN THE PATHOBIOLOGY OF OSTEOSARCOMA

***Jyotika Varshney*[1] *and Subbaya Subramanian*[1,2,*]**
[1]Department of Surgery, Division of Basic and Translational Research, University of Minnesota, Minneapolis, MN, US
[2]Masonic Cancer Center, University of Minnesota, Minneapolis, MN, US

ABSTRACT

Osteosarcoma is the most common primary bone malignancy affecting children, adolescents and young adults. Around 30% of patients with localized osteosarcoma and 70% of patients with metastasis will experience treatment failure within 5 years of diagnosis. Such a dismal outcome has remained static for the past 20 years leading to an urgent need to identify novel targets and therapeutic agents that will improve patients overall survival and minimize immediate and long-term side effects of current chemotherapeutic agents. Additionally, osteosarcoma is commonly found in canines, with approximately 10,000 new cases each year in the US. The complex biology of osteosarcoma and tumor heterogeneity makes it very difficult to identify effective actionable targets and therapeutic agents. This chapter will highlight the recent developments in our basic understanding of microRNA mediated gene regulations in osteosarcoma and discuss the potential for development of

[*] E-mail: subree@umn.edu; Tel: 612-626-4330; Fax: 612-626-7031.

microRNA-based prognostic biomarkers. Further, this chapter will analyze the recent development of preclinical evaluation of a novel agent Minnelide in the treatment of osteosarcoma and emphasize the prospects for combinatorial drug treatment in osteosarcoma.

INTRODUCTION: OSTEOSARCOMA, MICRORNAS, AND IMPROVING TREATMENT

Osteosarcoma is an aggressive malignant cancer that arises from primitive cells that are mesenchymal in origin [1]. Osteosarcoma is the eighth most commonly occurring pediatric cancer and is responsible for 20% of all bone cancers. Osteosarcoma is the most commonly occurring primary bone sarcoma that affects children and adolescents [1]. Rarely is it manifested in adults, making it have a bimodal onset. The incidence rates are estimated to be 5 cases per million per year in the United States (900 newly diagnosed cases per year). It is more commonly found in men (5.4 per million per year) than in women (4 per million per year) [2].

Osteosarcoma usually occurs in the metaphyseal region of long bones, with higher predilection to femur (42%) than tibia (19%) and humerus (10%). The remaining cases generally occur in the skull, jaw, and pelvis area [3].

Histologically, the characteristic feature of osteosarcoma is the presence of osteoid deposits within the tumor. The tumor cells appear to be very pleomorphic and may exhibit multinucleated, osteoclast-like giant cells [4].

Due to the chaotic karyotype and heterogeneous nature of osteosarcoma, understanding the molecular mechanisms of this cancer has been difficult [5]. Osteosarcoma is considered to be a differentiation disease that is caused by genetic changes that can disrupt osteoblast differentiation. Some of the osteosarcoma cases have familial disposition, where usually deletion of the 13q14 region is observed and leads to inactivation of the retinoblastoma gene [6]. Li-Fraumeni syndrome is another predisposing factor that contains germline *TP53* mutation that leads to osteosarcoma development [7]. Despite recent advances in surgery and combinatorial therapies, as discussed in more detail below, the survival rates remain unchanged. This disheartening outlook calls for an urgent need for a better and more clear understanding of the molecular mechanism of osteosarcoma in order to change the outcome of the disease in patients.

In recent years, it has been discovered that regulatory RNAs such as microRNAs (miRNAs) play a major role in osteosarcoma development and progression [8]. Given the need for better and clearer understanding of the molecular mechanism of osteosarcoma, it is essential to explore the role of regulatory RNAs such as miRNAs in osteosarcoma pathobiology. miRNAs are small, non-coding, regulatory RNAs that are 18-22 nucleotides in length. They are a component of the RNA interfering system and can either repress translation and/or cleave mRNA by base pairing to the 3′ untranslated region (3'UTR) of the target genes [9]. It is now estimated that more than 1400 miRNAs persist in the human genome. The function of miRNAs spans from regulation of critical biological processes in normal cells to proliferation in tumor cells. Moreover, these small non-coding miRNAs regulate more than 50% of the protein coding transcripts [10].

There is evidence that supports the contention that miRNAs are differentially regulated in normal and tumor cells, and it has been revealed that miRNAs can play a crucial role in the pathogenesis of cancer development and progression [11-13]. Additionally, miRNAs are highly conserved among various species, which suggests a potential role that miRNAs can play in diagnosis and prognosis of cancer, including osteosarcoma. For instance, in comparison with human osteosarcoma, dogs can more commonly acquire osteosarcoma, with said incidence being more than 10,000 cases per year with exquisite breed predilection [14]. The shorter life span, similar functioning and incidence of osteosarcoma, and extensive homology in genetic sequence and gene order between humans and dogs, make dogs a great model to study and to help researchers further understand the molecular mechanism in human osteosarcoma [15]. Recent findings involving canine osteosarcoma will be discussed below as well.

This chapter will analyze and explore the following topics:

1. *Role of miRNAs in osteosarcoma:* As touched on above, the chapter will survey various studies already conducted, as well as the authors' own studies of miRNAs in the context of osteosarcoma and other cancers.
2. *The perturbation of 14q32 miRNA/cMYC/miR-17-92 network:* This deregulated miRNA circuitry network is potentially a unifying molecular mechanism that could hold a better prognostic significance for osteosarcoma patients, which will be described in detail. We will also survey various prognostic markers in osteosarcoma, addressing the deficiencies and other gaps in these already-existing approaches.
3. *Current osteosarcoma therapies:* This chapter will survey current osteosarcoma therapies and other methods and discuss the benefits

and perhaps, at this point in the understanding of osteosarcoma, the necessity of a combinatorial approach to treating osteosarcoma patients.

4. *Minnelide and osteosarcoma:* Lastly, we will discuss the recent preclinical findings of a novel agent Minnelide, a pro-drug of Triptolide, and its potential in treating osteosarcoma patients.

In summary this chapter will attempt to provide a clearer understanding of the current science surrounding the topics of osteosarcoma prognosis and diagnosis, the molecular mechanism at play in osteosarcoma, the role miRNAs play in relation to these topics, and of the path to developing better approaches to treating osteosarcoma, and for further researching osteosarcoma as well as other forms of cancer.

ROLE OF MIRNAS IN OSTEOSARCOMA

The expression pattern of miRNAs can be clearly assessed by miRNA microarray approaches. Many studies have shown that there is a presence of differential expression patterns in various cancers, including osteosarcoma [16-19]. Sarver et al. have generated miRNA expression profiles for over 300 sarcoma tissue samples that represent 22 different sarcoma subtypes (including osteosarcoma), and have developed a Sarcoma MircoRNA Expression Database (S-MED) [14, 20]. Interestingly, out of all the sarcomas analyzed, osteosarcoma stood out as a single cluster distinct from various other sarcomas.

There are various other studies that have investigated the role of miRNAs in osteosarcoma using miRNA expression profiles [10, 18, 21-23]. It started when Maire et al. found differential miRNA expression profiles in 7 osteosarcoma samples that could target specific pathways compared to the normal bone [24]. Recently, Lulla et al. and Stabley et al. showed that there are more than 22 differentially expressed miRNAs as compared to osteoblasts [25, 26]. The miRNAs that are highly expressed include miR-135b, -150, -370, -542-5p, -652, and -654. For instance, miR-206 and -286 play an important role in osteoblast differentiation. Some of these miRNAs, such as miR-370, can target the Insulin receptor substrate-1 (IRS1) gene that interacts with Insulin-like growth factor 1 (IGF1R) gene, which is commonly overexpressed in osteosarcoma, suggesting miRNAs can directly influence key signaling pathways and differentiation of osteoblasts, resulting in osteosarcoma.

miRNAs can also target various tumor suppressor genes and affect their expression. For example, *TP53*, a common tumor suppressor that is expressed during DNA damage that leads to cell cycle arrest or apoptosis by dissociation from MDM2 is found mutated in more than 20% of osteosarcoma cases [7]. Among the several miRNAs that can target *TP53*, the highly conserved miR-34 family (miR-34a, -34b, and -34c) is one of the important components that induce G1 arrest and apoptosis via *CDK6*, *E2F3*, *Cyclin E2*, and *BCL2* in a TP53 dependent manner in osteosarcoma cells [27, 28]. According to various studies, miR-34 is significantly downregulated due to genetic and epigenetic alterations in primary osteosarcoma samples [29, 30].

Recently, our group identified that there is a significant downregulation of more than 40 miRNAs located in the 14q32 locus in various human osteosarcoma samples [16] and the miRNAs in this locus were conserved in canine and mice as well. Additionally, our group and various other studies found overexpression of clusters of miR-17-92 and its paralog miR-106b clusters that are located within introns of c13orf25 and *MCM7* respectively, suggesting an oncogenic role in osteosarcoma. Interestingly, transcription factors such as *E2F1, E2F2, E2F3* (components of the TGF-B pathway) and c*MYC* can activate both these miRNA clusters, and these transcription factors are amplified in the osteosarcoma as well [31-33].

A strong inverse correlation has also been identified between *PTEN*, and other tumor suppressor genes, and several members of the miR-17, -19, -130/301, and -26 families in osteosarcoma, when compared to normal bone [34]. This information is crucial because PTEN antagonizes signaling through the PI3K/ PTEN/ Akt pathway that promotes cell proliferation and inhibition of apoptosis.

Together, the above observations suggest that miRNAs play a crucial role in osteosarcoma progression, and they can behave either as a tumor suppressor or oncogene that can affect various target genes and contribute to development of osteosarcoma cancer.

THE PERTURBATION OF 14Q32 MIR-CMYC-MIR-17-92 NETWORK IN OSTEOSARCOMA

Osteosarcoma is characterized by various genetic and chromosomal aberrations. For instance, many tumors show DNA copy number amplification of *CD5L* and *RUNX2* at the 6p12 region and *cMYC* amplification at the 8q24 region, which are responsible for osteoblast differentiation [35-37]. Other common gene aberrations include mutations in *RB, TP53, BMPs,* and *MMPs* [38, 39]. But even with this information, little is known about the pathobiology of the disease itself.

The authors' group wanted to investigate the role of miRNAs in osteosarcoma and then identify any unifying mechanism that could hold a better prognostic and diagnostic significance. Their studies started with assessing *cMYC* expression in various osteosarcoma samples, and they made some unique and potentially significant findings and conclusions.

cMYC, a proto-oncogene, is amplified in about 30% of osteosarcoma patients, however the majority of osteosarcoma cases is characterized by overexpression of cMYC. The authors reasoned that *cMYC* expression was regulated by certain miRNAs. They identified a unique miRNA network involving 14q32 miRNAs, *cMYC*, and the miR-17-92 cluster. This network is novel in the sense that it has not been identified and/or analyzed before. The group performed a comprehensive expression profile of miRNAs on over 20 osteosarcoma tissues, and they observed that around 40 miRNAs in the 14q32 region were significantly downregulated (5 to 6 fold). In contrast to the 14q32 miRNAs cluster, the miR-17-92 cluster—especially miR-19a and -19b at the 13q32 region—showed significantly higher expression when compared with normal bone tissue samples. They validated such similar miRNA differential expressions in various osteosarcoma cell lines such as Saos-2, U2OS, and HOS, as compared to osteoblasts. Also, the team noticed that expression of 14q32 miRNAs were higher in differentiated osteoblasts (up to 4-fold) than the osteosarcoma cell lines (Figure 1).

To understand the function of the upregulated miR-17-92 cluster, the team performed a series of knockdown experiments. They found that blocking miR-18a and -20b with antimiRs in the cluster caused apoptosis, as compared to controls.

Similar results were observed when they blocked *cMYC* expression in osteosarcoma cell lines. These results suggest that osteosarcoma is oncogenically addicted to *cMYC* and that miR-17-92 expressions are essential for osteosarcoma cell proliferation. Also, restoration of the expression of 14q32 miRNAs (*miR-544, -369-3p, -134, and -382),* or a reduction of the miR-17–92 cluster by ectopic means resulted in induction of apoptosis in osteosarcoma cell lines.

The foregoing observations suggest a potential tumor suppressor role of 14q32 miRNAs and the regulation of *cMYC* and the miR-17-92 cluster with these 14q32 miRNAs.

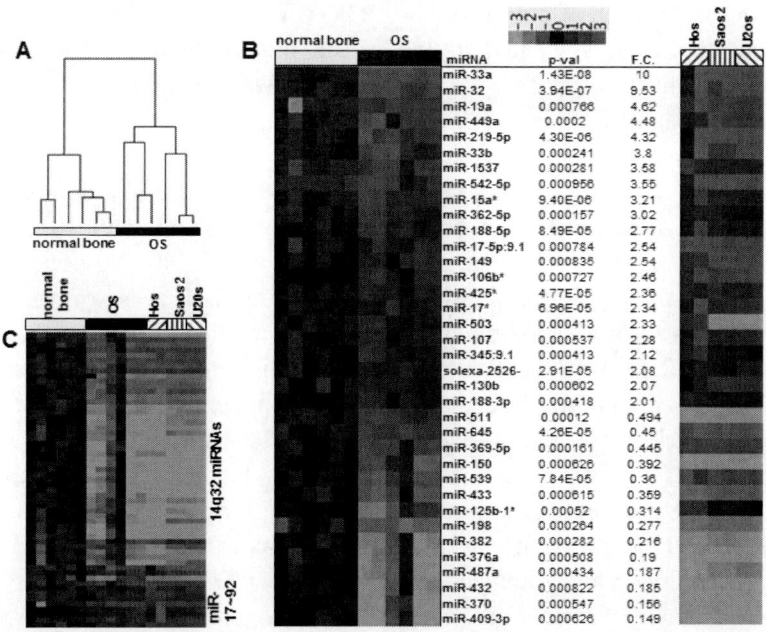

Figure 1. miRNA expression patterns in osteosarcoma. (A) Unsupervised hierarchical clustering of miRNA expression in osteosarcoma relative to normal bone tissues. (B) Differentially expressed miRNAs between normal bone tissue and osteosarcoma. The miRNA expression data for the OS cell lines Hos, Saos-2 and U2os relative to the expression in human osteoblasts is shown in the far right panel.

To validate the interaction between the 14q32 miRNAs (miR-544, -369-3p, -134, and -382) and *cMYC*, the team performed luciferase reporter assays with *cMYC* 3'UTR reporter construct, and they observed that the 14q32 miRNAs acted synergistically and suppressed reporter transcripts having the *cMYC* 3'UTR, and also that overexpression of the 14q32 miRNAs decreased cMYC protein expression.

Various studies have shown that *cMYC* transactivates the miR-17-92 cluster miRNAs that are an important component of many cancers including colon cancer, hepatoma, and leukemia. Investigating the *cMYC-miR-17-92* cluster in human osteosarcoma tissues further, the authors' group found that overexpression of the 14q32 miRNAs in osteosarcoma cells decreased transcript levels of miR-17-92 miRNAs leading to apoptosis. Further they showed that the pro-apoptotic effects of the 14q32 miRNAs are attenuated by exogenous expression of miR-17-92 or *cMYC* without the 3'UTR.

Next, the authors wanted to investigate the mechanism of significant downregulation of these 14q32 miRNAs. The comparative genomic hybridization analyses showed no DNA copy number change at the 14q32 region, which led to speculation of imprinting changes of this region in osteosarcoma. Previous studies in mice have shown that the homologous region of the *14q32* miRNA cluster is maternally expressed and related to the surrounding imprinted genes such as *Dlk1, Gtl2,* and *Rtl1* [40].

The *DLK-MEG3* region seems to be important, as it is also involved in Prader-Willi/Angelman syndromes (pUPD12 and pUPD14) [40]. In humans, three differentially methylated regions presumably control the corresponding DLK1-GTL2 region. *MEG3*, one of the components in this region, is maternally expressed, which is located upstream to the 14q32 miRNA clusters. *MEG3* was also expressed at significantly lower levels in osteosarcoma as compared to normal bone, suggesting a shared transcriptional mechanism that may regulate the expression of genes and miRNAs at the 14q32 locus. Also, *MEG3* can activate and stabilize tumor suppressor *TP53*, so it is likely that reduced *MEG3* expression may reduce the endogenous levels of *TP53* in osteosarcoma [41]. Based on this knowledge the authors' group investigated the possibility that downregulation of the 14q32 miRNAs was epigenetically controlled through DNA methylation and histone acetylation. They analyzed DNA methylation at the CpG regions of selected upstream 14q32 miRNAs (miR-127, -411, -431, and -432) using combined bisulfite restriction analyses (COBRA). The results suggested that there was no change in methylation patterns or relative hypomethylation patterns in osteosarcoma tumor samples as compared to normal bone. This suggests that DNA methylation may not be the primary reason of significant downregulation of these 14q32 miRNAs.

Next, the authors' assessed the histone acetylation in osteosarcoma cells (Saos-2) via ChIP assays. The ChIP arrays interpretation demonstrated significant deacetylation in histone (H3) proteins in samples that included human osteosarcoma cell lines as well as tissues.

Together, above experiments revealed a mechanistic role of 14q32 miRNAs and their tumor suppressor role in osteosarcoma, and how their loss may induce transformation of osteoblasts to osteosarcoma cells. These results suggest that downregulation of 14q32 miRNAs are necessary for apoptotic escape and thus for sustaining tumorigenesis in osteosarcoma. Additionally, DNA copy number analysis of osteosarcoma patient genomes showed that decreased expression of the 14q32 miRNAs in osteosarcoma is not due to the loss or deletion of the loci thereof, and hence may involve transcriptional and or epigenetic regulation. Further characterizations of these networks show decrease in histone acetylation. Also, the group identified a unifying mechanism that can potentially explain the regulation of *cMYC* in osteosarcoma. Therefore, the 14q32 miRNAs may not only be prognostically significant, but may also provide suitable targets for the development of more effective treatments of osteosarcoma.

PROGNOSTIC MARKERS IN OSTEOSARCOMA

There are various factors that can contribute to the prognosis of osteosarcoma [42]. Some of the factors include anatomical site, tumor size, age, stage, and histology, among others. Each of these factors and how it correlates with prognosis of osteosarcoma is discussed below.

It has been established that total surgical resection with negative margins is essential for achieving cure of non-metastatic osteosarcoma [43-45]. This gets quite challenging to achieve with axial osteosarcoma involving the spine, ribs, and pelvis due to anatomical constraints. Hence, axial tumors present with a worse prognosis (survival rate of 20-40%) than osteosarcoma of the extremity (survival rate of 60-70%), even if they are of comparable grade and stage [46, 47].

Another important factor that governs better prognosis of osteosarcoma is smaller tumor size, measured in terms of the gross tumor length, volume, or surface area. Studies have demonstrated that a tumor size of more than 10 centimeters has been consistently associated with poor outcome [48, 49]. However, due to variability in measuring tumor size, a single minimum cutoff value beyond which tumor size becomes significant is difficult to determine. In addition, it also becomes difficult to compare studies on tumor size because of use of different imaging modalities such as conventional radiography, CT scan, and MRI.

Age as a prognostic factor in osteosarcoma has been a very ambiguous subject to study. Two large retrospective studies showed that patients younger than 14 years and older than 40 years had inferior outcomes. In contrast to these studies, age was not a prognostic marker in the recently reported retrospective analysis on 2680 patients in ten centers worldwide [50-53]. This suggests that with better supportive care, age will no longer be an important prognostic factor.

The clinical stage in osteosarcoma is one of the strongest predictors of survival rate of osteosarcoma patients. There are two widely accepted staging systems in osteosarcoma: [1] the Musculoskeletal Tumor Society Staging System developed by Enneking et al. [54] and the American Joint Committee on Cancer (AJCC) staging system [55-60]. Various studies have shown that patients with metastatic disease have a worse outcome in comparison with patients with localized disease. Also, patients with pulmonary metastasis have a better outcome than patients with non-pulmonary metastasis. Patients with skip metastases (discontinuous lesions occurring in the same bone as the primary lesion) are associated with poor prognosis for as yet unknown reasons [61, 62]. It is worth noting that patients with stage 3 osteosarcoma (no metastasis, as per the AJCC classification), have an outcome similar to patients with stage 4 osteosarcoma (pulmonary metastasis).

Historically, it has been shown that chondroblastic osteosarcoma has a poor response to chemotherapy in comparison with other subtypes, and thus is associated with a poor outcome [63].

Patients who are eligible for limb salvage surgery have a higher risk of local recurrence but have osteosarcoma comparable with patients who undergo amputation [64, 65]. Patients who undergo amputation have large tumors and/or involvement of major neurovascular structures. These patients have inferior outcomes when compared with patients who underwent limb salvage surgery, due to the tumor size, aggressiveness, and difficulty in obtaining a negative margin, rather than due to the choice of amputation as a procedure. Therefore, limb salvage surgery is currently the preferred surgical procedure.

Elevated pre-therapy serum lactate dehydrogenase (LDH) levels were associated with decreased 5-year disease-free survival (DFS), when compared with patients with normal LDH (39.5% vs. 60%, respectively) [66-68].

Serum alkaline phosphate (SAP) levels are found elevated in increased osteoblastic activity as seen with fractures, physiological growth and osteosarcoma [69, 70]. Bacci et al. observed in extremity osteosarcoma that elevated SAP was found in 258 out of 560 patients and significantly correlated with poor DFS and osteosarcoma ($p = 0.002$) [71].

Another strong predictor to survival is response to chemotherapy. A tumor necrosis of more than 90% has been proposed as a cutoff for accepting a good response to chemotherapy and a better survival outcome [62, 72-74]. Approximately 20% of osteosarcoma patients in the West are presented with macrometastatic disease. Out of the remaining 80% of the osteosarcoma patient population, only 20% would be expected to survive if they are treated with surgery alone, suggesting that a significant number of non-metastatic patients have micrometastatic disease

High-dose methotrexate (HDMTX) can also be an important component of various regimens used for treating osteosarcoma [75-78]. The use of chemotherapy regimens that lack anthracyclines (doxorubicin) or platinum (cisplatinum) has been shown to be associated with inferior outcomes, confirming the important role played by these two agents in achieving a cure for osteosarcoma.

Tumor angiogenesis can play a major role in reflecting guarded prognosis [79]. Using antibodies against endothelial antigens such as CD31, CD34, factor 8, and VEGF can measure tumor angiogenesis. For instance, a study by Kaya et al. analyzed the serum VEGF level in patients with osteosarcoma and observed that a serum VEGF level more than 1000 pg/l was associated with worse osteosarcoma [80]. Also, a higher incidence of pulmonary metastasis has been shown to correlate with increased angiogenesis in osteosarcoma. However, there is no evidence that shows a correlation between angiogenesis and outcome in osteosarcoma. Additionally, Bajpai et al. observed that the degree of tumor angiogenesis in osteosarcoma correlated with the tumor grade and histological necrosis, which suggests that angiogenesis can be used as a surrogate marker for predicting tumor aggressiveness and response to chemotherapy [81].

14q32 miRNAs Are Potential Prognostic Markers

In addition to the above-mentioned factors for determining prognosis in osteosarcoma cases, miRNAs can also play a crucial role in determining the outcome of the disease.

Authors' group compared miRNA expression data in human tissues with an additional 16 human osteosarcoma tissue samples and a detailed clinical follow up with 37 canine osteosarcoma samples. As mentioned earlier, they observed a significant downregulation of 14q32 miRNAs compared to the other sarcoma types presented in the S-MED.

Additionally, they verified that these 14q32 miRNAs were highly correlated with each other using a correlation-based network analysis that was based on the miRNA expression levels as determined by microarray analyses. The high correlation of these 14q32 miRNAs suggests that an individual miRNA from this locus could represent the expression levels of most of the

14q32 miRNAs. On profiling the mRNA transcript levels of tumor samples that had miRNA profiles, they found expression changes in around 385 genes due to expression changes of miR-382. These gene expression level changes correlated with the poor survival rate of human patients.

This means that decrease in miR-382 expression led to increased expression of genes responsible for metastasis and lower survival rate of osteosarcoma patients (Figure 2). Similar results were observed in the orthologous miRNA 14q32 locus, CFA 8 in canine that was identified using the Entrez gene database. After mapping the miR-382 expression in 16 canine osteosarcoma samples, Sarver et al. observed that canine tumors with lower miR-382 levels correlated with increase gene expression of gene related to metastasis and shorter survival rates (Figure 3).

These results suggest that 14q32 miRNAs are conserved and have a potential prognostic significance in both human as well as canine osteosarcoma.

Current Osteosarcoma Drugs and Treatments

According to Dr. Fuchs, 10% of osteosarcoma patients require limb amputation, and currently the use of limb salvage is performed as a surgical alternative to amputation [82]. Limb salvage aims to extract cancerous cells while keeping the limb function intact [83].

However, the challenge of decreasing the recurrence of osteosarcoma remains unaltered. Osteosarcoma recurrence rates have been static since the 1970s, ranging between 10% and 20% [84]. The big question that yet remains to be answered is why it is still challenging to combat the cancer. Perhaps one of the reasons is that the osteosarcoma tumor is extremely heterogeneous, which makes testing new drugs extremely difficult.

Such deficiency in osteosarcoma therapies urgently calls for a better and clearer understanding of the molecular mechanism and progression of osteosarcoma tumors. This will necessarily involve understanding the crosstalk between different types of cells within the bone microenvironment and the interaction between tumor cells and stromal cells, endothelial cells, and macrophages [85].

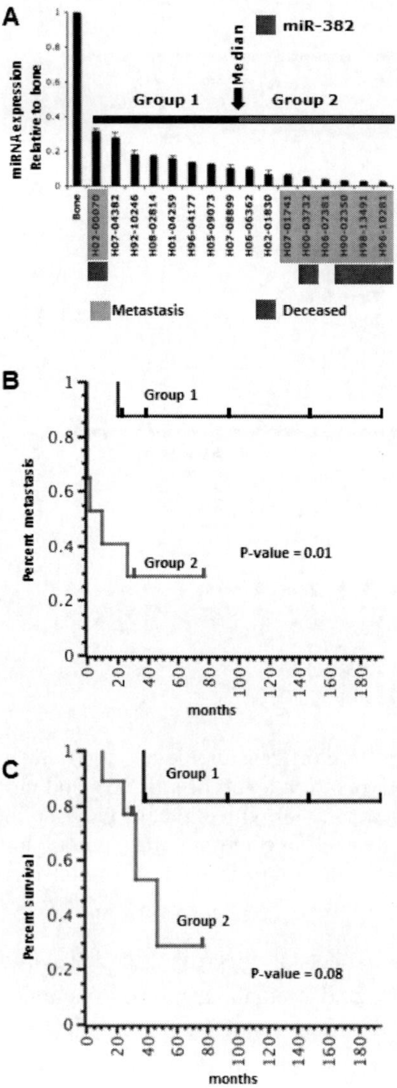

Figure adapted from Sarver et al., 2013.

Figure 2. 14q32 miRNA expression level, metastasis and outcome in human osteosarcoma. (A) miR-382 expression levels in osteosarcoma primary tumor samples with clinical follow-up information. (B and C) Kaplan-Meier analysis of metastasis in osteosarcoma patients based on miR-382 expression. Patients with lowest levels of miR-382 expression showed increased likelihood of metastasis and decreased likelihood of survival.

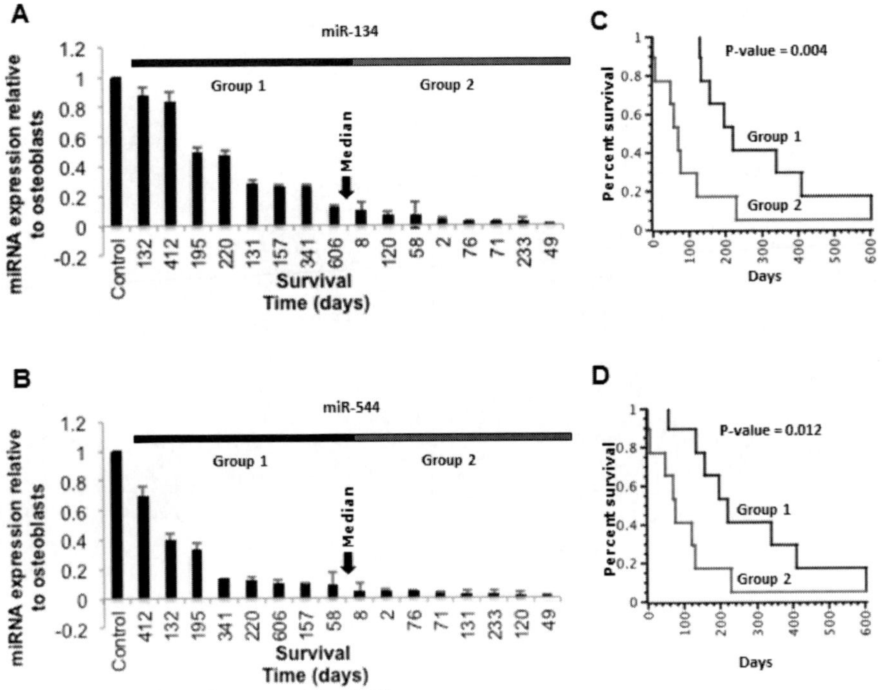

Figure adapted from Sarver et al., 2013.

Figure 3. 14q32 orthologous region transcript levels and outcome in canine osteosarcoma. (A and B) Expression levels of miR-134 and miR-544 in canine osteosarcoma primary tumor samples with clinical follow-up information. (C and D) Kaplan-Meier analysis of survival in osteosarcoma patients showing that dogs with lowest levels of miR-134 or miR-544 expression showed decreased likelihood of survival.

Another important aspect of this disease is to understand the cell that leaves the primary niche and metastasizes. For instance, genes involved with the macrophage activity play a crucial role in osteosarcoma metastasis [86]. The involvement of macrophages in metastasis could explain the beneficial effects of muramyl tripeptide (MTP) [87]. MTP improved 6-year survival rates from 70% to 78% by activating macrophages in osteosarcoma [88]. Another immunomodulatory approach is using GM-CSF, which can also stimulate macrophages that can prevent pulmonary recurrence [89].

Drugs that target other pathways fall under the class of SRC inhibitors, mTOR inhibitors, tyrosin kinase inhibitors, and RANKL inhibitors [90-92]. Saracatinib, a SRC inhibitor, could prevent adhesion and migration of osteosarcoma cells in vitro but had no effect on pulmonary metastases *in vivo*

[93]. Other tyrosine kinase inhibitors include Trastuzumab, an inhibitor of HER-2 receptors; Cituximab, an inhibitor of IGF1 receptors; Sorafenib, an inhibitor of VEGF receptors; and Osi-930, an inhibitor of multikinase receptors.

Another emerging class of drugs focuses on inhibiting osteoclast activity that plays a crucial role in the bone microenvironment [94]. A recent phase 2 study of the receptor activator of a nuclear factor-κb ligand (RANKL) inhibitor called Denosumab could prevent osteolysis and enhanced tumor response to other chemotherapeutic agents such as Ifosfamide [95]. Bisphosphonates constitute another class of drugs that tends to increase apoptosis in osteoclasts, which brings a correct balance in osteoblasts/ osteoclast ratio and eventually inhibits osteoclast-mediated angiogenesis [96].

In sum, the aforementioned drug studies suggest that one drug would not be able to cure osteosarcoma. The future therapeutics have to be designed in such a way that they target multiple pathways that can cause, contribute to, or otherwise result in osteosarcoma. And to that end, combinatorial drugs and treatments are essential.

COMBINATORIAL TREATMENT

Given the current understanding of the molecular mechanism of osteosarcoma, as well as the various shortcomings with standalone osteosarcoma drug therapies and treatments, it is apparent that there is an urgent need for combinatorial treatment of osteosarcoma. The authors' previous work, discussed above, has shown that there is an inverse correlation between expression of 14q32 miRNAs and *cMYC*. Furthermore, their work illustrated that the significant downregulation of 14q32 miRNAs is due to decreased histone acetylation.

Another study conducted by the same group demonstrated that using chromatin modifiers led to an increase in acetylation and an increase in 14q32 miRNAs, which were confirmed by western blots and ChIP [97]. Not only did the combination of the chromatin modifiers (5-Aza and 4-PBA) restore the expression of 14q32 miRNAs, but also they significantly changed the gene expression. On performing gene expression analyses of 13 osteosarcoma patient samples with 4 normal bones, and comparing this with the gene expression profile of drug treated and untreated Saos-2 cells, the microarray data identified 265 genes that were differentially expressed (greater than a 2-fold change, with p values less than 0.001). Also, the authors' group could replicate the same hypothesis using FDA approved chromatin modifiers such as SAHA (histone deacetylase inhibitor) and Zeb (DNA methylation inhibitor).

Next, they wanted to see if this same effect is also observed in canine osteosarcoma, as it was previously observed (discussed above) that 14q32 miRNAs are significantly downregulated in canines. Interestingly, they found that canine osteosarcoma cell lines with more "aggressive" gene expression profiles and shorter doubling times from both species were more sensitive to the effects of both compounds [98]. Thus, the results confirmed the authors' prediction that sensitivity to chromatin modification is directly related to specific patterns of genome-wide gene expression and downregulation of 14q32 miRNAs.

Minnelide and Osteosarcoma

Knowing that osteosarcoma is highly heterogenetic, it is necessary to find a novel drug that can target the proposed molecular mechanism of osteosarcoma.

Triptolide, a diterpene epoxide synthetic derivative from the Chinese plant *tryptergium wilfordii*, was identified in a small screen as a regulator of heat shock gene transcription.

This drug has been shown to inhibit cell proliferation and induce apoptosis mainly by downregulation of HSP70 levels [99]. However, in spite of these promising results, Triptolide was relatively ineffective for in vivo models, due to its being sparsely soluble in the body.

Resultantly, a group led by Dr. Saluja at the University of Minnesota developed a water-soluble prodrug of triptolode called Minnelide, and proceeded to demonstrate its true effectiveness in various preclinical models of pancreatic cancer, and has at present reached phase 1 trials [100]. The authors' group tested the effects of Triptolide and Minnelide *in vitro* and *in vivo* osteosarcoma models. The reason to test these two drugs was that there is a high elevation of HSP70 in osteosarcoma along with dysregulation of *cMYC* and *NF-κB* transcription factors responsible for osteosarcoma progression [101].

The authors' group observed that triptolide at doses as low as 100nM could induce cell death mediated by apoptosis in osteosarcoma cell lines, without any significant cell death in osteoblasts.

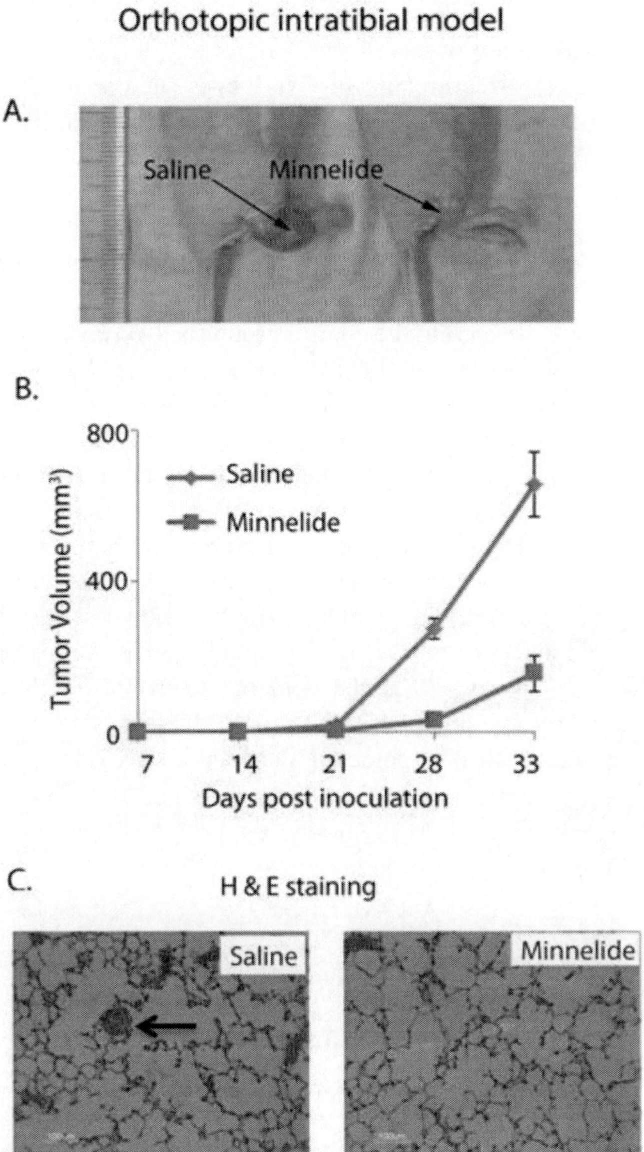

Figure adapted from Banerjee et al., 2013.

Figure 4. Minnelide treatment reduces tumor burden in an orthotopic mouse model of osteosarcoma. (A and B) Mice treated with Minnelide showed significantly decreased tumor size, late tumor onset and significantly reduced tumor progression. (C) HandE staining of lung tissue (10× mag). Minnelide decreased the formation of pulmonary micrometastasis.

These studies were confirmed by cell viability assays and caspase activity assays. Additionally, they observed that Triptolide (at 100nM) significantly reduced the levels of osteosarcoma survival genes such as *cMYC*, *β-catenin*, *cyclin D1*, *survivin*, and *RUNX2*. This suggests that triptolide has a potential role in inhibiting osteosarcoma cell proliferation by targeting various cell survival genes.

In further analyses of Minnelide (the soluble drug form of triptolide) in an osteosarcoma orthotopic mouse model (n=12), the authors' group observed significant decrease in tumor burden with insignificant presence of lung micrometastasis as compared to the control group (n=12) (Figure 4).

They also observed a significant decrease in the *NF-κB* activity in Minnelide mice tumor tissues and osteosarcoma cells, as compared to the untreated tissues and osteosarcoma cells.

Next, they assessed the role of Minnelide in osteosarcoma progression and metastasis in lung colonization mice models. Six weeks after starting Minnelide treatment in these mice, they noticed that the number of metastatic nodules in the treated group was significantly lower than the untreated group, and also that 3 out of 8 mice did not exhibit any lung nodules.

Therefore, the authors propose that Minnelide can be a novel therapeutic agent in osteosarcoma cases with the potential to increase survival rate by significant reduction of metastasis with only limited side effects. They consider this drug to have a potential therapeutic role in treating human osteosarcoma.

CONCLUSION

The discovery of miRNAs sheds new light on our basic understanding of gene regulation. It is now well established that miRNAs can fine-tune gene expression and maintain the functional balance of various gene networks. A single miRNA can regulate multiple (tens to hundreds) miRNA targets and, vice versa, several miRNAs can regulate a single miRNA [102-105]. Several studies have demonstrated the complexity of miRNA regulation of various genes interacting with multiple networks [106-108].

The complexity in gene regulation does not end in identifying and understanding the role of miRNAs. There are also other regulatory RNAs, such as long non-coding RNAs, competing endogenous RNAs, and piwi-interacting RNAs that along with miRNAs can affect the gene regulation and eventually various cellular networks and can lead to disease, including cancer.

To emphasize, gene expression can either be regulated in *cis* by enhancer sequences or in *trans* by genes that encode transcription factors (that act as activators or repressors) or RNA-binding proteins [109, 110].

Recently, several studies have demonstrated that non-coding RNA molecules can regulate gene expression in *trans* by acting as sponges of small regulatory RNAs such as miRNAs [111-113]. Together, these RNA molecules are called competing endogenous RNAs (ceRNAs) that constitute a major proportion of gene regulators. This concept of competitive target inhibition of miRNAs within a cell was first demonstrated by Phil Sharp's laboratory [114].

The identification of this level of gene regulation can explain the correlation between genome size and increase in species complexities. The extent of miRNA inhibition in such cases depends on the relative production and turnover rates of the miRNA and sponge RNA [116]. This idea of competitive target inhibition depicts another kind of unanticipated complexity in the network of RNA regulatory interactions.

Following this discovery, several other miRNAs were identified that could competitively inhibit regulatory small RNAs in prokaryotes [117-119]. Additionally, miRNA recognition elements ("MREs") that are present in coding and non-coding transcripts help in forming cross talk hubs for gene interactions, affecting the expression levels and activities of different ceRNAs. Decoding such cross talk between MREs and transcripts is critical to demarcate the intricacies in gene regulation, and we have just begun to unravel this complexity.

A remaining layer of complexity is generated by larger regulatory RNAs known as long noncoding RNAs ("lncRNAs"), which are longer than 200 nucleotides and fulfill a range of functions involving transcription, post-transcription, epigenetic regulation, both in the nucleus and the cytoplasm. It is now known that only one-fifth of transcription across the human genome is associated with protein-coding genes, which indicates that there are at least four times more lncRNAs than coding RNA sequences [120]. Moreover, the larger scale DNA sequencing projects such as FANTOM (Functional Annotation of Mammalian cDNA) are being undertaken to reveal the complexities of such transcription [121]. For instance, the FANTOM3 project has identified about 5,000 non-coding transcripts from around 10,000 distinct loci that contain various miRNA signatures such as 5' capping, splicing, and poly-adenylation, but have insignificant or no open reading frame (ORF) [121].

Recently, it has been shown that there are enhancers that could express lncRNAs, and these RNAs depicted an increase in concentration in a stimulus-dependent manner, suggesting that they might confer an additional layer of regulation in gene expression. The two studies that provided substantial evidence for a causal role in transcriptional activation for enhancer-associated lncRNAs were based on knockdown approaches to deplete the levels of several lncRNAs in human cells [109, 110]. Depletion of specific lncRNAs resulted in repression of neighboring protein-coding genes in a *cis* regulatory manner. Moreover, the above results of transcriptional activation could be reiterated in classical enhancer assays using heterologous reporters [109]. However, identifying such lncRNAs within various cDNA libraries still remains challenging, since it is difficult to distinguish protein-coding transcripts from non-coding transcripts.

We have just begun to identify such lncRNAs in osteosarcoma and the regulation thereof. One of the two recent discoveries of lncRNAs performed an expression profile of lncRNAs in osteosarcoma and compared it with paired adjacent noncancerous tissue using microarray analysis. It was found that there are 25,733 lncRNAs that were expressed in osteosarcoma; 403 lncRNAs were consistently over-regulated, and 798 lncRNAs were consistently under-regulated in all samples analyzed (>2.0-fold, $p < 0.05$) [122]. The other study described the role of one of the many lncRNAs, TUG1 and its associated transcript variants (n377360), in proliferation and apoptosis in one of the osteosarcoma cell lines (U2OS) [123]. These findings suggest that the role of such regulatory RNAs is still to be explored in depth.

The next step in understanding osteosarcoma biology is to apprehend the heterogeneity and aggressiveness of such cancer. Researchers already know that commercially available cell lines reflect different types of aggressiveness in vivo. A recent study led by Myklebost et al., demonstrated that osteosarcoma cell lines exhibited cancer-related phenotypes ranging from indolent to very aggressive [124]. Along with such observations, they discovered that several miRNAs were differentially expressed in highly aggressive osteosarcoma cell lines when compared with non-aggressive osteosarcoma cell lines. Notably, four genes (*COL1A2*, *KYNU*, *ACTG* and *NPPB*) were highly expressed in aggressive ostesoarcoma cell lines (HOS-143b), suggesting their role in osteosarcoma tumorigenesis. Also, in the same aggressive cell lines they found significant upregulation of miRNAs such as miR-135-5p, -146-5p and -155-5p which are predicted to have metastatic capacity in osteosarcoma [125]. This suggests that we as scientists cannot base our studies on just looking into one of the ostesoarcoma cell lines.

This brings us to another aspect of studying osteosarcoma: studying animal models. The challenge here is to find a model that can replicate human osteosarcoma's heterogeneity and aggressiveness. Dog models are among the best models to study osteosarcoma as they spontaneously develop the disease that closely resembles human osteosarcoma. The authors have shown that canine osteosarcoma shares similar genetic homology in terms of various genes and miRNAs as human osteosarcoma. Similarly many mouse models such as orthotopic mouse models, lung colonization models have also proven efficient in both mechanistic biological understanding of pathogenesis and preclinical evaluation of medical interventions in osteosarcoma. Most of these mouse models have been xenografts of human cells into immunocompromised mice that do not represent the right condition of the human body. Recent advances have been made in generating genetic mouse models that have been made able by genetic manipulation resulting in spontaneous occurrence and screening of the disease [126]. Authors' group in collaboration with other researchers at the University of Minnesota, have generated osteosarcoma mouse models using sleeping beauty based transposon system that causes random insertional mutagenesis in the mouse genome, specifically in osteoblasts, resulting in spontaneous osteosarcoma development. This model also helps us identify various driver genes that are oncogene or tumor suppressor in nature by using high throughput forward genetic screens. Therefore, such models can help us better understand the development of osteosarcoma tumor and metastasis.

The final portions of the foregoing chapter discussed the current and prospective therapeutics in osteosarcoma. As it is already known, in spite of use of conventional therapies such as surgical intervention and chemotherapy, 70% of osteosarcoma patients will succumb to death. This tells us that there is a need to understand and make use of unconventional medicine, one such practice being personalized medicine. Looking into and understanding individual cancer genomics through DNA sequencing and patient tumor analysis, researchers should aim to advance personalized medicine. This will help us differentiate patients on the basis of osteosarcoma subtypes and eventually lead to better survival rates. Such type of medicine is already being undertaken in various other cancers. For instance, the drug imatinib (Gleevec) is designed to inhibit an altered enzyme that is produced by a fused version of two genes found in chronic myelogenous leukemia [127]. Therefore, the future of cancer therapeutics most definitely relies on the type of genomic information generated by cancer genomics projects such as TCGA, which will drive research to develop similar treatment strategies that will be most effective for a given set of genomic changes [128].

The next "big thing" in the field of unconventional cancer therapy would be combinatorial treatment. As discussed above, the authors have found that there are more profound and effective therapeutic effects when two different drugs are combined. And such combinatorial therapies can become more robust when the drugs target two different pathways that are deregulated in osteosarcoma.

The authors' group is attempting to make use of such combinatorial therapeutics by combining the chromatin modifiers and Minnelide, as they correct epigenetic deregulation and *cMYC* overexpression in osteosarcoma, respectively (Figure 5).

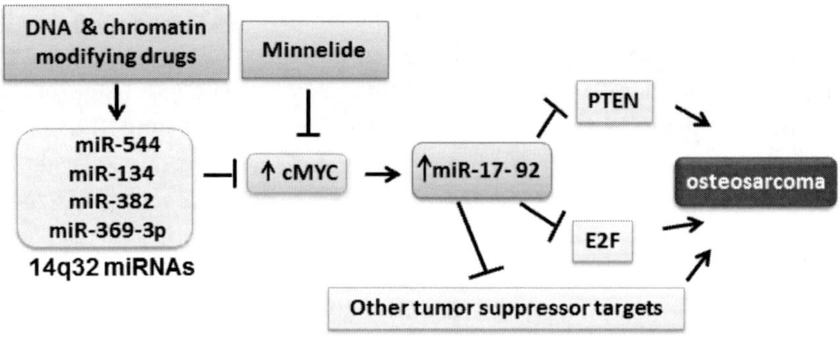

Figure 5. Schematic representation of 14q32 miRNA-cMYC-miR-17~92 gene regulatory network in OS. Downregulation of 14q32 miRNAs can potentially stabilize cMYC levels, leading to activation of miR-17-92 cluster miRNAs that in turn can target tumor suppressor genes and contribute to osteosarcoma.

Therefore, the future of osteosarcoma therapy lies in understanding the genomics of each individual patient and using drug therapy or the combination of drugs with conventional therapies that target these subtle but impactful mutations, with the end goal of individualized medicine.

Acknowledgment

We thank Drs. Ashok Saluja, Jaime Modiano and Aaron Sarver for helpful discussions and Jennie Walker Knoot for assisting in manuscript preparation. Due to the space restrictions we could not cite many other significant contributions made by numerous researchers and laboratories in this potentially important and rapidly progressing field. SS is supported by research grants funded by Department of Defense (W81XWH-10-1-0556), American Cancer Society Grant (RSG 13-381-01-RMC) University of Minnesota Academic Health Center, Masonic Cancer Center, the Wyckoff Rein in Sarcoma Foundation, Randy Shaver Foundation, Minnesota Medical Foundation and the Van Sloun Foundation.

REFERENCES

[1] Ottaviani G., Jaffe N. 2009. The epidemiology of osteosarcoma. *Cancer treatment and research,* 152:3-13.

[2] Smith M. A., Seibel N. L., Altekruse S. F., Ries L. A., Melbert D. L., O'Leary M., Smith F. O., Reaman G. H. 2010. Outcomes for children and adolescents with cancer: challenges for the twenty-first century. *Journal of clinical oncology: Official Journal of the American Society of Clinical Oncology*, 28:2625-2634.

[3] Mirabello L., Troisi R. J., Savage S. A. 2009. Osteosarcoma incidence and survival rates from 1973 to 2004: data from the Surveillance, Epidemiology, and End Results Program. *Cancer*, 115:1531-1543.

[4] Klein M. J., Siegal G. P. 2006. Osteosarcoma: anatomic and histologic variants. *American journal of clinical pathology*, 125:555-581.

[5] Lau C. C., Harris C. P., Lu X. Y., Perlaky L., Gogineni S., Chintagumpala M., Hicks J., Johnson M. E., Davino N. A., Huvos A. G., Meyers P. A., Healy J. H., Gorlick R., Rao P. H. 2004. Frequent amplification and rearrangement of chromosomal bands 6p12-p21 and 17p11.2 in osteosarcoma. *Genes, chromosomes and cancer*, 39:11-21.

[6] Kivela T., Tuppurainen K., Riikonen P., Vapalahti M. 2003. Retinoblastoma associated with chromosomal 13q14 deletion mosaicism. *Ophthalmology*, 110:1983-1988.

[7] Overholtzer M., Rao P. H., Favis R., Lu X. Y., Elowitz M. B., Barany F., Ladanyi M., Gorlick R., Levine A. J. 2003. The presence of p53 mutations in human osteosarcomas correlates with high levels of genomic instability. *Proceedings of the National Academy of Sciences of the United States of America*, 100:11547-11552.

[8] Jones K. B., Salah Z., Del Mare S., Galasso M., Gaudio E., Nuovo G. J., Lovat F., LeBlanc K., Palatini J., Randall R. L., Volinia S., Stein G. S., Croce C. M., Lian J. B., Aqeilan R. I. 2012. miRNA signatures associate with pathogenesis and progression of osteosarcoma. *Cancer research,* 72:1865-1877.

[9] Chen K., Rajewsky N. 2007. The evolution of gene regulation by transcription factors and microRNAs. Nature reviews. *Genetics,* 8:93-103.

[10] Kusenda B., Mraz M., Mayer J., Pospisilova S. 2006. MicroRNA biogenesis, functionality and cancer relevance. *Biomedical papers of the Medical Faculty of the University Palacky, Olomouc, Czechoslovakia,* 150:205-215.

[11] Vandenboom Ii T. G., Li Y., Philip P. A., Sarkar F. H. 2008. MicroRNA and Cancer: Tiny Molecules with Major Implications. *Current genomics,* 9:97-109.

[12] Shi M., Guo N. 2009. MicroRNA expression and its implications for the diagnosis and therapeutic strategies of breast cancer. *Cancer treatment reviews,* 35:328-334.

[13] Sassen S., Miska E. A., Caldas C. 2008. MicroRNA: implications for cancer. Virchows Archiv: *An International Journal of Pathology*, 452: 1-10.

[14] Sarver A. L., Thayanithy V., Scott M. C., Cleton-Jansen A. M., Hogendoorn P. C., Modiano J. F., Subramanian S. 2013. MicroRNAs at the human 14q32 locus have prognostic significance in osteosarcoma. *Orphanet Journal of Rare Diseases*, 8:7.

[15] Ostrander E. A., Wayne R. K. 2005. The canine genome. *Genome research*, 15:1706-1716.

[16] Thayanithy V., Sarver A. L., Kartha R. V., Li L., Angstadt A. Y., Breen M., Steer C. J., Modiano J. F., Subramanian S. 2012. Perturbation of 14q32 miRNAs-cMYC gene network in osteosarcoma. *Bone,* 50:171-181.

[17] Namlos H. M., Meza-Zepeda L. A., Baroy T., Ostensen I. H., Kresse S. H., Kuijjer M. L., Serra M., Burger H., Cleton-Jansen A. M., Myklebost O. 2012. Modulation of thc osteosarcoma expression phenotype by microRNAs. *PloS one*, 7:e48086.

[18] Kobayashi E., Hornicek F. J., Duan Z. 2012. MicroRNA Involvement in Osteosarcoma. *Sarcoma,* 2012:359739.

[19] Zhou G., Shi X., Zhang J., Wu S., Zhao J. 2013. MicroRNAs in osteosarcoma: from biological players to clinical contributors, a review. *The Journal of international medical research*, 41:1-12.

[20] Sarver A. L., Phalak R., Thayanithy V., Subramanian S. 2010. S-MED: sarcoma microRNA expression database. Laboratory investigation; *a journal of technical methods and pathology,* 90:753-761.

[21] DeSano J. T., Xu L. 2009. MicroRNA regulation of cancer stem cells and therapeutic implications. *The AAPS journal*, 11:682-692.

[22] Gattolliat C. H., Thomas L., Ciafre S. A., Meurice G., Le Teuff G., Job B., Richon C., Combaret V., Dessen P., Valteau-Couanet D., May E., Busson P., Douc-Rasy S., Benard J. 2011. Expression of miR-487b and miR-410 encoded by 14q32.31 locus is a prognostic marker in neuroblastoma. *British journal of cancer*, 105:1352-1361.

[23] Kelly A. D., Haibe-Kains B., Janeway K. A., Hill K. E., Howe E., Goldsmith J., Kurek K., Perez-Atayde A. R., Francoeur N., Fan J. B., April C., Schneider H., Gebhardt M. C., Culhane A., Quackenbush J., Spentzos D. 2013. MicroRNA paraffin-based studies in osteosarcoma reveal reproducible independent prognostic profiles at 14q32. *Genome medicine*, 5:2.

[24] Maire G., Martin J. W., Yoshimoto M., Chilton-MacNeill S., Zielenska M., Squire J. A. 2011. Analysis of miRNA-gene expression-genomic profiles reveals complex mechanisms of microRNA deregulation in osteosarcoma. *Cancer genetics*, 204:138-146.

[25] Lulla R. R., Costa F. F., Bischof J. M., Chou P. M., de F. B. M., Vanin E. F., Soares M. B. 2011. Identification of Differentially Expressed MicroRNAs in Osteosarcoma. *Sarcoma,* 2011:732690.

[26] Stabley D. L., Kamara, D., Holbrook, J., Sol-Church, K., Kolb, E. A., and McCahan, S. M. 2010. Digital gene expression of mirna in osteosarcoma xenografts: finding biological relevance in mirna high throughput sequencing data. *Journal of Biomolecular Techniques.*

[27] Chang T. C., Wentzel E. A., Kent O. A., Ramachandran K., Mullendore M., Lee K. H., Feldmann G., Yamakuchi M., Ferlito M., Lowenstein C. J., Arking D. E., Beer M. A., Maitra A., Mendell J. T. 2007. Transactivation of miR-34a by p53 broadly influences gene expression and promotes apoptosis. *Molecular cell*, 26:745-752.

[28] Mandke P., Wyatt N., Fraser J., Bates B., Berberich S. J., Markey M. P. 2012. MicroRNA-34a modulates MDM4 expression via a target site in the open reading frame. *PloS one,* 7:e42034.

[29] Doridot L., Houry D., Gaillard H., Chelbi S. T., Barbaux S., Vaiman D. 2013. miR-34a expression, epigenetic regulation, and function in human placental diseases. *Epigenetics: official journal of the DNA Methylation Society,* 9.

[30] Nalls D., Tang S. N., Rodova M., Srivastava R. K. Shankar S. 2011. Targeting epigenetic regulation of miR-34a for treatment of pancreatic cancer by inhibition of pancreatic cancer stem cells. *PloS one,* 6:e24099.

[31] Sylvestre Y., De Guire V., Querido E., Mukhopadhyay U. K., Bourdeau V., Major F., Ferbeyre G., Chartrand P. 2007. An E2F/miR-20a autoregulatory feedback loop. *The Journal of biological chemistry,* 282:2135-2143.

[32] Olive V., Jiang I., He L. 2010. mir-17-92, a cluster of miRNAs in the midst of the cancer network. *The international journal of biochemistry and cell biology,* 42:1348-1354.

[33] Li Y., Zhang H., Chen Y. 2011. MicroRNA-mediated positive feedback loop and optimized bistable switch in a cancer network Involving miR-17-92. *PloS one,* 6:e26302.

[34] Song M. S., Salmena L., Pandolfi P. P. 2012. The functions and regulation of the PTEN tumour suppressor. Nature reviews. *Molecular cell biology,* 13:283-296.

[35] Martin J. W., Zielenska M., Stein G. S., van Wijnen A. J., Squire J. A. 2011. The Role of RUNX2 in Osteosarcoma Oncogenesis. *Sarcoma,* 2011:282745.

[36] Lucero C. M., Vega O. A., Osorio M. M., Tapia J. C., Antonelli M., Stein G. S., van Wijnen A. J., Galindo M. A. 2013. The cancer-related transcription factor Runx2 modulates cell proliferation in human osteosarcoma cell lines. *Journal of cellular physiology*, 228:714-723.

[37] Han G., Wang Y., Bi W. 2012. C-Myc overexpression promotes osteosarcoma cell invasion via activation of MEK-ERK pathway. *Oncology research*, 20:149-156.

[38] Tang N., Song W. X., Luo J., Haydon R. C., He T. C. 2008. Osteosarcoma development and stem cell differentiation. *Clinical orthopaedics and related research,* 466:2114-2130.

[39] Broadhead M. L., Clark J. C., Myers D. E., Dass C. R., Choong P. F. 2011. The molecular pathogenesis of osteosarcoma: a review. *Sarcoma*, 2011:959248.

[40] Hagan J. P., O'Neill B. L., Stewart C. L., Kozlov S. V., Croce C. M. 2009. At least ten genes define the imprinted Dlk1-Dio3 cluster on mouse chromosome 12qF1. *PloS one*, 4:e4352.

[41] Zhou Y., Zhang X., Klibanski A. 2012. MEG3 noncoding RNA: a tumor suppressor. *Journal of molecular endocrinology*, 48:R45-53.

[42] Bakhshi S., Radhakrishnan V. 2010. Prognostic markers in osteosarcoma. *Expert review of anticancer therapy*, 10:271-287.

[43] Geller D. S., Gorlick R. 2010. Osteosarcoma: a review of diagnosis, management, and treatment strategies. *Clinical advances in hematology and oncology: HandO,* 8:705-718.

[44] Bruland O. S., Pihl A. 1997. On the current management of osteosarcoma. A critical evaluation and a proposal for a modified treatment strategy. *Eur. J. Cancer*, 33:1725-1731.

[45] Gonzalez-Herranz P., Burgos-Flores J., Ocete-Guzman J. G., Lopez-Mondejar J. A., Amaya S. 1995. The management of limb-length discrepancies in children after treatment of osteosarcoma and Ewing's sarcoma. *Journal of pediatric orthopedics*, 15:561-565.

[46] del Prever A. B., Fagioli F., Berta M., Bertoni F., Ferrari S., Mercuri M. 2005. Long-term survival in high-grade axial osteosarcoma with bone and lung metastases treated with chemotherapy only. *Journal of pediatric hematology/oncology,* 27:42-45.

[47] Lee J. A., Kim M. S., Koh J. S., Kim D. H., Lim J. S., Kong C. B., Song W. S., Cho W. H., Lee S. Y., Jeon D. G. 2010. Osteosarcoma of the flat bone. *Japanese journal of clinical oncology*, 40:47-53.

[48] Jaffe N., Jaffe D. M. 1996. Tumor size and prognosis in aggressively treated osteosarcoma. *Journal of clinical oncology: official journal of the American Society of Clinical Oncology*, 14:2399-2400.

[49] Bieling P., Rehan N., Winkler P., Helmke K., Maas R., Fuchs N., Bielack S., Heise U., Jurgens H., Treuner J., Romanowski R., Exner U., Kotz R., Winkler K. 1996. Tumor size and prognosis in aggressively treated osteosarcoma. *Journal of clinical oncology: official journal of the American Society of Clinical Oncology*, 14:848-858.

[50] Sternberg R. A., Pondenis H. C., Yang X., Mitchell M. A., O'Brien R. T., Garrett L. D., Helferich W. G., Hoffmann W. E., Fan T. M. 2013. Association between absolute tumor burden and serum bone-specific alkaline phosphatase in canine appendicular osteosarcoma. *Journal of veterinary internal medicine / American College of Veterinary Internal Medicine,* 27:955-963.

[51] Nahar N. N., Tague S. E., Wang J., Danley M., Garimella R., Anderson H. C. 2013. Histological characterization of bone marrow in ectopic bone, induced by devitalized Saos-2 human osteosarcoma cells. *International journal of clinical and experimental medicine*, 6:119-125.

[52] Endo M., Yoshida T., Yamamoto H., Ishii T., Setsu N., Kohashi K., Matsunobu T., Iwamoto Y., Oda Y. 2013. Low-grade central osteosarcoma arising from bone infarct. *Human pathology*, 44:1184-1189.

[53] Ueki H., Maeda N., Sekimizu M., Tsukushi S., Nishida Y., Horibe K. 2013. Osteosarcoma after bone marrow transplantation. *Journal of pediatric hematology/oncology*, 35:134-138.

[54] Ponce B. A., Thompson K. J., Rosenzweig S. D., Tate J. P., Sarver D. B., Thorpe J. B., 2nd, Sheppard E. D., Lopez R. R. 2013. Re-evaluation of pectoralis major height as an anatomic reference for humeral height in fracture hemiarthroplasty. *Journal of shoulder and elbow surgery / American Shoulder and Elbow Surgeons ... [et al.].*

[55] Bielack S., Carrle D., Casali P. G. 2009. Osteosarcoma: ESMO clinical recommendations for diagnosis, treatment and follow-up. *Annals of oncology: official journal of the European Society for Medical Oncology / ESMO,* 20 Suppl. 4:137-139.

[56] Bielack S., Carrle D., Jost L. 2008. Osteosarcoma: ESMO clinical recommendations for diagnosis, treatment and follow-up. *Annals of oncology: official journal of the European Society for Medical Oncology / ESMO,* 19 Suppl. 2:ii94-96.

[57] Saeter G. 2007. Osteosarcoma: ESMO clinical recommendations for diagnosis, treatment and follow-up. *Annals of oncology: official journal of the European Society for Medical Oncology / ESMO*, 18 Suppl. 2:ii77-78.

[58] Saeter G., Kloke O., Jelic S. 2005. ESMO Minimum Clinical Recommendations for diagnosis, treatment and follow-up of osteosarcoma. *Annals of oncology: official journal of the European Society for Medical Oncology / ESMO*, 16 Suppl. 1:i71-72.

[59] Saeter G. 2003. ESMO Minimum Clinical Recommendations for diagnosis, treatment and follow-up of osteosarcoma. *Annals of oncology: official journal of the European Society for Medical Oncology/ ESMO,* 14:1165-1166.

[60] Jawad M. U., Scully S. P. 2010. In brief: classifications in brief: enneking classification: benign and malignant tumors of the musculoskeletal system. *Clinical orthopaedics and related research*, 468:2000-2002.

[61] San-Julian M., Diaz-de-Rada P., Noain E., Sierrasesumaga L. 2003. Bone metastases from osteosarcoma. *International orthopaedics*, 27:117-120.

[62] Bacci G., Longhi A., Bertoni F., Briccoli A., Versari M., Pignotti E., Picci P. 2006. Bone metastases in osteosarcoma patients treated with neoadjuvant or adjuvant chemotherapy: the Rizzoli experience in 52 patients. *Acta orthopaedica*, 77:938-943.

[63] Sanerkin N. G. 1980. Definitions of osteosarcoma, chondrosarcoma, and fibrosarcoma of bone. *Cancer*, 46:178-185.

[64] Pan K. L., Chan W. H., Ong G. B., Premsenthil S., Zulkarnaen M., Norlida D., Abidin Z. 2012. Limb salvage in osteosarcoma using autoclaved tumor-bearing bone. *World journal of surgical oncology*, 10:105.

[65] Picci P., Bacci G., Ferrari S., Mercuri M. 1997. Neoadjuvant chemotherapy in malignant fibrous histiocytoma of bone and in osteosarcoma located in the extremities: analogies and differences between the two tumors. *Annals of oncology: official journal of the European Society for Medical Oncology / ESMO*, 8:1107-1115.

[66] Gavhed D., Akefeldt S. O., Osterlundh G., Laurencikas E., Hjorth L., Blennow K., Rosengren L., Henter J. I. 2009. Biomarkers in the cerebrospinal fluid and neurodegeneration in Langerhans cell histiocytosis. *Pediatric blood and cancer*, 53:1264-1270.

[67] Wang L., Park P., La Marca F., Than K., Rahman S., Lin C. Y. 2013. Bone formation induced by BMP-2 in human osteosarcoma cells. *International journal of oncology*, 43:1095-1102.

[68] Ghali J. K., Wikstrand J., Van Veldhuisen D. J., Fagerberg B., Goldstein S., Hjalmarson A., Johansson P., Kjekshus J., Ohlsson L., Samuelsson O., Waagstein F., Wedel H. 2009. The influence of renal function on clinical outcome and response to beta-blockade in systolic heart failure: insights from Metoprolol CR/XL Randomized Intervention Trial in Chronic HF (MERIT-HF). *Journal of cardiac failure*,15:310-318.

[69] Nagoya S., Uede T., Wada T., Ishii S., Yamawaki S., Kikuchi K. 1991. Detection of bone-type alkaline phosphatase by monoclonal antibodies reacting with human osteosarcoma-associated antigen. *Japanese journal of cancer research: Gann.*, 82:862-870.

[70] Troseid M., Arnesen H., Hjerkinn E. M., Seljeflot I. 2009. Serum levels of interleukin-18 are reduced by diet and n-3 fatty acid intervention in elderly high-risk men. *Metabolism: clinical and experimental*, 58:1543-1549.

[71] Bacci G., Picci P., Ferrari S., Orlandi M., Ruggieri P., Casadei R., Ferraro A., Biagini R., Battistini A. 1993. Prognostic significance of serum alkaline phosphatase measurements in patients with osteosarcoma treated with adjuvant or neoadjuvant chemotherapy. *Cancer,* 71:1224-1230.

[72] 1988. Age and dose of chemotherapy as major prognostic factors in a trial of adjuvant therapy of osteosarcoma combining two alternating drug combinations and early prophylactic lung irradiation. French Bone Tumor Study Group. *Cancer*, 61:1304-1311.

[73] Morello E., Buracco P., Martano M., Peirone B., Capurro C., Valazza A., Cotto D., Ferracini R., Sora M. 2001. Bone allografts and adjuvant cisplatin for the treatment of canine appendicular osteosarcoma in 18 dogs. *The Journal of small animal practice*, 42:61-66.

[74] Holzer G., Krepler P., Koschat M. A., Grampp S., Dominkus M., Kotz R. 2003. Bone mineral density in long-term survivors of highly malignant osteosarcoma. *The Journal of bone and joint surgery*, British volume, 85:231-237.

[75] Yoshikawa H., Takaoka K., Hamada H., Ono K. 1985. Clinical significance of bone morphogenetic activity in osteosarcoma. A study of 20 cases. *Cancer*, 56:1682-1687.

[76] Ambroszkiewicz J., Gajewska J., Klepacka T., Chelchowska M., Laskowska-Klita T., Wozniak W. 2010. Clinical utility of biochemical bone turnover markers in children and adolescents with osteosarcoma. *Advances in medical sciences*, 55:266-272.

[77] Ripamonti C., Avella M., Gnudi S., Figus E. 1993. [Effect of high and low doses of methotrexate (MTX) on bone mass in subjects treated for osteosarcoma of the limbs]. *Minerva medica*, 84:131-134.

[78] Wagener D. J., van Oosterom A. T., Mulder J. H., Somers R., Mouridsen H. T., Cortes Funes H., Thomas D., Sylvester R. 1986. Phase II study of low-dose methotrexate in advanced osteosarcoma followed by escalation after disease progression: a study of the Soft Tissue and Bone Sarcoma Group of the European Organization for Research on Treatment of Cancer. *Cancer treatment reports*, 70:615-618.

[79] Yang X., Wang Y. P., Liu F. X., Zeng K., Qian M. Q., Chen G., Shi L., Zhu G. X. 2013. Increased invasiveness of osteosarcoma mesenchymal stem cells induced by bone-morphogenetic protein-2. In vitro cellular and developmental biology. *Animal*, 49:270-278.

[80] Kaya M., Wada T., Akatsuka T., Kawaguchi S., Nagoya S., Shindoh M., Higashino F., Mezawa F., Okada F., Ishii S. 2000. Vascular endothelial growth factor expression in untreated osteosarcoma is predictive of pulmonary metastasis and poor prognosis. *Clinical cancer research: an official journal of the American Association for Cancer Research*, 6:572-577.

[81] Bajpai J., Gamanagatti S., Sharma M. C., Kumar R., Vishnubhatla S., Khan S. A., Rastogi S., Malhotra A., Bakhshi S. 2010. Noninvasive imaging surrogate of angiogenesis in osteosarcoma. *Pediatric blood and cancer,* 54:526-531.

[82] Yin K., Liao Q., Zhong D., Ding J., Niu B., Long Q., Ding D. 2012. Meta-analysis of limb salvage versus amputation for treating high-grade and localized osteosarcoma in patients with pathological fracture. *Experimental and therapeutic medicine*, 4:889-894.

[83] Mito J. K., Ferrer J. M., Brigman B. E., Lee C. L., Dodd R. D., Eward W. C., Marshall L. F., Cuneo K. C., Carter J. E., Ramasunder S., Kim Y., Lee W. D., Griffith L. G., Bawendi M. G., Kirsch D. G. 2012. Intraoperative detection and removal of microscopic residual sarcoma using wide-field imaging. *Cancer,* 118:5320-5330.

[84] Allison D. C., Carney S. C., Ahlmann E. R., Hendifar A., Chawla S., Fedenko A., Angeles C., Menendez L. R. 2012. A meta-analysis of osteosarcoma outcomes in the modern medical era. *Sarcoma,* 2012:704872.

[85] Andrews N. A. 2013. Osteosarcoma therapy: what is the way forward. *IBMS BoneKEy*, 10.

[86] Buddingh E. P., Kuijjer M. L., Duim R. A., Burger H., Agelopoulos K., Myklebost O., Serra M., Mertens F., Hogendoorn P. C., Lankester A. C., Cleton-Jansen A. M. 2011. Tumor-infiltrating macrophages are associated with metastasis suppression in high-grade osteosarcoma: a rationale for treatment with macrophage activating agents. *Clinical cancer research: an official journal of the American Association for Cancer Research*, 17:2110-2119.

[87] Meyers P. A., Schwartz C. L., Krailo M. D., Healey J. H., Bernstein M. L., Betcher D., Ferguson W. S., Gebhardt M. C. Goorin A. M., Harris M., Kleinerman E., Link M. P., Nadel H., Nieder M., Siegal G. P., Weiner M. A., Wells R. J., Womer R. B., Grier H. E. 2008. Osteosarcoma: the addition of muramyl tripeptide to chemotherapy improves overall survival--a report from the Children's Oncology Group. *Journal of clinical oncology: official journal of the American Society of Clinical Oncology*, 26:633-638.

[88] Chou A. J., Kleinerman E. S., Krailo M. D., Chen Z., Betcher D. L., Healey J. H., Conrad E. U., 3rd, Nieder M. L., Weiner M. A., Wells R. J., Womer R. B., Meyers P. A. 2009. Addition of muramyl tripeptide to chemotherapy for patients with newly diagnosed metastatic osteosarcoma: a report from the Children's Oncology Group. *Cancer,* 115:5339-5348.

[89] Arndt C. A., Koshkina N. V., Inwards C. Y., Hawkins D. S., Krailo M. D., Villaluna D., Anderson P. M., Goorin A. M., Blakely M. L., Bernstein M., Bell S. A., Ray K., Grendahl D. C., Marina N.,

Kleinerman E. S. 2010. Inhaled granulocyte-macrophage colony stimulating factor for first pulmonary recurrence of osteosarcoma: effects on disease-free survival and immunomodulation. a report from the Children's Oncology Group. *Clinical cancer research: an official journal of the American Association for Cancer Research*, 16: 4024-4030.

[90] Chawla S. P., Staddon A. P., Baker L. H., Schuetze S. M., Tolcher A. W., D'Amato G. Z., Blay J. Y., Mita M. M., Sankhala K. K., Berk L., Rivera V. M., Clackson T., Loewy J. W., Haluska F. G., Demetri G. D. 2012. Phase II study of the mammalian target of rapamycin inhibitor ridaforolimus in patients with advanced bone and soft tissue sarcomas. *Journal of clinical oncology: official journal of the American Society of Clinical Oncology*, 30:78-84.

[91] Ebb D., Meyers P., Grier H., Bernstein M., Gorlick R., Lipshultz S. E., Krailo M., Devidas M., Barkauskas D. A., Siegal G. P., Ferguson W. S., Letson G. D., Marcus K., Goorin A., Beardsley P., Marina N. 2012. Phase II trial of trastuzumab in combination with cytotoxic chemotherapy for treatment of metastatic osteosarcoma with human epidermal growth factor receptor 2 overexpression: a report from the children's oncology group. *Journal of clinical oncology: official journal of the American Society of Clinical Oncology*, 30:2545-2551.

[92] Yap T. A., Arkenau H. T., Camidge D. R., George S., Serkova N. J., Gwyther S. J., Spratlin J. L., Lal R., Spicer J., Desouza N. M., Leach M. O., Chick J., Poondru S., Boinpally R., Gedrich R., Brock K., Stephens A., Eckhardt S. G., Kaye S. B., Demetri G., Scurr M. 2013. First-in-human phase I trial of two schedules of OSI-930, a novel multikinase inhibitor, incorporating translational proof-of-mechanism studies. *Clinical cancer research: an official journal of the American Association for Cancer Research*, 19:909-919.

[93] Hingorani P., Zhang W., Gorlick R., Kolb EA. 2009. Inhibition of Src phosphorylation alters metastatic potential of osteosarcoma in vitro but not in vivo. *Clinical cancer research: an official journal of the American Association for Cancer Research*, 15:3416-3422.

[94] Rousseau J., Escriou V., Lamoureux F., Brion R., Chesneau J., Battaglia S., Amiaud J., Scherman D., Heymann D., Redini F., Trichet V. 2011. Formulated siRNAs targeting Rankl prevent osteolysis and enhance chemotherapeutic response in osteosarcoma models. *Journal of bone and mineral research: the official journal of the American Society for Bone and Mineral Research,* 26:2452-2462.

[95] Thomas D., Henshaw R., Skubitz K., Chawla S., Staddon A., Blay J. Y., Roudier M., Smith J., Ye Z., Sohn W., Dansey R., Jun S. 2010. Denosumab in patients with giant-cell tumour of bone: an open-label, phase 2 study. *The lancet oncology*, 11:275-280.

[96] Meyers P. A., Healey J. H., Chou A. J., Wexler L. H., Merola P. R., Morris C. D., Laquaglia M. P., Kellick M. G., Abramson S. J., Gorlick R. 2011. Addition of pamidronate to chemotherapy for the treatment of osteosarcoma. *Cancer*, 117:1736-1744.

[97] Thayanithy V., Park C., Sarver A. L., Kartha R. V., Korpela D. M., Graef A. J., Steer C. J., Modiano J. F., Subramanian S. 2012. Combinatorial treatment of DNA and chromatin-modifying drugs cause cell death in human and canine osteosarcoma cell lines. *PloS one,* 7:e43720.

[98] Scott M. C., Sarver A. L., Gavin K. J., Thayanithy V., Getzy D. M., Newman R. A., Cutter G. R., Lindblad-Toh K., Kisseberth W. C., Hunter L. E., Subramanian S., Breen M., Modiano J. F. 2011. Molecular subtypes of osteosarcoma identified by reducing tumor heterogeneity through an interspecies comparative approach. *Bone,* 49:356-367.

[99] Phillips P. A., Dudeja V., McCarroll J. A., Borja-Cacho D., Dawra R. K., Grizzle W. E., Vickers S. M., Saluja A. K. 2007. Triptolide induces pancreatic cancer cell death via inhibition of heat shock protein 70. *Cancer research*, 67:9407-9416.

[100] Chugh R., Sangwan V., Patil S. P., Dudeja V., Dawra R. K., Banerjee S., Schumacher R. J., Blazar B. R., Georg G. I., Vickers S. M., Saluja A. K. 2012. A preclinical evaluation of Minnelide as a therapeutic agent against pancreatic cancer. *Science translational medicine*, 4:156ra139.

[101] Banerjee S., Thayanithy V., Sangwan V., Mackenzie T. N., Saluja A. K., Subramanian S. 2013. Minnelide reduces tumor burden in preclinical models of osteosarcoma. *Cancer letters*, 335:412-420.

[102] Eulalio A., Huntzinger E., Izaurralde E. 2008. Getting to the Root of miRNA-Mediated Gene Silencing. *Cell,* 132:9-14.

[103] Bartel D. P. 2009. MicroRNAs: target recognition and regulatory functions. *Cell,* 136:215-233.

[104] Friedman R. C., Farh K. K., Burge C. B., Bartel D. P. 2009. Most mammalian mRNAs are conserved targets of microRNAs. *Genome research,* 19:92-105.

[105] Ebert M. S., Sharp P. A. 2012. Roles for microRNAs in conferring robustness to biological processes. *Cell*, 149:515-524.

[106] Sarver A., Li L., Subramanian S. 2010. MicroRNA miR-183 functions as an oncogene by targeting the transcription factor EGR1 and promoting tumor cell migration. *Can. Res.*, 70:9570-9580.

[107] Yang B., Lin H., Xiao J., Lu Y., Luo X., Li B., Zhang Y., Xu C., Bai Y., Wang H., Chen G., Wang Z. 2007. The muscle-specific microRNA miR-1 regulates cardiac arrhythmogenic potential by targeting GJA1 and KCNJ2. *Nature medicine*, 13:486-491.

[108] Hammond S. M. 2007. MicroRNAs as tumor suppressors. *Nature genetics,* 39:582-583.

[109] Orom U. A., Derrien T., Beringer M., Gumireddy K., Gardini A., Bussotti G., Lai F., Zytnicki M., Notredame C., Huang Q., Guigo R., Shiekhattar R. 2010. Long noncoding RNAs with enhancer-like function in human cells. *Cell,* 143:46-58.

[110] Wang X., Arai S., Song X., Reichart D., Du K., Pascual G., Tempst P., Rosenfeld M. G., Glass C. K., Kurokawa R. 2008. Induced ncRNAs allosterically modify RNA-binding proteins in cis to inhibit transcription. *Nature,* 454:126-130.

[111] Salmena L., Poliseno L., Tay Y., Kats L., Pandolfi P. P. 2011. A ceRNA hypothesis: the Rosetta Stone of a hidden RNA language? *Cell*, 146:353-358.

[112] Tay Y., Kats L., Salmena L., Weiss D., Tan S. M., Ala U., Karreth F., Poliseno L., Provero P., Di Cunto F., Lieberman J., Rigoutsos I., Pandolfi P. P. 2011. Coding-Independent Regulation of the Tumor Suppressor PTEN by Competing Endogenous mRNAs. *Cell,* 147:344-357.

[113] Karreth F. A., Tay Y., Perna D., Ala U., Tan S. M., Rust A. G., Denicola G., Webster K. A., Weiss D., Perez-Mancera P. A., Krauthammer M., Halaban R., Provero P., Adams D. J., Tuveson D. A., Pandolfi P. P. 2011. In Vivo Identification of Tumor- Suppressive PTEN ceRNAs in an Oncogenic BRAF-Induced Mouse Model of Melanoma. *Cell,* 147:382-395.

[114] Ebert M. S., Neilson J. R., Sharp P. A. 2007. MicroRNA sponges: competitive inhibitors of small RNAs in mammalian cells. *Nature methods,* 4:721-726.

[115] Franco-Zorrilla J. M., Valli A., Todesco M., Mateos I., Puga M. I., Rubio-Somoza I., Leyva A., Weigel D., Garcia J. A., Paz-Ares J. 2007. Target mimicry provides a new mechanism for regulation of microRNA activity. *Nature genetics*, 39:1033-1037.

[116] Chitwood D. H., Timmermans M. C. 2007. Target mimics modulate miRNAs. *Nature genetics*, 39:935-936.
[117] Figueroa-Bossi N., Valentini M., Malleret L., Fiorini F., Bossi L. 2009. Caught at its own game: regulatory small RNA inactivated by an inducible transcript mimicking its target. *Genes and development*, 23:2004-2015.
[118] Overgaard M., Johansen J., Moller-Jensen J., Valentin-Hansen P. 2009. Switching off small RNA regulation with trap-mRNA. *Molecular microbiology,* 73:790-800.
[119] Mandin P., Gottesman S. 2009. Regulating the regulator: an RNA decoy acts as an OFF switch for the regulation of an sRNA. *Genes and development,* 23:1981-1985.
[120] Kapranov P., St Laurent G., Raz T., Ozsolak F., Reynolds C. P., Sorensen P. H., Reaman G., Milos P., Arceci R. J., Thompson J. F., Triche T. J.. 2010. The majority of total nuclear-encoded non-ribosomal RNA in a human cell is 'dark matter' un-annotated RNA. *BMC biology*, 8:149.
[121] Carninci P., Kasukawa T., Katayama S., Gough J., Frith M. C., Maeda N., Oyama R., et al. *Science*, 309:1559-1563.
[122] Li J. P., Liu L. H., Li J., Chen Y., Jiang X. W., Ouyang Y. R., Liu Y. Q., Zhong H., Li H., Xiao T. 2013. Microarray expression profile of long noncoding RNAs in human osteosarcoma. *Biochemical and biophysical research communications,* 433:200-206.
[123] Zhang Q., Geng P. L., Yin P., Wang X. L., Jia J. P., Yao J. 2013. Down-regulation of long non-coding RNA TUG1 inhibits osteosarcoma cell proliferation and promotes apoptosis. *Asian Pacific journal of cancer prevention: APJCP,* 14:2311-2315.
[124] Lauvrak S. U., Munthe E., Kresse S. H., Stratford E. W., Namlos H. M., Meza-Zepeda L. A., Myklebost O. 2013. Functional characterisation of osteosarcoma cell lines and identification of mRNAs and miRNAs associated with aggressive cancer phenotypes. *British journal of cancer*, 109:2228-2236.
[125] Lauvrak S. U., Munthe E., Kresse S. H., Stratford E. W., Namlos H. M., Meza-Zepeda L. A., Myklebost O. 2013. Functional characterisation of osteosarcoma cell lines and identification of mRNAs and miRNAs associated with aggressive cancer phenotypes. *British journal of cancer.*
[126] Jones K. B. 2011. Osteosarcomagenesis: modeling cancer initiation in the mouse. *Sarcoma*, 2011:694136.

[127] Fausel C. 2007. Targeted chronic myeloid leukemia therapy: seeking a cure. *Journal of managed care pharmacy: JMCP,* 13:8-12.
[128] Chang K., Creighton C. J., Davis C., Donehower L., Drummond J., Wheeler D., Ally A., et al. 2013. The Cancer Genome Atlas Pan-Cancer analysis project. *Nature genetics*, 45:1113-1120.

In: Osteosarcoma
Editors: Edwin Choy

ISBN: 978-1-63321-052-3

Chapter 7

EMERGING SIGNALING PATHWAYS FOR FUTURE THERAPIES IN OSTEOSARCOMA: Wnt, NOTCH AND HEDGEHOG SIGNALING

Marco Mravic, Alan Nguyen, Michelle A. Scott D.D.S, M.B.A. and Aaron W. James*, M.D.

Department of Pathology & Laboratory Medicine, and Orthopedic Hospital Research Center, David Geffen School of Medicine, UCLA, Los Angeles, CA US

ABSTRACT

Introduction: The molecular alterations that induce sarcomagenesis are incompletely understood. This review will examine three important pathways in bone biology and their relation to the development of osteosarcoma: Wnt, Hedgehog and Notch signaling. We will briefly review basic signaling pathways, delineate what is known and yet unknown regarding their role in osteosarcoma formation and disease progression, and describe future treatment strategies.

---

* Coresponding author: Aaron W. James, M.D. Department of Pathology & Laboratory Medicine, University of California, Los Angeles, David Geffen School of Medicine, 10833 Le Conte Ave., A3-251 CHS, Los Angeles, California 90095, awjames@mednet.ucla.edu.

Results: Wnt, Hedgehog and Notch signaling have been examined as deregulated signaling pathways in osteosarcoma and potential molecular therapeutic targets. Canonical Wnt signaling activation has known roles in oncogenesis, and exogenous inhibition of Wnt signaling may have therapeutic benefit. For example, *FHL2 (*four and a half LIM domain 2) silencing reduces Wnt signaling and osteosarcoma tumorigenesis. Likewise, Wnt inhibition has been shown to sensitize osteosarcoma to chemotherapy, potentially via interaction with TWIST transcription factors. In the case of Hedgehog signaling, constitutive activation has been observed in various malignancies. Specific to osteosarcoma, Hedgehog receptors and downstream mediators show overexpression. In addition, inhibition of Smoothened (SMO) with pharmaceuticals and/or siRNA has led to diminished osteosarcoma cell proliferation *in vitro* and reduced osteosarcoma growth *in vivo*. Further studies have demonstrated the importance of GLI2 (glioma-associated oncogene homolog 2) Hedgehog signaling transduction for osteosarcoma growth. In the case of Notch signaling, aberrant upregulations of Notch signaling have been observed both in human osteosarcoma and *TP53* mutant mice osteosarcoma. Inhibition of Notch via either liposome transfection or small molecule delivery has resulted in reduced osteosarcoma cell proliferation and *in vivo* osteosarcoma growth. Moreover, Notch signaling and target gene *HES1 (*hairy and enhancer of split-1) have been associated with osteosarcoma invasion and metastasis.

Discussion: The role of Wnt, Hedgehog and Notch signaling in osteosarcoma is incompletely understood. All three pathways are fundamental in growth and patterning of the embryo, mesenchymal stem cell proliferation and differentiation, and skeletogenesis. The interest in manipulating these signaling pathways for chemotherapeutic purposes exceeds the scope of mesenchymal tumors, and includes epithelial and hematopoietic malignancies as well. Moreover, the interest in manipulating these signaling pathways, especially Wnt, is of tremendous interest to those researching osteoporosis. Potential cross over between fields may help in the rapid development of new, targeted therapies for osteosarcoma.

INTRODUCTION

The molecular alterations that induce osteosarcomagenesis are incompletely understood, and no singular genetic event has been found responsible for generating osteosarcomas. As a result, the manipulation of new and identified signaling pathways to treat osteosarcoma is a complex task. Thus, understanding the molecular basis determining relationships between tumor suppressor genes, oncogenes, and regulatory pathways is helpful in the early diagnosis of osteosarcoma, and integral to devising safe, therapeutic responses.

In particular, etiogenesis of osteosarcoma requires attention to three changes of gene and protein expression in sarcomagenesis. This review will focus on pathways involved in self-renewal, differentiation, and homeostasis of mesenchymal stem cells (MSC) and bone tissue—Wnt, Hedgehog, and Notch—and their roles in osteosarcoma and sarcomagenesis. Through their regulating growth and modulating genetic expression, components of the Wnt, Hedgehog, and Notch are feasible targets for gene therapy, pharmaceuticals, and other possible cancer treatments. We will review what is known about the molecular mechanisms driving these pathways' participation in micro- and macroscopic biological consequences leading to sarcomagenesis. Furthermore, we will highlight frontiers deserving of further exploration concerning Wnt, Hedgehog, and Notch signaling in sarcomagenesis that may improve and diversify the current treatment of osteosarcoma.

Wnt, Hedgehog and Notch Signaling in Cell and Bone Biology

Brief Review of Wnt Signaling

Although wingless-type MMTV integration site (Wnt) signaling was discovered through the identification of Wnt1 as a proto-oncogene, the Wnt signaling pathway has been shown to play diverse and essential roles in development, cell fate determination, self-renewal, and tissue morphogenesis [1]. Dysregulation of Wnt signaling, can leading to numerous disease states, including Parkinson's disease [2], retinopathy [3], osteoporosis [4], colon cancer [5], and melanoma [5]. Due to its myriad of cellular functions, there has been tremendous focus on characterizing the ligands, receptors, and effectors of the Wnt pathway. To date, there are 19 known Wnt ligands and over 15 receptors and co-receptors throughout seven protein families [1,6]. Wnt signaling pathways are either β-catenin dependent (the canonical Wnt pathway) or β-catenin independent.

In β-catenin dependent Wnt signaling, Wnt ligand proteins bind to the cysteine rich portion of Frizzled receptor (FRZ) family proteins, transmembrane G-protein coupled receptors, at the plasma membrane[1] (Figure 1).

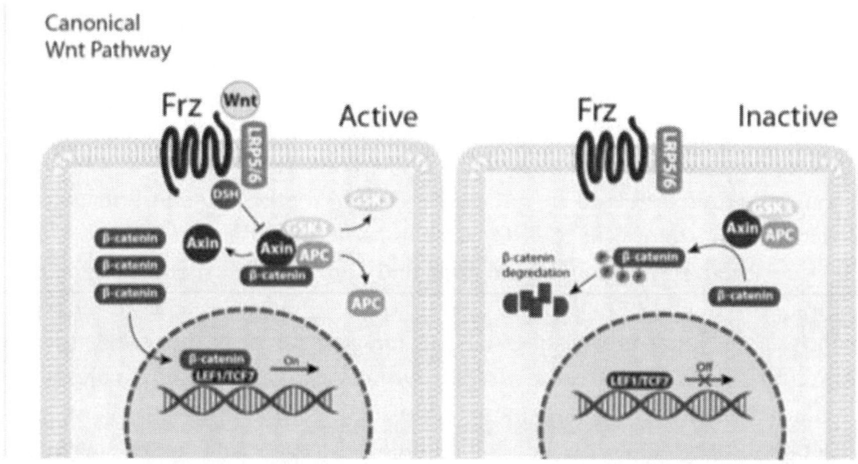

Figure 1. Simplified schematic of Wnt signaling transduction. The canonical Wnt pathway mediates gene expression through intracellular accumulation of β-catenin. Ligand binding to the Frizzled receptor (Frz) and LRP5/6 (lipoprotein receptor-related protein 5 or 6) co-receptor activates Disheveled (DSH), which dissociates the GSK/Axin/APC complex, preventing the phosphorylation of β-catenin, a tag for degradation. Following, increased stability of β-catenin leads to its accumulation in the cytosol, and translocation to the nucleus to activate LEF/TCF (lymphoid enhancer-binding factor/T cell factor) family transcription factors.

Although both canonical and non-canonical pathways activate the intracellular phosphoprotein Disheveled (DSH) directly downstream of FRZ proteins, only in the canonical pathway does DSH pair with transmembrane co-receptors low-density lipoprotein receptor (LRP) 5 and 6. Upon Wnt ligand binding, FRZ activates a DSH and LRP5/6 complex, which in turn disrupts a β-catenin cytosolic degradation complex, which requires the coordinated participation of Axin, GSK3 (glycogen synthase kinase 3), APC (Adenomatosis polyposis coli), and others [7]. The disassembly of this complex prevents GSK3 and Axin from tagging β-catenin for degradation via phosphorylation and promotes intercellular β-catenin stability [1,7]. Subsequential β-catenin accumulation allows for nuclear translocation and interaction with lymphoid enhancer-binding factor/T cell factor (LEF/TCF) family transcription factors [8]. By this mechanism, the canonical Wnt pathway modulates gene expression and is able to mediate MSC lineage determination [9] [see [10] for a more comprehensive review of Wnt signaling transduction].

The β-catenin independent, or non-canonical, pathway has two branches: the planar cell polarity (PCP) pathway and the Ca^{2+} pathway. Both non-canonical pathways share JNK (c-jun NH2-terminal kinase), Cam-KII (calmodulin kinase II), and PKC (protein kinase C), and both play a role in development, cell polarization, motility, and homeostasis [11]. A non-canonical Wnt ligand, such as Wnt5a, can stimulate osteogenic differentiation through the activation of both the PCP and Ca^{2+} pathways [12,13]. The PCP pathway is thought to interact with the cell's cytoskeleton influencing directionality and motility, while the presence of calcium in the cytosol activates calcium dependent enzymes, such as (CaMK)II and PKC [1,14]. Specifically, this calcium independent pathway uses FRZ co-receptors such as Ror2, which has a demonstrated role in osteogenesis both *in vitro* and *in vivo* [15,16].

Importance of Wnt Signaling in Bone Biology

In tissue maintenance and determining cell fate, the relationship between canonical Wnt signaling and bone mass is critical for promoting osteogenesis. Within the past decade, the Wnt/β-catenin signaling pathway's role in maintaining bone homeostasis has become well characterized. By mutating LRP5 upstream of β-catenin, it was shown that loss of function LRP5 mutations resulted in pseudo-glioma syndrome and a low bone mass phenotype; gain of function mutations in LRP5 led to a high bone mass (or osteosclerotic) phenotype [17–19]. Although the interaction between β-catenin and LRP5 has been proposed, only recently have the various roles of β-catenin through canonical Wnt signaling been verified as a regulator of both osteoblast and osteoclast function, in mature cells, as well as in the early stages of osteogenesis and postnatal development [20]. For example, reduced levels of β-catenin in mesenchymal progenitor cells arrests osteoblast development at an early stage, resulting in fetal skeletal defects [20–23]. Analogously, genetically induced β-catenin deficiencies in terminally differentiated osteoblasts can result in impaired maturation and mineralization, along with upregulation of an osteoclast differentiation factor, leading to significant bone resorption [24,25]. Inhibition of Wnt antagonists has also been explored as a treatment method, stimulating β-catenin dependent Wnt pathway activity to induce formation of new bone along with limiting bone resorption. By binding to co-receptors LRP5/6, Wnt antagonists Sclerostin and dickkopf-1 (DKK1) downregulate the accumulation of β-catenin, inhibiting β-catenin's influence on gene expression [26]. Introducing anti-Sclerostin and anti-DKK1, inhibitors of these antagonists, has shown the capacity to stimulate bone formation and increase bone mineral density, and are currently being tested as therapeutic agents for osteoporosis [27,28]. Phase II clinical trials have been completed for anti-Sclerostin using the humanized antibody romosozumab for osteoporotic bone loss [29], and press reports suggest that phase III trials are underway [30]. Likewise, phase II trials are underway using anti-DKK1 for multiple myeloma (31), during which anabolic bone activity was observed [32]. Small molecules can be used to the same end. A recent screening of over 2000 small molecules targeting the Wnt pathway activation is available for review [33]. Targeting β-catenin stability, GSK3 enzymatic activity, and LRP5/6 availability are possible routes to induce β-catenin nuclear translocation.

Brief Review of Hedgehog Signaling

In vertebrates, there are three homologues of the Drosophila Hedgehog (HH) protein: Sonic Hedgehog (SHH), Indian Hedgehog (IHH) and Desert Hedgehog (DHH). Although the role of DHH is limited to testis organogenesis [34], SHH and IHH are essential for proper embryogenesis. In skeletogenesis, SHH is involved in patterning the appendicular, axial, and facial skeleton, in addition to modulating vertebrate organogenesis [35,36]. IHH is closely related to SHH through gene duplication, and regulates chondrogenesis and endochondral bone formation [37]. The importance of HH signaling is exemplified with genetic mutations, which can lead to severe abnormalities, with holoprosencephaly being one of the most prevalent [38].

The HH pathway, conserved between the three homologs, becomes active through an autocatalytic cleavage from a 45kD to a 19kD protein, where the other protein has no known biologically relevance. Then, it is further processed by cholesterol addition to the C-terminus and palmitoyl addition to the N-terminus, increasing its hydrophobicity and membrane solubility [37,39] (Figure 2). This ligand leaves the cell via the Dispatched transmembrane protein to participate in paracrine signaling. The active HH protein interacts with the sterol sensing region of the 12-pass transmembrane receptor Patched (PTCH) on the target cell membrane. PTCH is a negative regulator of nearby seven pass transmembrane protein, Smoothened (SMO), and is internalized and directed to endosomal degradation at higher rates in the absence of SMO and in the presence of Wnt ligands [40]. SMO activity believed to be HH ligand independent, thus, PTCH is necessary for controlling HH activity. SMO leads to activation of downstream target genes via the transcription factor Gli (glioblastoma gene product) family: Gli1, Gli2, and Gli3. Gli1 expression has been a useful and reliable marker of HH signaling activity, acting as a target gene for the HH pathway [41,42].

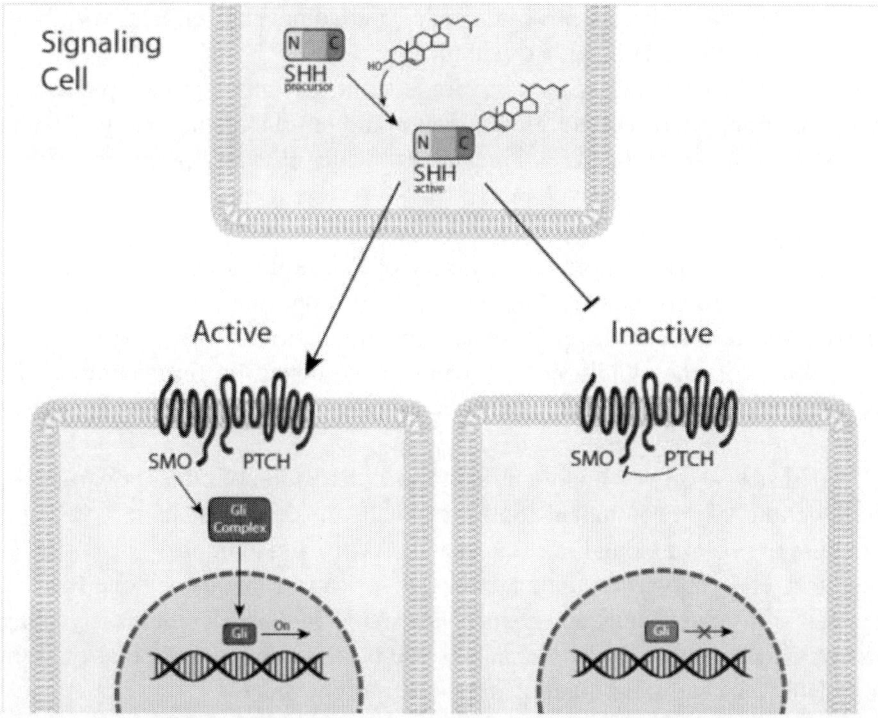

Figure 2. Simplified schematic of Hedgehog signaling transduction. Hedgehog (HH) precursors are post-translationally modified to include a cholesterol group, crucial to its binding to the Patched (PTCH) receptor on the receiving cell. Ligand binding to PTCH disrupts its inhibition of Smoothened (SMO), leading to the activation of Gli transcription factors.

Although it has not been documented completely, HH signaling may function primarily through the use of Gli transcription factors. As well, it is believed that HH signaling induces lineage commitment in MSC differentiation through Gli transcription factors [43].

Importance of Hedgehog Signaling in Bone Biology

In development as well as tissue maintenance, HH proteins play a crucial role in osteogenic linage commitment and differentiation, among a variety of other functions. In fact, SHH regulates osteoprogenitor cell differentiation by inducing osteogenic differentiation and antagonizing adipogenic differentiation in multiple mesenchymal cell types [44]. For example, exogenous N-terminal SHH was added to adipose derived stromal cells (ASC) to enhance osteoblast differentiation at the cost of adipogenesis, both *in vitro* and *in vivo* (45). Similar pro-osteogenic, anti-adipogenic effects have been observed with the IHH ligand as well [46].

The HH signaling pathway, important for mesodermal progenitor differentiation, interacts with growth factor and developmental pathways, and has roles in embryogenesis including mediating proliferations, tissue patterning, and organ development [47–49]. Ossification throughout the developing skeleton is greatly impaired in animals with disrupted SHH and IHH signaling. For example, the majority of *Shh* null mutant mice develop a cleft palate [50]. Similarly, *Ihh* null mice demonstrate severely shortened limbs (due to a defect in endochondral ossification) as well as a defect in ossification of the skull vault (owing to a defect in intramembranous ossification) [51]. Additionally, both *Ihh* and *Shh* null mice die in utero or at birth.

HH has also proved important in the vascularization of bone. In particular, introduction of recombinant SHH resulted in development of vascular structure of potential long bone transplants *in vitro* and to improve perfusion *in vivo* [52]. HH pathway is a potential target for cancer therapies, bone fracture healing and tissue engineering since it is integrated into complex signaling pathway coordinating functions such as cell proliferation, tissue polarity, stem cell maintenance, differentiation, and tissue morphogenesis.

Brief Review of Notch Signaling

Notch signaling plays a key role in cell proliferation and differentiation during embryonic development and throughout adult life. This pathway utilizes cell-cell interactions to mediate changes in gene expression, provoking an analogous signaling cascade in neighboring cells (Figure 3). Notch participates in numerous developmental mechanisms including angiogenesis, neurogenesis, myogenesis, and osteogenesis, among others [53]. In mammals, there are four single pass transmembrane Notch receptors, Notch1-4, that bind to five DSL (Delta/Serrate/LAG-2) family ligands on the membrane of the signaling cells: Delta-like (DLL) 1, DLL3, DLL4, Jagged1 and Jagged2 [54]. Notch receptors have a large extracellular domain, a transmembrane domain, and a smaller intercellular domain attached non-covalently. The extracellular domain, which activates upon ligand binding, contains approximately 30 EGF (epidermal growth factor) repeats, which have the propensity to bind to calcium, affecting ligand binding affinity and structure [55]. Upon activation, the receptor undergoes a sequential cleavage, freeing the intercellular domain from the transmembrane and extracellular domains, allowing it to localize in the nucleus to mediate transcriptional activity.

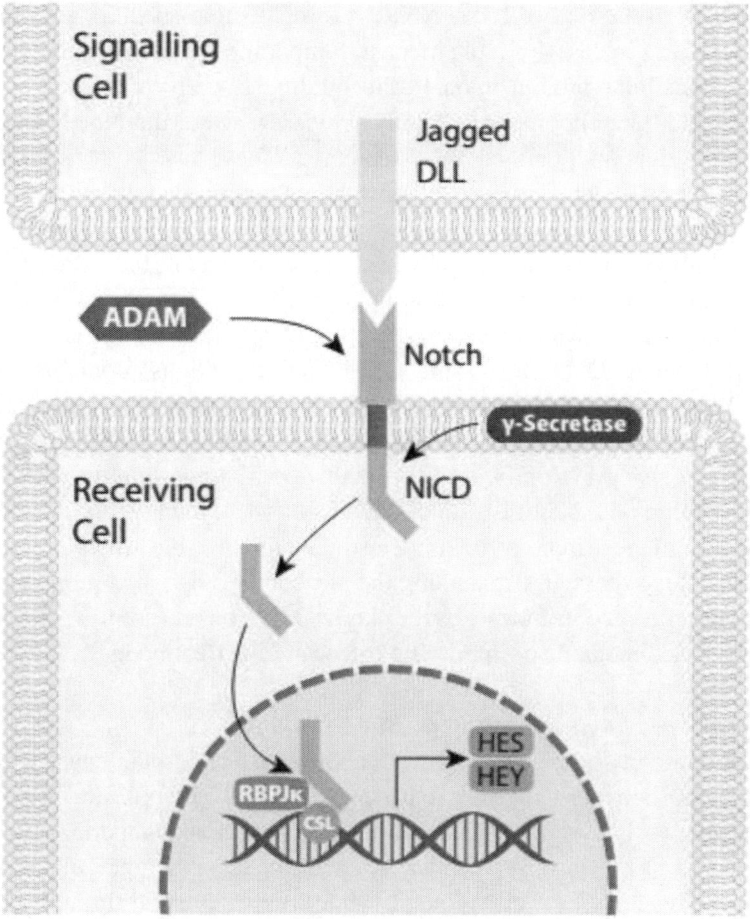

Figure 3. Simplified schematic of Notch signaling transduction. Binding to a Jagged or DLL (Delta-Like) protein ligand on the surface of the signaling cell induces the proteolytic cleavage of the Notch receptor. ADAM (A distintegrin and metalloprotease) family proteases cleave the extracellular domain, while γ-secretase liberates the Notch receptor intracellular domain (NICD) to bind to CSL (CBF1/RBPJ-kappa/Su (H)/Lag1) family of DNA-binding proteins activate HES (Hairy Enhancer of Split) and HEY (Hes related with YRPW motif)

There are many more molecules integral to these mechanisms which can be a source of dysfunction as a result of mutations, or be used as targets for chemotherapeutic drugs. The extracellular domain of Notch family receptors have a negative regulatory region (NRR), containing cysteine rich repeats and a heterodimerization domain, which prevent proteolytic cleavage in the absence of a ligand [55]. However, mutations or viral integration have shown to reduce the specificity of the NNR, leading to non-specific activation of Notch, resulting in cases of leukemia and lymphoma [55]. The initial cleavage of the extracellular protein upon ligand binding is performed by ADAM (a disintegrin and metalloprotease) family proteases, while the Notch receptor's intercellular domain liberated by γ-secretase. These two enzymes serve as potential points of interest in regulating the activation or inhibition of Notch signaling.

In addition to activating enzymes, other potential therapeutic targets include known Notch ligands. These ligands, typically membrane proteins on adjacent cells, are characterized by their DSL domains, having special EGF repeats known as DOS (Delta and OSM-11-like proteins) domains, and by having EGF repeats with the potential to bind calcium [55]. Alternatively, many non-canonical Notch ligands have been described. Although it seems that they are less prevalent within this pathway, it is possible that the lack of characterization and identification of unconventional Notch ligands has caused clinicians and researchers to underestimate their role in Notch-related pathology. Regardless, understanding the mechanisms by which non-canonical ligands function contributes to the knowledge base essential for Notch signaling-based methods of improving osteosarcoma treatments.

Importance of Notch Signaling in Bone Biology

Important in both development and stem cell maintenance, Notch signaling participates in the balance between osteoblastogenesis and osteoclastogenesis, which dictates the rate of bone mineralization and resorption. It has been observed that osteoclastogenesis is upregulated by the activation between DLL1 and Notch2, while it is suppressed through Jagged1 binding Notch1 [56]. Conversely, activated Notch proteins can induce osteogenic differentiation. The overexpression of Notch receptor intracellular domain (NICD) protein was shown to interact with BMP2 transcription factors Smad1 and induce osteogenic differentiation of vascular smooth muscle cells [57]. Canonical Notch target genes of the NICD protein are *HES* (Hairy Enhancer of Split) and *HEY* (Hes related with YRPW motif), encoding 7 and 3 proteins respectively. Upon arrival to the nucleus, NICD binds to a promoter complex from the CSL protein family, RBPJ (recombining binding protein suppressor of hairless) to activate HES and HEY gene expression [58]. Notch's relationship with these two genes is important in skeletal development (59). In fact, it was shown that Hey1 and NICD bind together to prevent Runt related transcription factor-2 (Runx2) from inducing osteoblast differentiation in mesenchymal progenitor cells [60]. Deregowski *et al.* observed that NICD overexpression blocked the pro-osteogenic effects of BMP2 or Wnt3a, but silencing HES1 with siRNA can negate NICD's influence, as observed in the bone marrow stromal cell line ST-2 [61]. BMP signaling transduction, specifically SMAD 1/5/8, were not affected by NICD expression. However, the β-catenin Wnt pathway was inhibited. Wnt inhibition is not surprising, as HES1 is known to recruit GRO (Groucho) and other repressors of Wnt transcriptional activator LEF1 [62], and GRO silencing alone by siRNA did not inhibit Wnt [61].

Notch is also known to balance cell differentiation and proliferation. Expression of micro-RNA 34c has been shown to target and downregulate expression of Notch 1 and 2, leading to reduced osteogenic differentiation [63]. Likewise, micro-RNA 34c induces osteoclastogenesis and osteoblast progenitors' proliferation [63]. As these Notch genes and proteins are essential in normal bone formation and development, identification of small molecules, proteins, nucleic acids, or other drugs and methods to manipulate their interactions and phenotypes may lead to improvements in Notch-based osteosarcoma treatments, as well as treating osteoporotic and developmental pathology.

Wnt, Hedgehog, and Notch Signaling in Osteosarcoma and Treatment

Importance of Wnt Signaling in Osteosarcoma

The aberrant activation of the canonical Wnt signaling in oncogenesis is relatively well documented [64]. Out of 44 high grade osteosarcoma patients' biopsies surveyed for mRNA, Hoang et al. detected LRP5 expression in 50% of samples, and found a correlation between LRP5 expression and β-catenin accumulation [65]. Likewise, Wnt inhibitory factor 1 (WIF-1) mRNA expression was significantly decreased in numerous osteosarcoma cell lines in comparison to normal human osteoblasts, which was attributed to WIF-1 promoter hypermethylation [66]. Dieudonné et al. reported that levels of pro-apoptotic membrane proteoglycan syndecan-2 are lower in osteosarcoma cells, and that LEF/TCF transcription factors are negative regulators of the Wnt pathway [67]. Similarly, TWIST, a basic helix-loop-helix transcription factor, is suspected to be a negative regulator of the canonical Wnt pathway, and is typically expressed in low levels in osteosarcoma [68]. Inducing overexpression of TWIST in vitro (in Saos-2 and MG-63 lines) led to a decrease in β-catenin, while knockout of TWIST with RNA interference

(RNAi) lead to increased levels of β-catenin [68]. Manipulation of TWIST expression in Saos-2 osteosarcoma cells also led to altered sensitivity to cisplatin induced apoptosis, where TWIST RNAi increased resistance to apoptosis, whereas TWIST overexpression lead to increased susceptibility to apoptosis [68]. Only one study has found inactive Wnt signaling in osteosarcoma to our knowledge: Cai et al. observed the lack nuclear β-catenin in 90% of over 50 osteosarcoma biopsies stained, and increased mRNA levels of the Wnt inhibitor DKK1 in vitro (observed in MG-63, SJSA-1, and HOS cell lines) [69]. However, abundant evidence points towards an active Wnt signaling pathway in osteosarcomas [70].

Thus, investigated treatment methods commonly target Wnt machinery and regulators to inhibit and downregulate Wnt signaling activity [71]. To reduce β-catenin dependent Wnt pathway activity, Brun et al. used in vitro RNA interference (RNAi) in the osteosarcoma cell line K7M2 to knockdown a widely used transcription factor FHL2 (four and a half LIM domains protein 2). This was found to reduce proliferation and caspase activity in the presence and absence of Wnt ligand, Wnt3a [72]. It is known that activating the Wnt pathway can inhibit apoptosis [73], which can be counterproductive in combination with chemotherapeutic drugs [72]. For example, small molecule niclosamide was effective in degrading LRP6 to disable ligand binding in prostate and breast cancer cells, which inactivated Wnt, inhibited proliferation, and induced apoptosis [74]. As well, Jin et al. utilized sulfated polysaccharide degraded iota-carrageenan both inactivate the β-catenin dependent Wnt pathway, associated with induction of apoptosis of osteosarcoma cells [75]. Another small molecule, Wnt antagonist PKF115-584, was used to restore the cytotoxicity of common chemotherapeutic doxorubicin in resistant U2OS cells, likely through the decrease of TCF transcriptional activity and rescue of syndecan-2 expression levels [76]. Conversely, the resistance to apoptosis of osteosarcoma cell line MG-63 upon treatment with doxorubicin was shown to be enhanced by siRNA knockdown of β-catenin [77]. Although this reduced sensitivity does not necessarily correlate with the activity or inhibition of the Wnt pathway, it brought to light a previously unknown interaction of β-catenin with NF-κβ (nuclear factor kappa-light-chain-enhancer of activated B cells) signaling in apoptosis [77]. Thus, whether Wnt inhibition can directly induce apoptosis is not well documented, and if so, the precise mechanisms remain unknown. Regardless, previous research has suggested that Wnt pathway inhibition has anti-proliferative, pro-apoptotic effects in osteosarcoma cells.

Importance of Hedgehog Signaling in Osteosarcoma

Inappropriate activation of the HH pathway is thought to lead to tumorigenesis and acceleration of tumor growth in a variety of cancers and tissues. Constitutive activation of Hedgehog signaling has been observed in various tumor types, including basal cell carcinoma [78], and osteochondroma [79], among others. For this reason, HH signaling is being actively explored as a target of pharmaceutical treatments of osteosarcomas [80]. Three methods have been proposed by which HH signaling leads to tumor formation [81]. Ligand independent HH activation can occur through the mutation of PTCH or SMO, allowing SMO to remain active. Second, autocrine or juxtacrine HH activation can occur through ectopic Gli or PTCH expression and through elevated expression of HH ligands. Thirdly, paracrine, ligand dependent HH activation can occur through ectopic expression or mutations in HH machinery transferred from the stroma supporting the tumor. In response to Wnt activating GIN (GSK3β inhibitor), there was no significant induction of HH signaling detected by Gli-luciferase reporter activity, although GSK3β is thought to participate in HH, suggesting that Wnt is downstream from HH [69].

In human osteosarcoma biopsies and in osteosarcoma cell lines (including HOS, 143B, MG63, and Saos-2 cells), HH ligands (*IHH, SHH*), receptors (*SMO, PTCH1*), and downstream transcriptional activators, (*Gli1, Gli2*), have shown increased mRNA expression, as compared to normal osteoblasts [82]. *In vitro* siRNA knockdown of *Gli2* resulted in decreased proliferation and decreased cell viability, as well as increased sensitivity to chemotherapeutic drugs, in osteosarcoma cell lines U2OS and KHOS [83]. In line with these findings, SMO inhibition using both small hairpin RNA (shRNA) interference and cyclopamine, a steroidal veratrum alkaloid, slowed proliferation, reduced *m*RNA transcripts of cell cycle transcription factors, and hindered colony formation in a soft agar assay *in vitro* using 143B and HOS lines [82]. These authors went on to show that *in vivo* growth and proliferation of transplanted 143B cells was hampered by *SMO* shRNA when placed in nude mice. This was observed by tumor burden and a significant reduction in Ki67 (30% reduction in *SMO* shRNA tumors) [82]. In aggregate, these preclinical studies suggest that methods of inhibiting HH signaling, including RNAi and small molecule inhibition, may have future therapeutic promise for osteosarcoma. However, the HH antagonist cyclopamine may have limited therapeutic potential due to side effects of skin ulceration and teratogenic effects [84,85].

In contrast to cyclopamine, arsenic trioxide (ATO), an FDA approved drug for leukemia (Trisenox®), has shown promise in both *in vitro* and *in vivo* studies in osteosarcoma. ATO likely induces apoptosis through oxidative stress, since treatment increases intracellular reactive oxygen species levels and ATO's therapeutic effect can be reduced when combined with antioxidant n-acetyl cysteine [86]. Upon *in vitro* treatment of p53 deficient MG63 cells, a dose dependent apoptotic response to ATO was observed [86]. To increase dose length, consistency, and efficiency, Li *et al.* explored time-dependent drug delivery of ATO, and used magnetic ATO nanoparticles encapsulated in poly(lactic acid) (PLA) to achieve inhibition of tumor growth similar to using ATO alone [87]. Similarly, Nakamura *et al.* was able to downregulate the overexpression of HH markers *Gli1, Gli2*, and *PTCH*, characteristic of osteosarcoma cell lines (143B, Saos-2, U2OS, and HsOs), by treatment with ATO [88]. As well, *in vivo* ATO injections in immune-deficient mice with 143B xenografts significantly reduced tumor size by about 300% after eight weeks [89]. These studies suggest that the success of ATO in osteosarcoma treatment stems from its ability to shut down the HH pathway via Gli1 / Gli2 silencing. Other therapeutic morphological changes in osteosarcoma cells resulting from ATO include induction of apoptosis and remodeling of the extracellular matrix, which reported affects these cells performance in motility, invasion, and cell adhesion assays, which are properties relevant to metastasis [90]. Overall, blocking the HH signaling pathway through targeting cell surface receptors PTCH or SMO results in reduced Gli1 / Gli2 transcriptional activity, hindering osteosarcoma growth and inducing apoptosis. Further development of specific and safe pharmaceuticals targeting the HH signaling pathway may yield to improved therapies for osteosarcoma.

Importance of Notch Signaling in Osteosarcoma

Similar to the Wnt and HH pathways, inhibition of canonical Notch signaling may switch gene expression towards a phenotype that is more susceptible to becoming cancerous, that is, reverting towards a more embryonic, proliferative phenotype. Upregulations of various components of Notch signaling have been observed in human osteosarcoma samples, including *Jagged1, Notch1, Notch2, HES1*, and *HEY2*. These findings have also been recapitulated in mouse osteosarcoma driven by *TP53* mutations [91,92]. Inhibition of Notch signaling was achieved *in vitro* via γ-secretase inhibitor XX (GSIX), which prevents NICD translocation, in HOS and 143B cell lines. This inhibition resulted in a significant reduction of *HES1* mRNA, retarding *in vitro* tumor growth and increasing the percentage of cells arrested in the G1 phase [92]. In fact, *HES1* mRNA expression has been shown to have an inverse correlation with survival in a 16 patient study [94]. However, GSIX did not significantly contribute to additional cell death [92]. *In vivo*, Tanaka *et al.* also used GSIX to significantly reduce proliferation (Ki67 index) and slowed tumor growth in a nude mouse model with injected 143B cells [92]. Likewise, use of the small molecule Curcumin alone or in combination with *Notch1* siRNA inhibited Notch signaling, and reduced osteosarcoma cell proliferation and cell invasion *in vitro* [93].

Additional Notch components known to be upregulated in osteosarcoma have been targeted to repress osteosarcoma growth and metastasis. Small molecule inhibitors of the enzyme complex histone deacetylase MS-275 and trichostatin, currently used to treat seizures and proposed for cancer therapy, have shown pro-apoptotic effects in osteosarcoma cell lines and tumor size regression in mice with osteosarcoma lung metastasis [95,96]. However, one such histone diacetylase inhibitor Valproate, was show to increase *HES1* expression in non-invasive Saos-2 cells at clinically relevant dosages, leading to a paradoxical 250-fold increase in invasion in a matrigel assay [94]. To confirm HES1 expression was correlated to invasiveness and metastatic potential, invasive OS-187 cells were transfected with a dominant negative form of the Mastermind-like gene MAM (dnMAM), which inhibited HES1, leading to an over 50% reduction in matrigel invasion. Thus, *HES1* upregulation plays a major role in osteosarcoma cell invasion / metastasis, and may be the primary pathway blocked by γ-secretase inhibitors, mentioned above. Although *HES1* expression is reduced downstream from γ-secretase inhibition [94], other methods of *HES1* downregulation deserve focus. Likewise, overexpression of NICD1 inhibitor *Deltex1*, was shown to reduce invasion of the OS 187 cell line *in vitro* [97]. Interestingly, this effect was reversed by *HES1* overexpression. In fact, HES1 is known to repress expression of *Deltex1*. This interaction is believed to occur through HES1's recruitment of co-repressor GRO and other co-repressors. In fact, a HES1 binding site within the promoter region of *Deltex1* has been identified, confirming this relationship [97]. Although expression of *Deltex1* is the likely consequence of downregulation of HES1 after γ-secretase inhibition, increasing Deltex1 levels in itself may be an alternate route to inhibition of Notch signaling. However, the most prevalent Notch-based osteosarcoma treatments currently being pursued target γ-secretase.

Many clinical trials inhibiting Notch are underway, primarily for pancreatic tumors [98]. In fact, combinatorial Phase Ib/II clinical trials using small molecule inhibition of γ-secretase, downregulating Notch signaling, with SMO inhibitor vismodegib, downregulating HH transcription factors Gli1 and Gli2, to treat any type of advanced or metastatic sarcoma began in 2010, and has been ongoing through 2013 [99]. Although the latter option of targeting γ-secretase may later become a clinically relevant osteosarcoma treatment, the success of supplementing Curcumin, and possibly chemotherapeutic drugs, with RNAi showing potential as well.

CONCLUSION

Wnt, Hedgehog and Notch signaling are essential for development, tissue morphogenesis, cell proliferation, and differentiation. Improper function or regulation of these pathways is antecedent to a variety of diseases, including osteosarcoma. In designing therapeutics, manipulation of these pathways has shown potential for success to treat not only mesenchymal malignancies (sarcomas), but also epithelial, neural, and hematopoietic malignancies. However, there is an incomplete understanding of the key mechanisms by which these pathways become deleterious.

As mentioned previously, a single genetic event leading to sarcomagenesis is not usually identifiable. For example, interconnectivity of Wnt and Notch signaling was highlighted in one study showing that exposing osteosarcoma cell lines to a specific Wnt ligand, Wnt10b, activated Notch signaling while another, Wnt3a, did not [100]. Thus, documenting the interconnectivity and regulation of these pathways, all guiding proliferation, apoptosis, and differentiation, requires further focus. Nevertheless, we have presented a sample of the varying degrees of success achieved by targeting Wnt, Hedgehog, and Notch machinery, slowing tumor growth, inducing apoptosis of osteosarcomas, and preventing disease progression. Studies to date suggest that therapies designed to inhibit Wnt, Hedgehog, and/or Notch signaling may hold success in treating osteosarcoma. Such therapies may also demonstrate benefit for malignancies of other origins as well as bone diseases, including osteoporotic bone loss.

ACKNOWLEDGEMENTS, FUNDING, AND CONFLICTS OF INTEREST

MM is supported by NIH MARC T34 GM008563.

REFERENCES

[1] Rao TP, Kühl M. An updated overview on Wnt signaling pathways: a prelude for more. *Circ. Res*. 2010 Jun 25;106(12):1798–806.

[2] Berwick DC, Harvey K. The importance of Wnt signalling for neurodegeneration in Parkinson's disease. *Biochem. Soc. Trans.* 2012 Oct 1;40(5):1123–8.

[3] Chen J, Stahl A, Krah NM, Seaward MR, Dennison RJ, Sapieha P, et al. Wnt signaling mediates pathological vascular growth in proliferative retinopathy. *Circulation.* 2011 Oct 25;124(17):1871–81.

[4] Maeda K, Takahashi N, Kobayashi Y. Roles of Wnt signals in bone resorption during physiological and pathological states. *J. Mol. Med. Berl. Ger*. 2013 Jan;91(1):15–23.

[5] Morin PJ, Sparks AB, Korinek V, Barker N, Clevers H, Vogelstein B, et al. Activation of beta-catenin-Tcf signaling in colon cancer by mutations in beta-catenin or APC. *Science*. 1997 Mar 21;275(5307):1787–90.

[6] Niehrs C. The complex world of WNT receptor signalling. *Nat. Rev. Mol. Cell Biol.* 2012 Dec;13(12):767–79.

[7] MacDonald BT, Tamai K, He X. Wnt/beta-catenin signaling: components, mechanisms, and diseases. *Dev. Cell.* 2009 Jul;17(1):9–26.

[8] Pandur P, Maurus D, Kühl M. Increasingly complex: new players enter the Wnt signaling network. *BioEssays News Rev. Mol. Cell Dev. Biol.* 2002 Oct;24(10):881–4.

[9] Etheridge SL, Spencer GJ, Heath DJ, Genever PG. Expression profiling and functional analysis of wnt signaling mechanisms in mesenchymal stem cells. *Stem Cells Dayt Ohio.* 2004;22(5):849–60.

[10] Kim W, Kim M, Jho E. Wnt/β-catenin signalling: from plasma membrane to nucleus. *Biochem. J.* 2013 Feb 15;450(1):9–21.

[11] Davis LA, Zur Nieden NI. Mesodermal fate decisions of a stem cell: the Wnt switch. *Cell Mol. Life Sci. CMLS.* 2008 Sep;65(17):2658–74.

[12] Boland GM, Perkins G, Hall DJ, Tuan RS. Wnt 3a promotes proliferation and suppresses osteogenic differentiation of adult human mesenchymal stem cells. *J. Cell Biochem*. 2004 Dec 15;93(6):1210–30.

[13] Kobayashi Y. [Roles of Wnt signaling in bone metabolism]. *Clin. Calcium.* 2012 Nov;22(11):1701–6.

[14] Komiya Y, Habas R. Wnt signal transduction pathways. *Organogenesis.* 2008 Apr;4(2):68–75.

[15] Liu Y, Ross JF, Bodine PVN, Billiard J. Homodimerization of Ror2 tyrosine kinase receptor induces 14-3-3(beta) phosphorylation and

promotes osteoblast differentiation and bone formation. *Mol. Endocrinol. Baltim. Md.* 2007 Dec;21(12):3050–61.

[16] Liu Y, Bhat RA, Seestaller-Wehr LM, Fukayama S, Mangine A, Moran RA, et al. The orphan receptor tyrosine kinase Ror2 promotes osteoblast differentiation and enhances ex vivo bone formation. *Mol. Endocrinol. Baltim. Md.* 2007 Feb;21(2):376–87.

[17] Boyden LM, Mao J, Belsky J, Mitzner L, Farhi A, Mitnick MA, et al. High bone density due to a mutation in LDL-receptor-related protein 5. *N. Engl. J. Med.* 2002 May 16;346(20):1513–21.

[18] Gong Y, Slee RB, Fukai N, Rawadi G, Roman-Roman S, Reginato AM, et al. LDL receptor-related protein 5 (LRP5) affects bone accrual and eye development. *Cell.* 2001 Nov 16;107(4):513–23.

[19] Little RD, Carulli JP, Del Mastro RG, Dupuis J, Osborne M, Folz C, et al. A mutation in the LDL receptor-related protein 5 gene results in the autosomal dominant high-bone-mass trait. *Am. J. Hum. Genet.* 2002 Jan;70(1):11–9.

[20] Chen J, Long F. β-catenin promotes bone formation and suppresses bone resorption in postnatal growing mice. *J. Bone Miner Res. Off J. Am. Soc. Bone Miner Res.* 2013 May;28(5):1160–9.

[21] Day TF, Guo X, Garrett-Beal L, Yang Y. Wnt/β-Catenin Signaling in Mesenchymal Progenitors Controls Osteoblast and Chondrocyte Differentiation during Vertebrate Skeletogenesis. *Dev. Cell.* 2005 May 1;8(5):739–50.

[22] Hill TP, Später D, Taketo MM, Birchmeier W, Hartmann C. Canonical Wnt/beta-catenin signaling prevents osteoblasts from differentiating into chondrocytes. *Dev. Cell.* 2005 May;8(5):727–38.

[23] Hu H, Hilton MJ, Tu X, Yu K, Ornitz DM, Long F. Sequential roles of Hedgehog and Wnt signaling in osteoblast development. *Dev. Camb. Engl.* 2005 Jan;132(1):49–60.

[24] Glass DA 2nd, Bialek P, Ahn JD, Starbuck M, Patel MS, Clevers H, et al. Canonical Wnt signaling in differentiated osteoblasts controls osteoclast differentiation. *Dev. Cell.* 2005 May;8(5):751–64.

[25] Holmen SL, Zylstra CR, Mukherjee A, Sigler RE, Faugere M-C, Bouxsein ML, et al. Essential role of beta-catenin in postnatal bone acquisition. *J. Biol. Chem.* 2005 Jun 3;280(22):21162–8.

[26] Gatti D, Viapiana O, Fracassi E, Idolazzi L, Dartizio C, Povino MR, et al. Sclerostin and DKK1 in postmenopausal osteoporosis treated with denosumab. *J. Bone Miner Res. Off J. Am. Soc. Bone Miner Res.* 2012 Nov;27(11):2259–63.

[27] Lim V, Clarke BL. New therapeutic targets for osteoporosis: beyond denosumab. *Maturitas.* 2012 Nov;73(3):269–72.

[28] Padhi D, Jang G, Stouch B, Fang L, Posvar E. Single-dose, placebo-controlled, randomized study of AMG 785, a sclerostin monoclonal antibody. *J. Bone Miner Res. Off J. Am Soc. Bone Miner Res.* 2011 Jan;26(1):19–26.

[29] National Institutes of Health; Amgen A. Study To Assess Fracture Healing With Sclerostin Antibody [Internet]. Bethesda (MD): National Library of Medicine (US).; 2013. Report No.: NCT01081678. Available from: http://clinicaltrials.gov/ct2/show/record/NCT01081678 NLM

[30] Grogan K. UCB and Amgen bone-building drug goes into Phase III. Pharma Online [Internet]. 2012 Apr 4 [cited 2013 Jun 20]; Available from: http://www.pharmatimes.com/article/12-04-04/UCB_and_ Amgen _bone-building_drug_goes_into_Phase_III.aspx

[31] National Institutes of Health; Novartis. Study of BHQ880 in Patients With High Risk Smoldering Multiple Myeloma [Internet]. Bethesda (MD): National Library of Medicine (US).; 2013. Report No.: NCT01302886. Available from: http://clinicaltrials.gov/ct2/ show/study/ NCT01302886

[32] Munshi NC et al. Early Evidence of Anabolic Bone Activity of BHQ880, a Fully Human Anti-DKK1 Neutralizing Antibody: Results of a Phase 2 Study in Previously Untreated Patients with Smoldering Multiple Myeloma At Risk for Progression [Internet]. Atlanta, GA; 2012 [cited 2013 Jun 20]. Available from: https://ash.confex.com/ash/2012/ webprogram/Paper48568.html

[33] Verkaar F, van der Stelt M, Blankesteijn WM, van der Doelen AA, Zaman GJR. Discovery of Novel Small Molecule Activators of β-Catenin Signaling. PLoS ONE. 2011 Apr 29;6(4):e19185.

[34] Yao HH-C, Whoriskey W, Capel B. Desert Hedgehog/Patched 1 signaling specifies fetal Leydig cell fate in testis organogenesis. *Genes Dev.* 2002 Jun 1;16(11):1433–40.

[35] Riddle RD, Johnson RL, Laufer E, Tabin C. Sonic hedgehog mediates the polarizing activity of the ZPA. *Cell.* 1993 Dec 31;75(7):1401–16.

[36] Ruat M, Roudaut H, Ferent J, Traiffort E. Hedgehog trafficking, cilia and brain functions. *Differentiation.* 2012 Feb;83(2):S97–S104.

[37] Bitgood MJ, McMahon AP. Hedgehog and Bmp genes are coexpressed at many diverse sites of cell-cell interaction in the mouse embryo. *Dev. Biol.* 1995 Nov;172(1):126–38.

[38] Nanni L, Ming JE, Bocian M, Steinhaus K, Bianchi DW, Die-Smulders C, et al. The mutational spectrum of the sonic hedgehog gene in holoprosencephaly: SHH mutations cause a significant proportion of autosomal dominant holoprosencephaly. *Hum. Mol. Genet.* 1999 Dec;8(13):2479–88.

[39] Chamoun Z, Mann RK, Nellen D, von Kessler DP, Bellotto M, Beachy PA, et al. Skinny hedgehog, an acyltransferase required for palmitoylation and activity of the hedgehog signal. *Science.* 2001 Sep 14;293(5537):2080–4.

[40] Incardona JP, Gruenberg J, Roelink H. Sonic hedgehog induces the segregation of patched and smoothened in endosomes. *Curr. Biol. CB.* 2002 Jun 25;12(12):983–95.

[41] Hooper JE, Scott MP. Communicating with Hedgehogs. Nat Rev Mol Cell Biol. 2005 Apr;6(4):306–17.

[42] Ruiz i Altaba A, Mas C, Stecca B. The Gli code: an information nexus regulating cell fate, stemness and cancer. *Trends Cell Biol.* 2007 Sep;17(9):438–47.

[43] Hojo H, Ohba S, Taniguchi K, Shirai M, Yano F, Saito T, et al. Hedgehog-Gli activators direct osteo-chondrogenic function of bone morphogenetic protein toward osteogenesis in the perichondrium. *J. Biol. Chem.* 2013 Apr 5;288(14):9924–32.

[44] James AW, Leucht P, Levi B, Carre AL, Xu Y, Helms JA, et al. Sonic Hedgehog influences the balance of osteogenesis and adipogenesis in mouse adipose-derived stromal cells. *Tissue Eng.* Part A. 2010 Aug;16(8):2605–16.

[45] James AW, Pang S, Askarinam A, Corselli M, Zara JN, Goyal R, et al. Additive effects of sonic hedgehog and Nell-1 signaling in osteogenic versus adipogenic differentiation of human adipose-derived stromal cells. *Stem Cells Dev.* 2012 Aug 10;21(12):2170–8.

[46] Day TF, Yang Y. Wnt and hedgehog signaling pathways in bone development. *J. Bone Joint Surg. Am.* 2008 Feb;90 Suppl 1:19–24.

[47] Ingham PW, McMahon AP. Hedgehog signaling in animal development: paradigms and principles. *Genes Dev.* 2001 Dec 1;15(23):3059–87.

[48] Murray JC, Schutte BC. Cleft palate: players, pathways, and pursuits. *J. Clin Invest.* 2004 Jun 15;113(12):1676–8.

[49] Pan A, Chang L, Nguyen A, James AW. A review of hedgehog signaling in cranial bone development. *Front Physiol.* 2013;4:61.

[50] Rice R, Spencer-Dene B, Connor EC, Gritli-Linde A, McMahon AP, Dickson C, et al. Disruption of Fgf10/Fgfr2b-coordinated epithelial-

mesenchymal interactions causes cleft palate. *J. Clin. Invest.* 2004 Jun;113(12):1692–700.

[51] Lenton K, James AW, Manu A, Brugmann SA, Birker D, Nelson ER, et al. Indian hedgehog positively regulates calvarial ossification and modulates bone morphogenetic protein signaling. *Genes* New York N 2000. 2011 Oct;49(10):784–96.

[52] Rivron NC, Raiss CC, Liu J, Nandakumar A, Sticht C, Gretz N, et al. Sonic Hedgehog-activated engineered blood vessels enhance bone tissue formation. *Proc. Natl. Acad. Sci. U S A.* 2012 Mar 20;109(12):4413–8.

[53] Artavanis-Tsakonas S, Rand MD, Lake RJ. Notch signaling: cell fate control and signal integration in development. *Science.* 1999 Apr 30;284(5415):770–6.

[54] Radtke F, MacDonald HR, Tacchini-Cottier F. Regulation of innate and adaptive immunity by *Notch. Nat. Rev. Immunol.* 2013 Jun;13(6):427–37.

[55] Kopan R, Ilagan MXG. The canonical Notch signaling pathway: unfolding the activation mechanism. *Cell.* 2009 Apr 17;137(2):216–33.

[56] Sekine C, Koyanagi A, Koyama N, Hozumi K, Chiba S, Yagita H. Differential regulation of osteoclastogenesis by Notch2/Delta-like 1 and Notch1/Jagged1 axes. *Arthritis Res. Ther.* 2012;14(2):R45.

[57] Shimizu T, Tanaka T, Iso T, Matsui H, Ooyama Y, Kawai-Kowase K, et al. Notch signaling pathway enhances bone morphogenetic protein 2 (BMP2) responsiveness of Msx2 gene to induce osteogenic differentiation and mineralization of vascular smooth muscle cells. *J. Biol Chem.* 2011 May 27;286(21):19138–48.

[58] Miele L. Transcription factor RBPJ/CSL: A genome-wide look at transcriptional regulation. *Proc. Natl. Acad. Sci.* 2011 Sep 6;108 (36): 14715–6.

[59] Zanotti S, Canalis E. Notch regulation of bone development and remodeling and related skeletal disorders. *Calcif. Tissue Int.* 2012 Feb;90(2):69–75.

[60] Hilton MJ, Tu X, Wu X, Bai S, Zhao H, Kobayashi T, et al. Notch signaling maintains bone marrow mesenchymal progenitors by suppressing osteoblast differentiation. *Nat. Med.* 2008 Mar;14(3):306–14.

[61] Deregowski V, Gazzerro E, Priest L, Rydziel S, Canalis E. Notch 1 Overexpression Inhibits Osteoblastogenesis by Suppressing Wnt/β-Catenin but Not Bone Morphogenetic Protein Signaling. *J. Biol. Chem.* 2006 Mar 10;281(10):6203–10.

[62] McLarren KW, Theriault FM, Stifani S. Association with the Nuclear Matrix and Interaction with Groucho and RUNX Proteins Regulate the Transcription Repression Activity of the Basic Helix Loop Helix Factor Hes1. *J. Biol. Chem.* 2001 Jan 12;276(2):1578–84.

[63] Bae Y, Yang T, Zeng H-C, Campeau PM, Chen Y, Bertin T, et al. miRNA-34c regulates Notch signaling during bone development. *Hum. Mol. Genet.* 2012 Jul 1;21(13):2991–3000.

[64] Peifer M, Polakis P. Wnt Signaling in Oncogenesis and Embryogenesis--a Look Outside the Nucleus. *Science.* 2000 Mar 3;287(5458):1606–9.

[65] Hoang BH, Kubo T, Healey JH, Sowers R, Mazza B, Yang R, et al. Expression of LDL receptor-related protein 5 (LRP5) as a novel marker for disease progression in high-grade osteosarcoma. *Int. J. Cancer J. Int. Cancer.* 2004 Mar;109(1):106–11.

[66] Rubin EM, Guo Y, Tu K, Xie J, Zi X, Hoang BH. Wnt inhibitory factor 1 decreases tumorigenesis and metastasis in osteosarcoma. *Mol. Cancer Ther.* 2010 Mar;9(3):731–41.

[67] Dieudonné F-X, Marion A, Haÿ E, Marie PJ, Modrowski D. High Wnt signaling represses the proapoptotic proteoglycan syndecan-2 in osteosarcoma cells. *Cancer Res.* 2010 Jul 1;70(13):5399–408.

[68] Wu J, Liao Q, He H, Zhong D, Yin K. TWIST interacts with β-catenin signaling on osteosarcoma cell survival against cisplatin. *Mol. Carcinog.* 2012 Dec 31;

[69] Cai Y, Mohseny AB, Karperien M, Hogendoorn PCW, Zhou G, Cleton-Jansen A-M. Inactive Wnt/beta-catenin pathway in conventional high-grade osteosarcoma. *J. Pathol.* 2010 Jan;220(1):24–33.

[70] McQueen P, Ghaffar S, Guo Y, Rubin EM, Zi X, Hoang BH. The Wnt signaling pathway: implications for therapy in osteosarcoma. *Expert Rev. Anticancer. Ther.* 2011 Aug;11(8):1223–32.

[71] Yang J, Zhang W. New molecular insights into osteosarcoma targeted therapy. *Curr. Opin. Oncol.* 2013 Jul;25(4):398–406.

[72] Brun J, Dieudonné F-X, Marty C, Müller J, Schüle R, Patiño-García A, et al. FHL2 Silencing Reduces Wnt Signaling and Osteosarcoma Tumorigenesis In Vitro and In Vivo. *PLoS ONE.* 2013 Jan 28;8(1):e55034.

[73] Pećina-Šlaus N. Wnt signal transduction pathway and apoptosis: a review. *Cancer Cell Int.* 2010 Jun 30;10(1):22.

[74] Lu W, Lin C, Roberts MJ, Waud WR, Piazza GA, Li Y. Niclosamide Suppresses Cancer Cell Growth By Inducing Wnt Co-Receptor LRP6

Degradation and Inhibiting the Wnt/β-Catenin Pathway. *PLoS ONE*. 2011 Dec 16;6(12):e29290.

[75] Jin Z, Han Y-X, Han X-R. Degraded iota-carrageenan can induce apoptosis in human osteosarcoma cells via the Wnt/β-catenin signaling pathway. *Nutr. Cancer*. 2013;65(1):126–31.

[76] Dieudonné F-X, Marion A, Marie PJ, Modrowski D. Targeted inhibition of T-cell factor activity promotes syndecan-2 expression and sensitization to doxorubicin in osteosarcoma cells and bone tumors in mice. *J. Bone Miner Res. Off J. Am. Soc. Bone Miner Res.* 2012 Oct;27(10):2118–29.

[77] Zhang F, Chen A, Chen J, Yu T, Guo F. SiRNA-mediated silencing of beta-catenin suppresses invasion and chemosensitivity to doxorubicin in MG-63 osteosarcoma cells. *Asian Pac. J. Cancer Prev. APJCP*. 2011;12(1):239–45.

[78] Cirrone F, Harris CS. Vismodegib and the hedgehog pathway: a new treatment for basal cell carcinoma. *Clin. Ther.* 2012 Oct;34(10):2039–50.

[79] Jones KB, Morcuende JA. Of hedgehogs and hereditary bone tumors: re-examination of the pathogenesis of osteochondromas. *Iowa Orthop J.* 2003;23:87–95.

[80] Ando K, Heymann M-F, Stresing V, Mori K, Rédini F, Heymann D. Current Therapeutic Strategies and Novel Approaches in Osteosarcoma. *Cancers*. 2013 May 24;5(2):591–616.

[81] Gupta S, Takebe N, LoRusso P. Targeting the Hedgehog pathway in cancer. *Ther. Adv. Med. Oncol.* 2010 Jul;2(4):237–50.

[82] Hirotsu M, Setoguchi T, Sasaki H, Matsunoshita Y, Gao H, Nagao H, et al. Smoothened as a new therapeutic target for human osteosarcoma. *Mol. Cancer*. 2010;9:5.

[83] Yang W, Liu X, Choy E, Mankin H, Hornicek FJ, Duan Z. Targeting hedgehog-GLI-2 pathway in osteosarcoma. *J. Orthop. Res. Off Publ. Orthop. Res. Soc. 2013* Mar;31(3):502–9.

[84] Warzecha J, Dinges D, Kaszap B, Henrich D, Marzi I, Seebach C. Effect of the Hedgehog-inhibitor cyclopamine on mice with osteosarcoma pulmonary metastases. *Int. J. Mol. Med.* 2012 Mar;29(3):423–7.

[85] U.S. Environmental Protection Agency. Chemical Summary: cyclopamine (4449-51-8) [Internet]. Aggregated Computational Toxicology Resource; Report No.: 4449-51-8. Available from: http://actor.epa.gov/actor/GenericChemicalPdfServlet;jsessionid=4BC5F0E2FDB63FFED573F306026D9181?casrn=4449-51-8.

[86] Wang Y, Wei Y, Zhang H, Shi Y, Li Y, Li R. Arsenic trioxide induces apoptosis of p53 null osteosarcoma MG63 cells through the inhibition of catalase. *Med. Oncol. Northwood Lond. Engl.* 2012 Jun;29(2):1328–34.

[87] Li X-S, Li W-Q, Wang W-B. Using targeted magnetic arsenic trioxide nanoparticles for osteosarcoma treatment. *Cancer Biother Radiopharm.* 2007 Dec;22(6):772–8.

[88] Nakamura S, Nagano S, Nagao H, Ishidou Y, Yokouchi M, Abematsu M, et al. Arsenic Trioxide Prevents Osteosarcoma Growth by Inhibition of GLI Transcription via DNA Damage Accumulation. *PLoS ONE.* 2013 Jul 8;8(7):e69466.

[89] Beauchamp EM, Ringer L, Bulut G, Sajwan KP, Hall MD, Lee Y-C, et al. Arsenic trioxide inhibits human cancer cell growth and tumor development in mice by blocking Hedgehog/GLI pathway. *J. Clin. Invest.* 2011 Jan;121(1):148–60.

[90] Tingting R, Wei G, Changliang P, Xinchang L, Yi Y. Arsenic trioxide inhibits osteosarcoma cell invasiveness via MAPK signaling pathway. *Cancer Biol. Ther.* 2010 Aug 1;10(3):251–7.

[91] Engin F, Bertin T, Ma O, Jiang MM, Wang L, Sutton RE, et al. Notch signaling contributes to the pathogenesis of human osteosarcomas. *Hum. Mol. Genet.* 2009 Apr 15;18(8):1464–70.

[92] Tanaka M, Setoguchi T, Hirotsu M, Gao H, Sasaki H, Matsunoshita Y, et al. Inhibition of Notch pathway prevents osteosarcoma growth by cell cycle regulation. *Br. J. Cancer.* 2009 Jun 16;100(12):1957–65.

[93] Li Y, Zhang J, Ma D, Zhang L, Si M, Yin H, et al. Curcumin inhibits proliferation and invasion of osteosarcoma cells through inactivation of Notch-1 signaling. *FEBS J.* 2012 Jun;279(12):2247–59.

[94] Hughes DPM. How the NOTCH pathway contributes to the ability of osteosarcoma cells to metastasize. Cancer Treat Res. 2009;152:479–96.

[95] Cheng D-D, Yang Q-C, Zhang Z-C, Yang C-X, Liu Y-W. Antitumor activity of histone deacetylase inhibitor trichostatin A in osteosarcoma cells. *Asian Pac. J. Cancer Prev. APJCP.* 2012;13(4):1395–9.

[96] Rao-Bindal K, Koshkina NV, Stewart J, Kleinerman ES. The histone deacetylase inhibitor, MS-275 (entinostat), downregulates c-FLIP, sensitizes osteosarcoma cells to FasL, and induces the regression of osteosarcoma lung metastases. *Curr. Cancer Drug Targets.* 2013 May;13(4):411–22.

[97] Zhang P, Yang Y, Nolo R, Zweidler-McKay PA, Hughes DPM. Regulation of NOTCH Signaling by Reciprocal Inhibition of HES1 and

Deltex 1 and its Role in Osteosarcoma Invasiveness. *Oncogene.* 2010 May 20;29(20):2916–26.

[98] Liss AS, Thayer SP. Therapeutic targeting of pancreatic stroma. In: Grippo PJ, Munshi HG, editors. Pancreat Cancer Tumor Microenviron [Internet]. Trivandrum (India): Transworld Research Network; 2012 [cited 2013 Jul 16]. Available from: http://www.ncbi.nlm.nih.gov/books/NBK98931/

[99] National Institutes of Health; National Cancer Society. Vismodegib and Gamma-Secretase/Notch Signalling Pathway Inhibitor RO4929097 in Treating Patients With Advanced or Metastatic Sarcoma [Internet]. Bethesda (MD): National Library of Medicine (US).; 2013. Report No.: NCT01154452. Available from: http://clinicaltrials.gov/ct2/show/record/NCT01154452

[100] Mödder UI, Oursler MJ, Khosla S, Monroe DG. Wnt10b activates the Wnt, notch, and NFκB pathways in U2OS osteosarcoma cells. *J. Cell Biochem.* 2011 May;112(5):1392–402.

Reviewed by:

Benjamin Levi, MD
Department of Surgery
University of Michigan
blevi@umich.edu

In: Osteosarcoma
Editors: Edwin Choy
ISBN: 978-1-63321-052-3

Chapter 8

EMERGING ROLES OF PROTEIN KINASES IN OSTEOSARCOMA AND POTENTIAL NOVEL THERAPEUTIC STRATEGIES

Eiji Osaka[1,2*], Francis J. Hornicek[1,2], Xiaoqian Yang[1,2] and Zhenfeng Duan[1,2]

[1]Department of Orthopaedic Surgery, Massachusetts General Hospital, Boston, MA, US

[2]Sarcoma Biology Laboratory, Center for Sarcoma and Connective Tissue Oncology, Massachusst General Hospital, Boston, MA, US

ABSTRACT

Osteosarcoma is the most common primary malignant tumors of bone in young adults and adolescents. Current treatment protocols for osteosarcoma include wide surgical resection of the primary lesion and chemotherapy. While chemotherapy significantly improved overall survival, patient survival has been at a plateau for many years. In fact, there has been no significant progress in improving the survival rate of osteosarcoma patients for almost three decades. In addition, despite chemotherapy involving several agents, one-third of patients with

---

* Address: 55 Fruit Street, GRJ-11-1106, Boston, MA 02114; Tel: 617-724-3144, E-mail:eosaka@med.nihon-u.ac.jp. Correspondence to: Zhenfeng Duan; E-mail: ZDUAN@mgh.harvard.edu.

osteosarcoma develop local recurrence or distant metastasis. If such patients have tumors refractory to multiple-agent treatment, the average survival period after recurrence is less than 1 year. Therefore, there is an urgent need to develop new therapeutic approaches for osteosarcoma. Protein kinases play important roles in regulating cellular functions in tumors, including proliferation/cell cycle regulation, cell metabolism, survival/apoptosis, DNA damage repair, cell motility, and drug resistance. Targeting specific kinases with small-molecule inhibitors has revolutionized the treatment of a select group of cancers. Several groups including us have been made intensive efforts to search for potential therapeutic kinase targets in osteosarcoma. Kinases, such as polo-like kinase 1 (PLK1), minibrain-related kinase (MIRK), insulin-like growth factor 1 receptor (IGF-1R), ROCK1, CDK11, PI3K, AKT, PDGFR, and mTOR, have been found to be highly expressed and activated in osteosarcomas. Additionally, some of these kinse expressions are known to correlate with the outcomes of patients. These findings suggest the potential utility of kinases as drug targets for novel therapeutic interventions in osteosarcoma. In this chapter, we will present recent advances in the development of protein kinases and their emerging roles in osteosarcoma treatment, as well as potential novel therapeutic strategies.

1. INTRODUCTION

Osteosarcoma is the most common primary malignant tumors of bone and occurs mostly in young adults and adolescents between 10 and 20 years of age. It is believed that osteosarcoma arises from mesenchymal bone forming tissue and its most characteristic histological feature is the production of malignant osteoid [1, 2]. The standard treatment of osteosarcoma involves aggressive surgical resection of the primary lesion and systemic chemotherapy. Multi-agent chemotherapy including doxorubicin, cisplatin, ifosfamide and methotrexate has dramatically improved overall survival [3]. Despite these multidisciplinary treatments, the survival rate remains at approximately 60-70% [4]. Patient survival has been at a plateau for many years in osteosarcoma and there has been no significant progress in improving the survival rate of patients for almost three decades [5]. In addition, despite chemotherapy with several agents, almost one-third of patients with osteosarcoma develop local recurrence or distant metastasis [6]. If such patients have tumors refractory to multi-agent treatment, the average survival period after recurrence is usually less than 1 year [7]. Thus, there is an urgent need to develop new therapeutic approaches for osteosarcoma patients [8].

Protein kinases play important roles in regulating cellular functions in tumors, including proliferation/cell cycle regulation, cell metabolism, survival/apoptosis, DNA damage repair, cell motility, and drug resistance. Therapeutic targeting of protein kinases has been proved to be effective against many cancers. Imatinib (Gleevec) and gefitinib have dramatically changed management and improved the outcomes in patients with chronic myelogenous leukemia (CML) and lung cancer [9, 10]. Therefore, protein kinase inhibitors have been proven effective against defined sarcoma subtypes such as gastrointestinal stromal tumors (GIST) and dermatofibrosarcoma protuberans (DFSP) [11, 12]. To date, several protein kinase inhibitors have been pre-clinically and clinically evaluated for osteosarcoma.

This chapter will present recent studies on the emerging roles of kinase in osteosarcoma, and in the development of agents targeting protein kinases as well as novel therapeutic strategies for osteosarcoma.

2. Protein Kinase

Kinases are involved in almost every signal transduction pathway. More than 600 protein kinase existed in human genomes known as "kinome" [13]. A protein kinase is a type of enzyme that phosphorylates tyrosine or serine/threonine residues in the target protein, using ATP. The human kinome phosphorylate 250,000 or more sites of proteins [14-16]. In general, there are two types of human kinases: tyrosine kinase (TK) family and serine/threonine kinase (STK) family (Table 1).

2.1. Tyrosine Kinase (TK) Family

Tyrosine kinases (TKs) are classified as receptor tyrosine kinases (RTKs), such as IGFR, PDGFR, EGFR, FGFR, IR, and VEGFR, and non-receptor tyrosine kinases (NRTKs) that lack transmembrane domains such as SRC, ABL, FAK and Janus kinase (Table 1). TKs exist in the cytosol, nucleus, and inner surface of the plasma membrane [17]. The RTKs play roles not only as cell surface transmembrane receptors, but also as enzymes with kinase activity [18]. All RTKs have a similar structure and consist of a ligand binding region in the extracellular domain, a single pass transmembrane hydrophobic helix and a cytoplasmic TK domain. After receiving a signal, RTKs are activated by autophosphorylation and trigger downstream intracellular signaling pathways.

Table 1. Protein kinase classification

Tyrosine kinase family	TK group	RTKs	IGFR, PDGFR, EGFR, FGFR, IR, VEGFR
		NRTKs	Src, Abl, Csk, FAK,JAK
Serine/threonine kinase family	STE group		Ste7, Ste11, Ste20
	CK1 group		CK1, VRK, TTBK, TTBKL
	AGC group		Akt, S6K, SGK, PDL1, ROCK, PKA, PKC, PKG
	CAMK group		CAMKI, CAMKII, CAMKL, MAPKAPK, DAPK, PSK, RAD53
	CMGC group		MAPK, CDK, CDKL, CK2, DYRK, GSK, CLK
	RGC group		ANPα, ANPβ
	TKL group		MLK, RAF, STKR, LRRK, LISK, IRAK, RIPK
	Other group		Aur, Bub, Bud32, CAMKK, CDC7, Haspin, IRE, WEE, NKF, PLK
	Atypical group		PDHK, NDK, PyK

TK: Tyrosine kinase, STE: Sterile, CK1: Cell Kinase 1, AGC: cAMP-dependent protein kinase/protein kinase G/protein kinase C extended, CAMK: Calcium/Calmodulin regulated kinases, CMGC: Cyclin-dependent Kinases and other close relatives, RGC: Receptor Guanylate Cyclases, TKL: Tyrosine Kinase Like, RTK:receptor tyrosine kinases, NRTK: non-receptor tyrosine kinases.

Although NRTKs contribute to diverse activation mechanisms, some of these NRTKs are phosphorylated and activated by RTKs, and play a transducing role for downstream signaling molecules from activated RTK. TKs serve as important mediators of various signal transduction processes such as cell proliferation, differentiation, migration, metabolism and programmed cell death [19, 20].

2.2. Serine/Threonine Kinase (STK) Family

The STK family is classified into nine groups: STE (Sterile), CK1 (Cell kinase I), AGC (cAMP-dependent protein kinase/protein kinase G/protein kinase C extended), CAMK (Calcium/Calmodulin regulated kinases), CMGC (Cyclin-dependent kinases and other close relatives), RGC (Receptor guanylate cyclases), TKL (Tyrosine kinase like), other group and atypical group (Table 1) [21-26].

The STE group is involved in the Mitogen-activated protein kinases (MAPK) pathway. STE7 (MAP2Ks or MEKs) kinases are part of the MAPK signaling cascades and they are activated by *STE11* (MAP3K) and phosphorylate *MAPK* kinases. The CK1 group regulates signal transduction pathways, isoforms of which are mainly involved in Wnt signaling and circadian rhythms [21, 22]. The AGC group is regulated by the second messenger of cAMP, cGMP and lipids, and involves various core intracellular signaling kinases and regulates critical biological processes such as growth, differentiation and survival [21, 24]. The CAMK group is activated by binding of calcium/calmodulin complexes. This group is classified as specialized CAMK, consisting of a myosin light chain kinase and a multifunctional CAMK [23]. There are mainly two groups of key proteins in CMGC, MAPK and CDK (cyclin-dependent kinases), which are involved in regulation of the cell cycle and the MAPK pathway which functions in various biological processes, including growth, proliferation, differentiation, migration, apoptosis and survival [21, 25]. The RGC group generates the cGMP as a second messenger. In turn, these induce inactivation of a particular kinase domain, resulting in regulation of functions such as dauer stage formation. However, the functions of most RGC proteins remain unknown [21]. The TKL group consists of receptor kinases [21]. Although the Other group is clearly eukaryotic protein kinases, these kinases cannot be easily classified into the other groups [26]. The Atypical group contains kinases which display little or no sequence similarity to eukaryotic protein kinase domains [26].

Almost every member of the STK family except for TKL is a non-receptor kinase and regulates various cellular functions such as stress responses, proliferation, differentiation, apoptosis, metabolism and embryonic development [23].

2.3. Protein Kinases as Therapeutic Targets in Cancer

Protein kinases play important roles in almost every aspects of cellular behaviors including those for metabolism, transcription, cell cycle progression, cytoskeletal rearrangement and cell movement, apoptosis, and differentiation, and which are thus widely investigated as drug targets [27-29]. Recently, therapeutic targeting of protein kinases has proved to be effective in many cancers. For instance, agents such as imatinib, BCR-ABL, PDGFRs and c-KIT inhibitor, and gefitinib, EGFR inhibitor, inhibit tumor growth by antagonizing specific survival kinases.

The prototypical TK inhibitor (TKI), imatinib, has dramatically changed management and improved the outcomes of patients with Philadelphia chromosome-positive CML [9]. CML is a clonal myeloproliferative hematopoietic stem cell disorder that is characterized by a t(9;22) translocation that produces a shortened chromosome 22, the so-called Philadelphia chromosome. This translocation induces in the expression of BCR-ABL fusion oncoproteins [30]. Abnormal interactions of the BCR-ABL oncoprotein activate the Ras–mitogen-activated protein kinase (MAPK), the Janus-activated kinase (JAK) / signal transducer and activator of transcription proteins (STAT) pathway, and the phosphoinositide 3-kinase (PI3K)/AKT pathway. As a result, they lead to increased proliferation, transcriptional activity and inhibition of apoptosis [31]. The BCR-ABL inhibitor, imatinib, is remarkably effective and improves the survival outcomes of CML patients [9]. Other studies have shown that imatinib is also effective for c-KIT positive patients with other solid tumors such as GIST and DFSP [11, 12]. The TK known as c-KIT is overexpressed in more than 95% of GISTs, with many exhibiting mutations that increase kinase activity. The use of TKI against c-KIT has dramatically impacted treatment because stable disease or partial responses can be induced in many patients, thereby increasing survival [32, 33].

In non-small cell lung carcinoma (NSCLC), 40-80% of patients overexpress the epidermal growth factor receptor (EGFR) which plays important roles in tumorigenesis [10]. EGFR activation induces MAPK, and the PI3K/AKT and JAK/STAT pathways. Therefore, EGFR inhibitors have efficacy in NSCLC patients with EGRF overexpression, prolonging their survival [34].

The aberrant expression of human epidermal growth factor receptor (HER2) has been correlated with breast cancer development [35]. Similarly, aberrant expression of EGFR has been found in many other malignant neoplasms such as pancreatic adenocarcinoma and NSCLC [36, 37]. Therapeutic targets of HER2 have been developed and have improved survival in patients with HER2 overexpression [35-37].

Recently, crizotinib, a small molecule inhibitor of RTKs, specifically target ALK and c-MET (hepatocyte growth factor receptor), has been highlighted in lung cancer. Crizotinib has been shown to yield clinical benefits such as an objective response rate and progression-free survival in cases with advanced NSCLC [38].

There have been more than 100 clinical trials of TKIs, as therapeutic agents in various cancers including osteosarcoma. The strategies for applying these therapeutic agents include monoclonal antibodies (mAB) and small molecular drugs.

3. Protein Kinase Involvement in Osteosarcoma

Targeting specific kinases with small-molecule inhibitors has revolutionized the treatment of a select group of cancers as described above. Several groups including us have made intensive efforts to search for potential therapeutic kinase targets in osteosarcoma. Some kinases such as polo-like kinase 1 (PLK1), minibrain-related kinase (MIRK), insulin-like growth factor 1 receptor (IGF-1R), ROCK1, CDK11, PI3K, AKT, PDGFR (platelet derived growth factor receptor), and mammalian target of rapamycin (mTOR) have been found to be highly expressed and activated in osteosarcomas. These findings suggest the potential utility of these kinases as drug targets for therapeutic intervention in osteosarcoma. Additionally, some of these expressions are known to correlate with patient outcomes. Moreover, protein kinases that have been implicated in osteosarcoma treatment include IGF-1R [39, 40], PDGFR-A [41], and mTOR [42, 43]. The TKI imatinib demonstrated little evidence of efficacy in a 2008 study on osteosarcoma [44]. Recently, numerous protein kinase inhibitors have been pre-clinically and clinically evaluated for osteosarcoma. Figure 1 and Table 2 show intracellular signal transduction and therapeutic targets of kinaeses in osteosarcoma, including RTKs, intracellular signaling pathways associated protein kinases.

3.1. Signaling Pathways of Receptor Tyrosine Kinases

To date, more than 50 RTKs belonging to at least 18 receptor families of kinases have been identified. RTKs have a transmembrane structure and consist of an extracellular ligand-binding domain and an intracellular TK domain (Figure 1). After receiving a signal, RTKs are activated by autophosphorylation. Subsequently, RTK activity promotes intracellular signal transduction and activates downstream signaling pathways. RTKs, such as IGF-1R, PDGFR and EGFR, have been implicated in the tumorigenesis of osteosarcoma [45]. Recent studies have shown therapeutic targets of RTKs to yield improvements in both quality of life and long-term survival [46, 47].

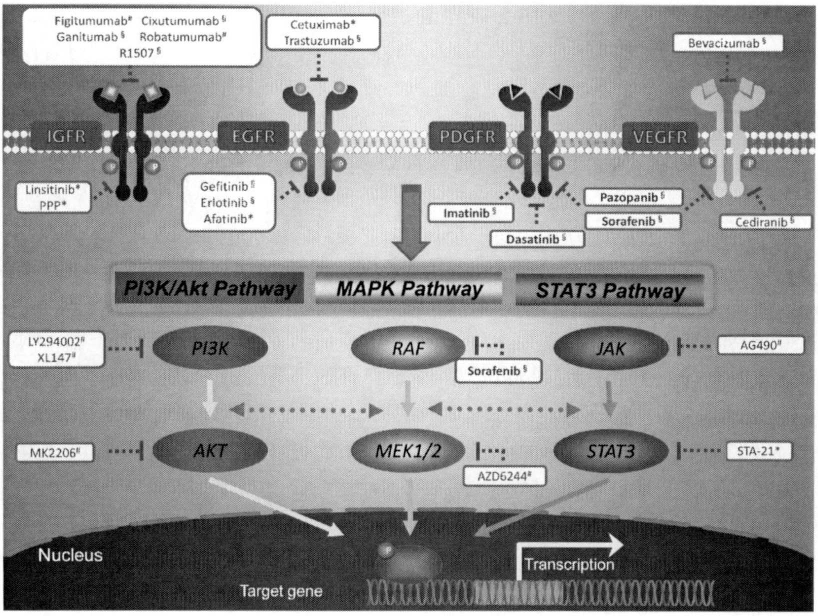

*: Studied *in vitro*, #: Studied both *in vitro* and *in vivo*, §: Developed into clinical trials.

Figure 1. Intracellular Signal Transduction of TRK and potential target sites in osteosarcoma. Intracellular signal transduction and therapeutic targets in osteosarcoma, including RTKs and intracellular signaling pathways. RTK activates three major downstream signaling pathways, including the PI3K/AKT, STAT3 and MAPK pathways. Though often acting independently, there is significant cross-talk and overlap among these pathways. Bold represent multi-kinase inhibitors include:Imatinib: BCR-ABL, PDGFRs, c-KIT, **Sorafenib**: Raf-1, FGFR, VEGFR-2, VEGFR-3, PDGFR-β, RET, FLT-3, c-KIT, Dasatinib: Abl/Src, c-Kit, PDGFR, Ephrin, Pazopanib: VEGFR-1, -2, and -3, PDGFR-α, -β, c-KIT.

3.1.1. Expression of Insulin-Like Growth Factor Receptor (IGFR) in Osteosarcoma and Its Potential as a Therapeutic Target

IGFRs consist of the IGF receptor type 1 (IGF-1R) and the IGF receptor type 2 (IGF-2R). IGF-1R is expressed on the cell surface, as holoreceptors comprised of two extracellular α-subunits, ligand binding domains, and two transmembrane TK β-subunits. Upon binding with ligands to the extracellular parts of the receptor, such as IGF-1 or IGF-2 which are peptides synthesized mainly by the liver and are major stimulators of tissue and cellular growth [48], the receptor is activated and the intracellular TK domain is phosphorylated. Activation of the TK domain induces phosphorylation of several substrates, e.g. the insulin receptor substrate proteins (IRS-1, 2, 3 and 4) which constitute a signal regulatory protein family.

Mainly three signal transduction pathways are triggered after activation of IRS-1. One is the Ras–Raf–MAPK pathway. The other is PI3K/AKT and JAK/Stat3 pathway (Figure 1). The IGF-1R signaling pathway plays important roles in protecting cells from apoptosis and in promoting transcription, proliferation and cell growth [49]. Therefore, IGF-1R is an increasingly attractive target for cancer treatment [50].

The IGF-1R is one of the protein kinases recognized as a potential therapeutic target in osteosarcoma and has been extensively studied. IGF signaling is involved in osteogenesis and bone homeostasis in normal bone [51]. IGF-1R has been shown to be overexpressed and recognized as having a biologically relevant role in various human malignant neoplasms including osteosarcoma [52, 53]. Therapeutically, however, IGF-1R has been difficult to target in cancers because it is structurally similar to the insulin receptor (IR). Thus, there are toxicities associated with nonspecific inhibition. Recently, small molecules and monoclonal antibodies without excessive toxicity for IGF-1R have been developed. Recent study reported lentivirus-mediated RNAi regulation suppressed osteosarcoma cell growth rates *in vitro* and reduced tumorigenicity *in vivo* [53]. Moreover, down-regulation of IGF-1R not only arrested cells in the G0/G1 phase of the cell cycle but also induced apoptosis via the activation of Caspase-3 [54]. Furthermore, the inhibition of IGF-1R combined with CDDP or DTX treatment synergistically suppressed the growth of osteosarcoma cells not only *in vitro* but also *in vivo* [55]. Linsitinib (OSI-906) is a selective small molecule dual kinase inhibitor of both IR and IGF-1R[56]. Clinical trials of linsitinib are now being started by OSI Pharmaceuticals. There is a phase III trial underway for adrenocortical carcinoma (NCT00924989) and a phase I/II clinical trial for ovarian cancer (NCT00889382). In osteosarcoma, linsitinib has been shown to exert a strong inhibitory effect on proliferation in 3 of 4 osteosarcoma cell lines in preclinical studies [49]. Cyclolignan picropodophyllin (PPP) inhibits IGF-1R activation, thereby inhibiting the PI3K/AKT pathway. PPP leads to apoptosis of cancer cells and reduces cell motility *in vitro*, and tumor regression has been observed in various xenografted models [57]. Our study revealed PPP to significantly inhibit IGF-1R expression and activation in both chemotherapy-sensitive and chemotherapy-resistant osteosarcoma cell lines [58]. Recently, treatments with mAbs directed toward IGF-1R, such as Figitumumab, Cixutumumab (IMC-A12), Ganitumab, Sch717454 (Robatumumab) and R1507, have emerged as an effective option for osteosarcoma. Cixutumumab (IMC-A12), a human immunoglobulin G 1/λ monoclonal antibody binding IGF-1R, inhibits IGF/IR expression by blocking interactions with IGF-1 and IGF-2 ligands. Now, Cixutumumab has been developed for clinical trials in osteosarcoma (NCT01614795, NCT00831844 and NCT00609141). A phase II trial of Cixutumumab was performed by a multicenter, open-label for chemotherapy-refractory bone and soft-tissue sarcomas (NCT01016015). Although there were no complete responses, three of 24 with osteosarcoma had partial responses [59]. SCH717454, a humanized neutralizing anti-IGF-1R antibody, is being evaluated for patients with *relapsed osteosarcoma* in a phase II trial (NCT00617890) and has exhibited high response activity in four of six osteosarcoma xenograft models [60, 61]. Moreover, clinical trials are starting for several other mAbs of EGFR, including ganitumab (AMG479, NCT00563680) and R1507. R1507 induced inhibition of tumor growth and improvement in event –free survival in osteosarcoma xenograft tumour models [62]. A phase II trial of R 1507 has shown two of 4 with osteosarcoma had stable disease and others had progression disease for chemotherapy-refractory bone and soft-tissue sarcomas (NCT00642941) [61].

3.1.2. Expression of Platelet-Derived Growth Factor Receptor (PDGFR) in Osteosarcoma and Its Potential as a Therapeutic Target

Platelet-derived growth factor (PDGF) consists of four polypeptides designated A, B, C and D [63, 64], and is the main mitogen in serum for mesenchymal cells (Figure 1). PDGFs promote cell migration, proliferation, and survival by binding to PDGFRs which have two isoforms: PDGFRα and PDGFRβ [65, 66]. The activations of PDGFRα and PDGFRβ both overlap numerous signaling pathways, but they have different expression patterns and physiological roles. PDGFRα signaling plays an important role in the embryogenesis of organs such as the lungs, intestine, skin, testis, kidneys, neuroprotective tissues and bones. PDGFRβ signaling is as an essential regulator of the formation of new vessels and collagen production [67]. Both PDGFRα and PDGFRβ are involved in several signaling pathways, such as Ras-MAPK, PI3K/AKT and PLC-γ, which in turn function in multiple cellular and developmental responses [67]. Therefore, mutations of PDGF and PDGRF correlate with the pathogenesis, invasion, and distant metastasis of many cancers including osteosarcoma.

The expressions of PDGF and PDGFR correlate with a poor prognosis and distant metastasis in many cancers such as Ewing sarcoma, lung carcinoma, breast cancer, ovarian cancer, chondrosarcoma and osteosarcoma [68-73]. PDGF stimulates proliferation and differentiation of osteoblasts and osteoclasts [74]. A recent retrospective study demonstrated, immunohistochemically, that approximately 86% and 81% of human osteosarcoma samples express PDGF and PDGFR, respectively [73]. Moreover, 38% of 37 osteosarcomas expressed PDGF and PDGFR immunohistochemically. Both were expressed in 30% of cases, and PDGF-positive tumors showed higher proliferation than PDGF-negative tumors. Therefore, PDGF expression plays an important role as a mediator of cell proliferation control, through an autocrine mechanism, in osteosarcomas [75].

Imatinib is a TKI not only target BCR-ABL but also inhibit PDGFRs and c-KIT [76, 77]. Imatinib has been shown to inhibit PDGF-mediated proliferation of osteosarcoma cell lines *in vitro* [78]. However, *in vivo*, imatinib had no significant effect on tumor size of osteosarcoma, as demonstrated by the lack of any difference between treatment and control mice [78]. A phase II trial of imatinib was performed by a children's oncology group for refractory or relapsed solid tumors including osteosarcoma (NCT00030667). However, there were no objective responses for treatment with imatinib [44]. In other phase II trial of imatinib (NCT0031915), a clinical benefit response was achieved in five of 27 with osteosarcoma [79]. Despite these findings, clinical trials are now assessing imatinib as an osteosarcoma treatment (NCT00154388).

Dasatinib inhibits a dual Abl/Src TK and also inhibits c-KIT, PDGFR and Ephrin receptors. Dasatinib has been approved for the treatment of imatinib-resistant CML and Philadelphia chromosome-positive acute lymphocytic leukemia. Dasatinib exerted an effect on BCR–ABL mutations and imatinib-resistant malignancies [80]. Dasatinib is currently being evaluated for patients with advanced sarcoma in a phase II trial (NCT00464620) and has exhibited intermediate response activity in two of five osteosarcoma xenograft models [81]. Dasatinib in combination with ipilimumab (NCT01643278), carboplatin, etoposide and ifosfamide (NCT00788125) is also being clinically investigated.

3.1.3. Expression of Epidermal Growth Factor Receptor (EGFR) in Osteosarcoma and Its Potential as a Therapeutic Target

Epidermal growth factor (EGF) involves in cell growth [82]. There are four EGF receptors (EGFRs) designated ErbB1/EGFR/HER1, ErbB2/HER2/Neu, ErbB3/HER3 and ErbB4/HER4, which constitute the ErbB family of RTK and consist of an extracellular ligand-binding domain and an intracellular TK domain separated by a transmembrane region [83]. Many normal epithelial tissues such as skin, hair follicles and the gastrointestinal tract constitutively express EGFR, which plays important roles in normal cell function [84].

EGFRs selectivity promote autophosphorylation via the binding of ligands such as EGF, transforming growth factor-α (TGF-α), amphiregulin, heparin-binding EGF-like growth factor, betacellulin or epiregulin [85]. Subsequently, TK activity promotes an intracellular signal transduction process and thereby activates three major downstream signaling pathways, including the KRAS/RAF/MEK/MARK, PI3K/AKT and JAK/STAT pathways (Figure 1). Deregulation of these pathways contributes to cell proliferation, survival, invasion, metastasis and angiogenesis in many cancers including osteosarcoma [86, 87].

EGFRs contribute mainly to various signaling cascades that modulate cell proliferation, survival, adhesion, motility, invasion, differentiation and angiogenesis in cancers. Many studies have reported overexpression of EGFR in cancers, including NSCLC, colon, breast, and ovarian tumors, as well as squamous cell carcinoma of the head and neck. Overexpression of EGFR was reported to be strongly associated with aggressive cancers and a poor prognosis [85]. Therefore, several therapies targeting EGFRs, including the anti-EGFR mAB cetuximab, and the TKIs gefitinib and erlotinib, have been pre-clinically and clinically evaluated as treatments for various cancers [88-92]. Several studies have reported expression of EGFR in 40-81% of osteosarcoma tumor tissues [75, 93-95]. EGFR inhibitors effectively suppressed the growth of osteosarcoma cells i*n vitro* [96, 97]. However, the impact of EGFR expression on prognosis is controversial. EGFR did not correlate significantly with OS in osteosarcoma patients [93, 96, 98]. These findings were probably due to the small sample size and selection bias, and that the role of EGFR in osteosarcoma might differ from its role in other cancers. However, other study reported EGFR to be associated with a good clinical outcome [99].

Gefitinib and erlotinib are orally bioavailable, small-molecule TKI which specifically target EGFR signaling. These agents dramatically improve progression-free survival as compared with conventional standard chemotherapy for lung cancer and are currently being evaluated in numerous clinical trials for several tumors [100]. In a previous study, gefitinib and afatinib (BIBW2992) were showed not effective against osteosarcoma cells *in vitro*. However, EGFR is expressed in osteosarcoma cells, such that further studies are necessary to explore the potential of other therapeutic agents targeting EGFR. Therapeutic agents targeting EGFR are now being launched. A phase I trial clinical trial of erlotinib is underway (NCT00077454) in osteosarcoma [101].

Recently, treatment with a mAb directed toward EGFR, such as trastuzumab or cetuximab, has emerged as an effective treatment option. HER2 is overexpressed in various cancers including osteosarcoma, and this overexpression has been reported to predict therapeutic resistance and to be associated with poor outcomes. Trastuzumab, a humanized monoclonal antibody binding to HER2, is dramatically effective and improves both disease-free survival and overall survival in patients with HER2-positive breast cancer [102]. HER2 was overexpressed in 42% of patient with osteosarcomas, and that high expression levels correlated strongly with metastasis and poor outcomes [103]. A phase II trial (NCT00023998) investigated the efficacy of trastuzumab with standard chemotherapy for patients with HER2-positive metastatic osteosarcoma. However, survival outcomes were poor and there was no significant difference between HER2-positive and HER2-negative osteosarcoma patients [104].

Cetuximab, which is an immunoglobulin G (IgG1) human–mouse chimeric mAB, competitively inhibits the TK domain of EGFR by blocking dimerization and ligand-induced receptor signaling [105]. The cytolytic potential of resting natural killer cells can be potentiated and directed toward osteosarcoma cells with cetuximab [106]. Therefore, they concluded that immunotherapy with cetuximab might be regarded as a novel treatment strategy for the management of advanced osteosarcoma.

Moreover, several therapies targeting EGFR are used in clinical settings, including TKI such as dacomitinib (PF00299804), neratinib (HKI-272) and lapatinib [107-109]. These TKIs are currently being investigated as ErbB family inhibitors that target EGFR, HER2, and HER4 in other cancers. It is hoped that more research will be conducted using these inhibitors in osteosarcoma.

3.2. Intracellular Signaling Pathways

RTKs are selectivity promoted upon phosphorylation via binding to extracellular stimuli. The resultant TK activity promotes intracellular signal transduction and activates three major downstream signaling pathways, including the PI3K/AKT, STAT3 and MAPK pathways (Figure 1). Although often acting independently, there is significant cross-talk and overlap among these pathways. It is therefore necessary to inhibit more than one signaling cascade to achieve therapeutic intervention targets in cancers including osteosarcoma. These pathways are frequently dysregulated because of the genetic changes associated with malignant transformation. Intracellular signaling pathways are involved in various biological processes, including growth, proliferation, differentiation, migration, apoptosis and survival. Therefore, the dysregulation of these pathways correlates with tumorigenesis in many cancers including osteosarcoma. These findings suggest the potential utility of kinases as drug targets for osteosarcoma therapy. Herein, we present on overview of the PI3K/AKT, STAT3, and MAPK pathways and these therapeutic targets in osteosarcoma (Table 2).

Table 2. List of potential protein kinases involved osteosarcoma and currently clinical trails

Drug	Other name	Target protein kinases	Identified ID from Clinical Trials.gov Refer
Figitumumab[#]		IGFR	-
Cixutumumab[§]		IGFR	NCT01016015, NCT01614795, NCT00831844, 183NCT00720174, NCT00668148, NCT00609141
Ganitumab[§]	AMG479	IGFR	NCT00563680
Robatumumab[#]	Sch717454	IGFR	-
R 1507[§]		IGFR	NCT00642941
Linsitinib*	OSI-906	IGFR	-
Cyclolignan picropodophyllin (PPP)*		IGFR	-
Imatinib[§]		BCR-ABL, PDGFRs, c-KIT	NCT0031915, NCT00030667, NCT00062205, NCT00154388
Cetuximab*		EGFR	-
Trastuzumab[§]		EGFR	NST00023998, NCT00005033
Gefitinib[§]		EGFR	NCT00132158
Erlotinib[§]		EGFR	NCT00077454
Afatinib *	BIBW2992	EGFR	-
LY294002[#]		PI3K	-
XL147[#]	SAR245408	PI3K	-
MK2206[#]		Akt	-
Sirolimus[§]	Rapamycin	mTORC1	NCT00743509, NCT01331135, NCT01522820
Temsirolimus[§]	CCI-779	mTORC1	NCT01016015, NCT01204450, NCT00949325
Ridaforolimus[§]	AP23573, MK-8669, formerly	mTORC1	NCT00538239, NCT00093080

Drug	Other name	Target protein kinases	Identified ID from Clinical Trials.gov Refer
	deforolimus		
Everolimus§	RAD001	mTOR	NCT01804374, NCT01216826,NCT01830153
AZD6244#		MEK1/2	-
AG490#		JAK	-
SU6656*		Src	-
Saracatinib§		Src	NCT00752206
STA-21*		SH2 domain	-
Roscovitine#	Seliciclib	CDK1,2,7,9	-
Flavopiridol§	Alvocidib	CDK1,2,4,6	NCT00012181
Dinaciclib*	SCH 727965	CDK1,2,9	-
BI 2536#		PLK1	-
Alisertib§	MLN8237	Aurora kinases	NCT01154816
MK-8776#		CHK1	-
MK1775#		WEE1	-
Bevacizumab§		VEGF	NCT00667342, NCT00516295, NCT01492673
Cediranib §	AZD2171	VEGF	NCT00502060
Dasatinib§		Abl/Src, c-Kit, PDGFR, Ephrin	NCT00464620, NCT01643278, NCT00788125
Sorafenib§	BAY 43-9006	Raf-1, FGFR, VEGFR-2, VEGFR-3, PDGFR-β, RET, FLT-3, c-KIT	NCT00889057, NCT00330421, NCT01518413, NCT01804374, NCT00880542, NCT01518413
Pazopanib§		VEGFR-1, -2, and -3, PDGFR-α, -β, c-KIT	NCT01130623

Source used; clinicaltrials.gov.
*: *in vitro*, #: *in vivo*, §:clinical trials.

3.2.1. Phosphoinositide-3 Kinases (PI3K)/Akt Pathway as a Therapeutic Target in Osteosarcoma

PI3K belong to the family of lipid kinases that phosphorylate the hydroxyl group at the 3'-position of inositol rings, which transduce the signaling pathways involved in biological processes such as proliferation, growth, apoptosis and cytoskeleton rearrangement.

PI3Ks are stimulated by cell surface RTK such as EGFR, IR/ IRS-1, HER2, ErbB-3, IGF-1R, PDGFR and fibroblast growth factor receptor (FGFR), cell adhesion molecules such as integrins, G protein-coupled receptors (GPCRs) and oncogenes such as Ras, c-Met, and c-KIT [110]. PI3K phosphorylates phosphatidylinositol-4, 5-disphosphate (PIP2) to form phosphatidylinositol-3, 4, 5-trisphosphate (PIP3), which is a critical second cellular messenger that recruits AKT for activation of growth, proliferation and survival signaling [111]. Phosphatase and tensin homolog (PTEN), which modulates the tumor suppressor, regulates the dephosphorylation of PIP3 (Figure 2). Regulation of the PI3K/AKT pathway is controlled by PTEN, as well as the lipid phosphatases SHIP1 and SHIP2. PIP3 directly binds to the PH domain in AKT and phosphoinositide-dependent kinase 1 (PDK1) at the plasma membrane and recruits these proteins to the cell membrane. Subsequently, PDK1 phosphorylates AKT. The three isoforms of AKT are AKT1, AKT2 and AKT3, which exist in most tissues.

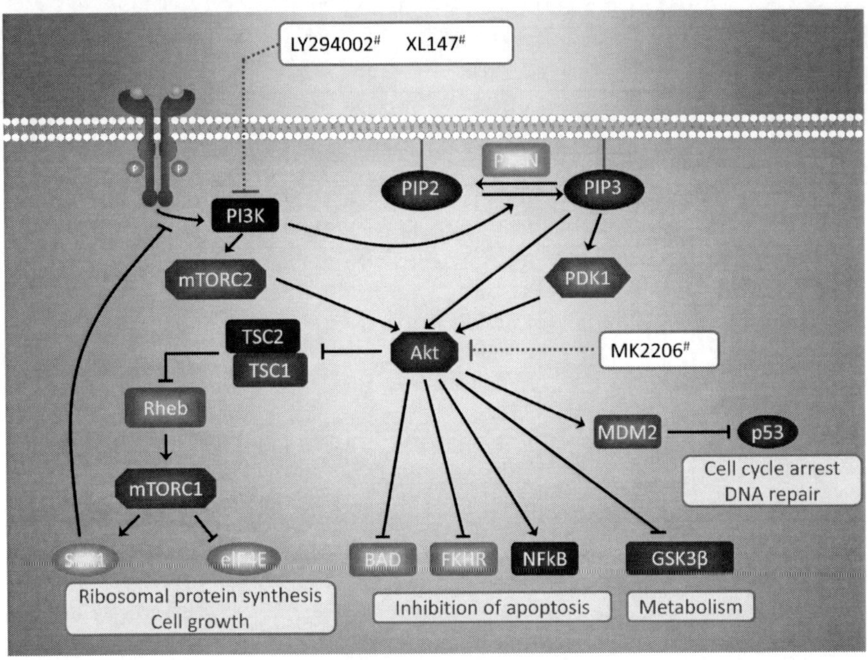

#: Studied both in vitro and in vivo.

Figure 2. Details of PI3K/AKT signaling pathway and potential target sites in osteosarcoma. PI3Ks are stimulated by cell surface RTK. PI3K phosphorylates PIP2 to form PIP3. PTEN regulates the dephosphorylation of PIP3. Regulation of the PI3K/AKT pathway is controlled by PTEN. PIP3 directly binds to AKT and PDK1. Subsequently, PDK1 phosphorylates AKT. AKT is activated and stimulates various biological processes.

AKT is activated and stimulates various downstream signaling proteins, such as mTOR, S6K1 and eIF4E, which induce ribosomal protein synthesis and cell growth, inhibition of BAD (a pro-apoptotic protein of the *Bcl-2* family) and FKHR (forkhead transcription factor Foxo1), and activation of nuclear factor kappa beta which suppresses apoptosis, activates GSK3β which promotes metabolism, and activates MDM2 (mMouse double minute 2 homolog) which induces cell-cycle arrest and DNA repair mediated by p53 [112].

The PI3K/AKT pathway is constitutively activated in various cancers. Activation mechanisms of this pathway include loss of tumor suppressor PTEN function [113], amplification or mutation of PI3K or AKT, and activation of cell surface RTKs. These genomic aberrations promote tumorigenesis via upregulation of the PI3K/AKT pathway. This pathway is notable as a therapeutic target in cancer because many malignancies contribute to initiation and maintenance by stimulating its downstream substrates.

Loss of tumor suppressor PTEN function constitutively activates of the PI3K/AKT pathway and increases cell proliferation, cell survival, migration and metastasis [113], and is found in many different cancers including osteosarcoma. PTEN was identified in 19 of 28 (68%) osteosarcoma tumor samples using immunohistochemistry. Loss of PTEN is a common occurrence in osteosarcomas and identified a correlation between EGFR amplification and loss of PTEN [96]. Loss of PTEN function in cancers is involved in pathogenesis, invasion and metastasis and PTEN expression levels may be a good prognostic marker for various cancers including osteosarcoma.

Mutation of PIK3CA, the gene encoding the p110α catalytic subunit of PI3K, increases the activity of PI3K *in vitro*, and the expression of p110α mutants in cells induces AKT activation in the absence of growth factor stimulation. This mutation subsequently leads to oncogenesis. Hotspot mutations are frequently observed either in the helical domain (E545K and E542K) or in the kinase domain (H1047R). Mutations of the PIK3CA gene are common in various cancers, including breast, endometrial, colorectal, urinary tract and ovarian tumors [114]. Furthermore, there were three mutations in PIK3CA (H1047R, E545K and H701P) in osteosarcomas [115]. Amplification of PIK3CA is also very frequently found in head and neck tumors, squamous cell lung carcinoma, gastric and cervical cancers, and is associated with poor survival rates [116-118].

LY294002, a PI3K inhibitor, competitively binds ATP and has enormous potential for targeting the ATP-binding site of p110. LY294002 exhibited the effect on the cell cycle distribution and apoptosis of osteosarcoma cancer stem-like cells (CSCs) *in vitro*, and which may represent a potential strategy for managing human osteosarcoma employing CSCs [119].

Several PI3K inhibitors, including XL147, PX-866, BKM120, GDC0941, GSK2126458, CH5132799, and ATU027, have been discovered and these are now advancing from the preclinical phase to clinical trials for the treatment of various cancers except osteosarcoma [120]. Further studies are needed to validate PI3K inhibitors as a treatment for osteosarcomas.

Amplifications of AKT have been reported in various malignancies including pancreatic, ovarian, and head and neck cancers. A recent study revealed a somatic mutation in the PH domain of AKT1 in breast, colorectal and ovarian cancers. The PH domain mutation prolongs AKT activation and constitutive association with the plasma membrane [118]. Amplification of AKT2 has been found in lymphomas, as well as in ovarian and pancreatic cancers. Mutation of AKT2 has also been found in colorectal cancers [110].

In clinical development, AKT inhibitors are classified as either ATP-competitive or allosteric. ATP-competitive AKT inhibitors such as AZD5363 are pan-AKT kinase inhibitors. Allosteric AKT inhibitors such as MK2206 bind to the PH domain of AKT. Activation of AKT is disrupted due to conformational changes [120]. Several AKT inhibitors are now advancing from the preclinical phase to clinical trials for the treatment of various cancers.

Amplification and/or mutations of AKT indicate a potential role for AKT inhibitors in therapeutic targeting. However, it is as yet unclear whether these amplifications or mutations have any significant effects on the clinical outcomes of osteosarcoma patients.

3.2.2. Mammalian Target of Rapamycin (MTOR) Pathway as a Therapeutic Target in Osteosarcoma

mTOR is a serine/threonine kinase belonging to the PI3K protein family. The mTOR pathway is activated by not only growth factors but also nutrients and immune signals (Figure 3). mTOR is present two distinct multi-protein complexes termed mTOR complex 1 (mTORC1) and mTORC2. These complexes are differentially stimulated by distinct extracellular and intracellular signals. These signals activate the PI3K/AKT pathway. Activated AKT in turn activates mTOR through inhibition of the mTORC1 repression factor Tuberous Sclerosis Complex (TSC), comprised of TSC1 and TSC2. These TSCs inhibit the GTP-binding protein Rheb. In turn, Rheb activates mTORC1 [121]. Four proteins, mammalian lethal with regulatory-associated protein of mTOR (Raptor), SEC13 protein 8 (mLST8), proline-rich AKT substrate of 40 kDa (PRAS40), and DEP domain-containing mTOR-interacting protein (DEPTOR), are the components of mTORC1.

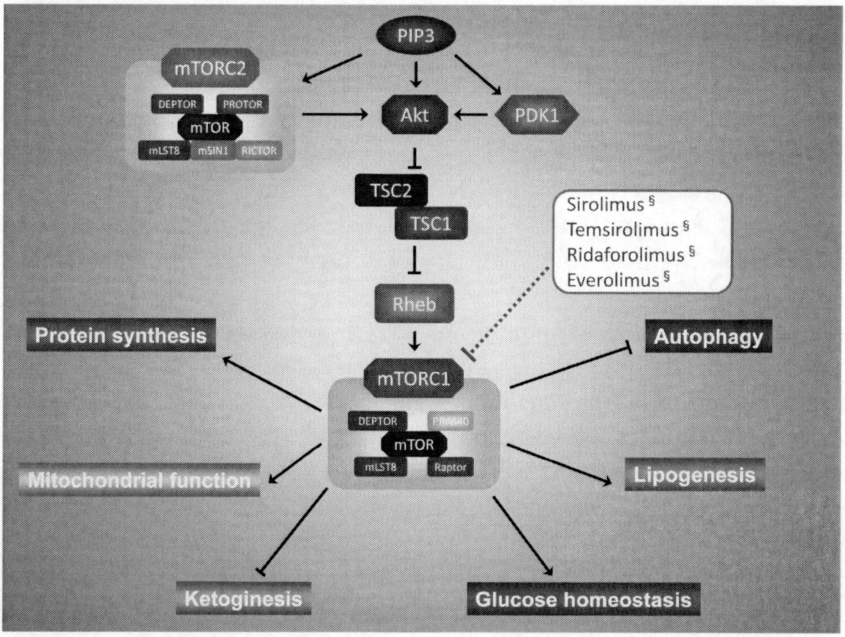

§: Developed into clinical trials.

Figure 3. mTOR pathway and potential target sites in osteosarcoma. The mTOR pathway activates the PI3K/AKT pathway. Activated AKT in turn activates mTOR through inhibition of TSC1/2. These TSCs inhibit Rheb. In turn, Rheb activates mTORC1. mTORC1 regulates protein translation. AKT is also phosphorylated by mTORC2. Several mTOR inhibitor blocks the mTOR pathway by directly binding mTORC1, potentially exerting immunosuppressive and anti-proliferative effects.

As mTORC1 regulates protein translation by phosphorylating S6 kinase (S6K) and eIF4E-binding proteins (4E-BPs), it controls cell growth, proliferation and metabolic processes. The five proteins in mTORC2 are raptor-independent companion of TOR (RICTOR), mLST8, DEPTOR, mammalian stress-activated protein kinase interacting protein 1 (mSIN1) and the protein observed with RICTOR (PROTOR). AKT and serum and glucocorticoid-inducible kinase (SGK), which regulates cell survival and proliferation, are phosphorylated by mTORC2 [122].

Activation of the mTOR pathway is a common finding in various cancers because this pathway is regulated via others, such as the PI3K/AKT pathway, mainly by upstream signals. Moreover, constitutive activation of the mTOR pathway renders tumors refractory to therapy, and is a poor prognostic factor for various cancers [123]. Thus, inhibition of mTOR might be a good therapeutic strategy for targeting cancerous tissues and cells.

Recent studies revealed the mTOR pathway to play important roles in osteosarcoma, and showed immunohistochemically that the mTOR/p70S6K pathway is activated in osteosarcoma. In addition, overexpressions of mTOR and p70S6K proteins correlated significantly with surgical stage, metastasis pattern and percentage of dead cells in osteosarcoma. These factors had a significant influence on OS and DFS. High levels of mTOR and p70S6K proteins were associated with significantly poorer outcomes of osteosarcoma cases [124].

Rapamycin (sirolimus) inhibits the mTOR pathway by directly binding mTORC1, potentially exerting immunosuppressive and anti-proliferative effects, while mTORC2 is generally insensitive to rapamycin. Several mTOR inhibitors, including rapamycin (sirolimus), and the rapamycin analogues temsirolimus (CCI-779) and ridaforolimus (AP23573, MK-8669, formerly deforolimus), have been studied in phase I/II clinical trials for advanced solid tumors [125, 126].

Rapamycin inhibited proliferation of osteosarcoma cells *in vitro* and also inhibited the growth of xenografts of osteosarcoma cell lines *in vivo* [127]. In a phase II trial (NCT00093080), ridaforolimus has a promising clinical benefit and progression-free survival rates in advanced sarcoma [128]. A phase III randomized, double-blind, placebo-controlled trial of ridaforolimus was performed by the Sarcoma Multi-Center Clinical Evaluation of the Efficacy of Ridaforolimus (SUCCEED) for metastatic soft-tissue sarcomas and metastatic bone sarcoma (NCT00538239). Treatment with ridaforolimus decreased the target lesion size, prolonged progression-free survival and improved median overall survival. Ridaforolimus treatment reduced the risk of disease progression or death by 28% in patients with metastatic soft tissue or bone sarcomas [129]. Everolimus (RAD001), an orally available mTOR inhibitor, has been developed for a phase II trials in patients with osteosarcoma (NCT01830153, NCT01216826). Everolimus showed inhibition of tumor growth in patients with bone and soft-tissue sarcoma after failure of previously chemotherapy [130].

Further benefits of mTOR inhibitors as single-dose therapy (NCT01216826, NCT01331135) and as multi-agent regimens (NCT00743509, NCT01804374) in the treatment of osteosarcoma patients are now being investigated.

3.2.3. Mitogen-Activated Protein Kinase (MAPK) Pathway as a Therapeutic Target in Osteosarcoma

Mitogen-activated protein kinases (MAPKs) are a family of hierarchically and widely-conserved serine/threonine kinases. MAPK pathways are comprised of a three-tier module activated through a phosphorylation cascade. The MAPKs are phosphorylated and activated by dual specificity MAPK kinases (MAPKK). In turn, the MAPKKs are phosphorylated and activated by MAPKK kinases (MAPKKKs). The MAPKKKs are activated by interaction with a family of small GTPases and/or other protein kinases, connecting the MAPK module to various extracellular signals including cytokines and growth factors. MAPKs phosphorylate their target proteins, which include transcription factors. Hence, MAPKs play important roles in various gene regulatory processes (Figure 4). There are three major MAPK pathways: MAPK/ERK (extracellular signal-regulated protein kinase), JNK (c-Jun N-terminal kinase), and p38 [131].

The MAPK/ERK pathway is classically referred to as the MAPK pathway. This pathway consists of Ras, Raf, MAPK/ERK kinase (MEK) and ERK. The MAPK/ERK pathway is activated by numerous extracellular signals including growth factors and mitogens binding to RTK. Numerous extracellular signals lead to the recruitment of GDP/GTP exchange factors, growth-factor-receptor bound protein 2 (Grp2) and Sons of Sevenless (SOS) to the plasma membrane where Ras resides, and thereby promote the activation of Ras. Activated Ras binds to Raf, serving as a control of molecular switches in cellular signal transduction. Rafs (Raf-1, B-Raf and A-Raf) activate MEK1 and MEK2. MEK1 and MEK2 activate ERK1 and ERK2 upon phosphorylation. In turn, activated ERKs induce the phosphorylation of nuclear and cytoplasmic target proteins such as transcription factors and cytoskeletal proteins. The MAPK/ERK pathway controls an array of biological processes including proliferation, differentiation, survival, migration, angiogenesis and chromatin remodeling [132].

The JNK pathway is strongly activated by heat, oxidative stress, inflammatory cytokines, UV radiation, growth factors, DNA damage, certain G-protein coupled receptors and serum. The JNK pathway includes Racs, Rhos and Cdc42s. MEK kinase (MEKK) 1 and MEKK4, MLK2 and MLK3, ASK1, TAK1 and Tpl2 activate MEK4 and MEK7. MEK 4 and MEK7 activate JNK (JNK1, JNK2 and JNK3). In turn, activated JNKs induce apoptosis, inflammation, cytokine production and metabolic processes [133].

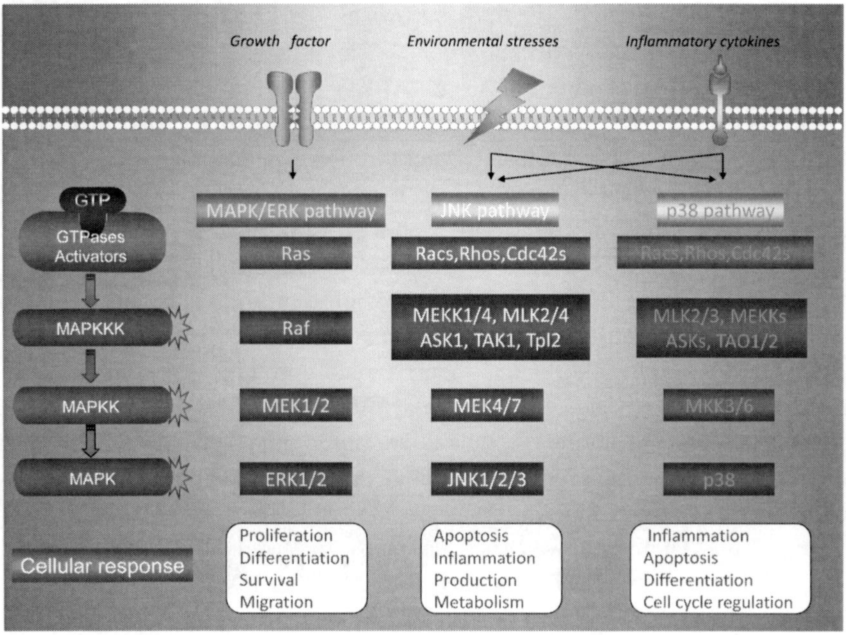

Figure 4. MAPK pathway. MAPK pathways are comprised of a three-tier module activated through a phosphorylation cascade. The MAPKs are phosphorylated and activated by dual specificity MAPKK. In turn, the MAPKKs are phosphorylated and activated by MAPKKKs. The MAPKKKs are activated by interaction with a family of small GTPases and/or other protein kinases, connecting the MAPK module to various extracellular signals including cytokines and growth factors. MAPKs phosphorylate their target proteins, which include transcription factors. There are three major MAPK pathways: MAPK/ERK, JNK, and p38.

The p38 pathway is activated by environmental stress factors such as heat, osmotic and oxidative stresses, ionizing radiation and ischemia-induced vaso-activation, and inflammatory cytokines. The p38 pathway was found in 2007 to include the Rho family GTPases Cdc42 and Rac (Johnson and Nakamura). MLK2 and MLK3, MEKKs, ASKs, TAK1, and TAO1 and TAO2 activate MKK3 and MKK6. MKK3 and MKK6 activate p38 (p38a, p38b, p38g, and p38d). In turn, activated p38 induces inflammation, apoptosis, and cell differentiation, as well as regulating the cell cycle [134].

MAPK pathways are involved in various biological processes, including growth, proliferation, differentiation, migration, apoptosis and survival. Therefore, dysregulation of MAPK pathways correlates with tumorigenesis in many cancers including osteosarcoma.

Dysregulation of the MAPK pathway is commonly identified in a variety of cancers. Aberrant activation of the Ras/Raf/MEK/MAP kinase pathway is involved in tumorigenesis in various malignancies including osteosarcoma [135].

The RAS family has three isofroms: H-, N-, and K-Ras. RAS gene mutations have been investigated in various cancers including osteosarcomas. RAS gene mutations constitutively lead to the activation of downstream effectors such as Raf, PI3K, and Ral-Guanine Nucleotide Dissociation Stimulator, which is a guanine nucleotide exchange factor for the small GTPase Ral. Indeed, RAS gene mutations are found in more than 30% of cancers [136]. However, in a study of osteosarcoma, the *K-ras* gene was mutated in 12% of cases, while the *N-ras* gene was mutated in only one of 28 cases and *H-ras* gene was not mutated in osteosarcoma [137-139]. Moreover, amplification of Raf-1 was identified in osteosarcoma [140]. The ERK1/2, MCL-1 and ERM pathways were activated in approximately 70% of cases and in all osteosarcoma cell lines, and has a promising therapeutic targets for osteosarcoma. Moreover, a mutation of the B-Raf gene was found in 4 of 30 osteosarcoma patients [141]. Sorafenib (BAY 43-9006) is a multi-kinase inhibitor, and inhibits the RAF/MEK/ERK pathway via inhibition of Raf-1. Furthermore, sorafenib also targets several RTK such as FGFR, VEGFR-2, VEGFR-3, PDGFR-β, RET, FLT-3 and c-KIT. Sorafenib inhibits the ERK1/2, MCL-1 and ERM pathways, thereby blocking angiogenesis and tumor activity *in vitro* and *in vivo* [141]. Sorafenib has exhibited intermediate response activity in four of five osteosarcoma xenograft models [142]. In a phase II trial of sorafenib (NCT00889057), a clinical benefit response was achieved in ten of 35 with osteosarcoma [143]. Sorafenib is also being clinically investigated in combination with everolimus (NCT01804374), ifosfamide (NCT00880542) and irinotecan (NCT01518413).

AZD6244 is a MEK1/2 inhibitor and its efficacy for the inhibition of tumor growth was investigated in the Pediatric Preclinical Testing Program. AZD6244 showed intermediate activity in three of six osteosarcoma xenograft models [144]. However, clinical trials of AZD6244 for osteosarcomas have not yet begun.

Many growth factor receptors including IGF-1R, EGFR, VEGFR, and PDGFR associated with osteosarcoma biology activate the MAPK/ERK pathway, and targeting this pathway may have utility in designing novel therapeutic interventions for osteosarcoma.

3.2.4. Signal Transducers and Activators of Transcription 3 (STAT3) Pathway as a Therapeutic Target in Osteosarcoma

STAT3 is one of seven members of the STAT transcription factor family. STAT3 modulates the transcription factors for genes including anti-apoptotic proteins such as bcl-2, Bcl-xL, survivin and Mcl-1, cell cycle regulatory molecules such as Cyclin D1/D2, p21, and p27 and mitochondrial apoptosis pathway-related proteins such as Bax, Bak, Cytochrome c and Caspase3 (Figure 5). Thus, STAT3 is involved in the regulation of biological processes including proliferation, apoptosis, development, cell differentiation, inflammation, angiogenesis, metastasis, and immune responses.

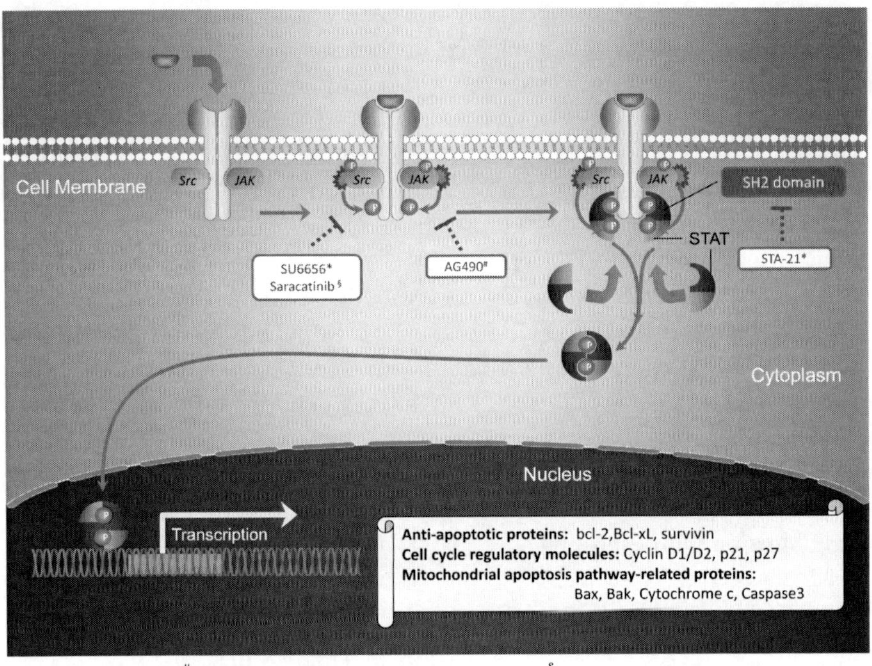

*: Studied in vitro, #: Studied both in vitro and in vivo, §: Developed into clinical trials.

Figure 5. STAT3 pathway and potential target sites in osteosarcoma. Ligand binding to the membrane receptor triggers receptor dimerization of the cytoplasmic domain and activation of JAK proteins. The cytoplasmic STATs are recruited to the phosphorylated receptor through their SH2 domain. STATs are phosphorylated by JAK and then dimerized. The STAT3 dimer is then translocated into the nucleus by importins. In the nucleus, active STAT will specifically bind to consensus DNA sequences at an interferon-gamma activated site, thereby modulating the transcription factors of target genes.

STAT proteins are regulated by RTKs such as EGFR, TGF-α, PDGFR, and colony stimulating factor-1R, and cytokines such as interleukin (IL)-6, LIF (leukemia inhibitory factor), CT-1, CNTF (ciliary neurotrophic factor), IL-10, IL-11, and oncostatin M. In addition, the Src family of kinases (SFKs), which includes Src, Lck, Hck, Lyn, Fyn, and Fgr, either activates STAT3 directly or stimulates downstream factors involved in the activation of RTKs or GPCRs such as the angiotensin II receptor. Ligand binding to the membrane receptor triggers receptor dimerization of the cytoplasmic domain and activation of JAK proteins. The JAK family has four members, JAK1, JAK2, JAK3, and tyrosine kinase 2. Of these, JAK2 has been implicated as the major player in STAT3 phosphorylation. The cytoplasmic STATs are recruited to the phosphorylated receptor through their SH2 domain. STATs are phosphorylated by JAK at tyrosine 705 and then dimerized. The STAT3 dimer is then translocated into the nucleus by importins. In the nucleus, active STAT will specifically bind to consensus DNA sequences at an interferon-gamma activated site, thereby modulating the transcription factors of target genes [145]. Downstream JAKs also induce activation of the Ras/Raf/ MAPK and PI3K/AKT pathways [146].

In many cancers, an imbalance among signaling pathways leads to constitutive activation of STAT3 that is sufficient to induce tumorigenesis, apoptosis and resistance to chemotherapy. Constitutive activation of STAT3 is increasingly recognized as loss of function of the negative regulators in various types of cancer including osteosarcoma. Disruption of the STAT3 pathway inhibits the growth and apoptosis of tumor cell lines and inhibits tumor growth in mouse xenograft cancer models [145]. Anti-apoptotic proteins such as BCL-xL, MCL-1 and survivin were shown to be up-regulated in osteosarcoma [147]. Moreover, these data showed that cell lines and 88% of tissues overexpressed pSTAT3 in osteosarcoma, and the staining level of pSTAT3 correlated with poor outcomes [147]. High levels of activated STAT3 expression have been associated with poor outcomes for many cancer patients, including those with renal cell carcinoma, colorectal cancer, ovarian carcinoma, gastric carcinoma, intestinal-type gastric adenocarcinoma, cervical squamous-cell carcinoma, epithelial ovarian carcinoma and osteosarcoma. Therefore, the STAT3 pathway is a potential therapeutic target.

Recent studies have demonstrated the biological effects of upstream kinases of the STAT3 pathway or direct STAT inhibition in various cancers. The therapeutic target of the upstream kinase of the STAT3 pathway has been inhibition of JAK using AG490, and Src inhibitors such as SU6656. Inhibitors of JAK have been pre-clinically and clinically evaluated as cancer treatments.

AG490 inhibits the phosphorylation of JAK2 and STAT3 in osteosarcoma [148]. Src inhibitors also showed promise for STAT3 inhibition *in vitro*. The Src inhibitor, SU6656, blocks constitutively active STAT3 in osteosarcoma cell lines, thereby providing a potential target for therapeutic intervention [149].

Therapeutic agents targeting direct STAT inhibition have been reported to suppress STAT3 activity in cancers. Target sites for STAT3 inhibition have been identified and include direct inhibition of the SH2 domain of the kinases Src or JAK and blocking dimerization, inhibition of the DBD domain for binding of STAT3 to DNA, and inhibition of the transcriptional activity of STAT3 with the N-terminal domain [150]. STA-21 is a small molecule inhibitor that directly inhibits the SH2 domain of STAT3 and thereby blocks dimerization. Treatment with STA-21 induced apoptosis in osteosarcoma cells *in vitro*. Inhibition of the STAT3 pathway may thus be an effective treatment strategy for osteosarcoma [151].

Recently, clinical trials for Src inhibitors, such as Saracatinib, have been recruiting by the Sarcoma Alliance for Research through Collaboration in a phase II trial for osteosarcoma (NCT00752206). However, other therapeutic targets in the STAT3 pathway have not been sufficiently studied to allow clinical trials for osteosarcoma. Current studies are, however, demonstrating the potential utility of such therapeutic interventions for osteosarcoma.

3.3. Cell Cycle Kinases as a Therapeutic Target in Osteosarcoma

Cell division is manipulated by protein kinases in mammalian cells. Cyclin-dependent kinases (CDKs) are key cell cycle regulatory proteins the activation of which is modulated by several activators such as cyclins and inhibitors such as members of the inhibitor of CDK4 (INK4) family including INK4A (p16), INK4B (p15), INK4C (p18) and INK4D (p19), which inhibit CDK4 and CDK6, and the Cip/Kip family including p21 (Waf1, Cip1), p27 (Cip2), and p57 (Kip2), which suppress CDK2 activity. CDKs are heterodimeric protein kinases composed of a catalytic subunit ("CDK") and a regulatory subunit ("Cyclin"). These complexes regulate cell cycle progression and transcription. In the mammalian genome, CDKs have been directly implicated in the cell cycle, with CDK1, CDK2, CDK3, CDK4, CDK6, and CDK7 being involved, and in transcription with CDK7, CDK8 and CDK9 being involved, as well as in neuronal functions involving CDK5 and CDK11. CDKs regulate cell cycle progression through the four sequential phases of this cycle, and are essential for driving each of the phases, i.e. G1 (CDK4, CDK6 and CDK2), S (CDK2), M and G2 (CDK1).

Cyclin D (D1, D2 and D3) binds to and thereby activates CDK4 and CDK6 during the G1 phase, in which the cell prepares to initiate DNA synthesis. The cyclin D-CDK4/6 complex leads to partial inactivation of pocket proteins such as retinoblastoma protein (Rb), Rbl1 (p107) and Rbl2 (p130), resulting in dissociation and thereby activation of E2F transcription factors. E2F transcription factors initiate both cyclin E and CDK2. Cyclin E (with E1 and E2 forms) binds to and activates CDK2 from the G1 through the S phase. The cyclin E–CDK2 complex leads to complete inactivation of pocket proteins, and is essential for promoting entry into the S phase and DNA synthesis (Figure 6). Subsequently, cyclin A binds to CDK2, in turn activating this complex from the S phase to the G2 phase. Cyclin B binds with CDK1, which is known as cell division control protein 2 (CDC2), and this complex, which is the key regulatory protein for mitotic entry, promotes progression during the G2–M transition and mitosis. Moreover, PLK1 and Aurora kinase A are involved in centrosome maturation and spindle formation throughout mitosis. During the G2-M transition, PLK1 phosphorylates cyclin B-CDK1. CDC25 is dephosphorylated, reversing the inhibitory phosphorylation of CDK. Consequently, CDK1 is activated for entry into the mitotic process.

PLK1 phosphorylates the positive regulator CDC25 and inhibits the negative regulators WEE1 and membrane-associated CDK1-inhibitory kinase, thereby promoting the activation of CDK1 (Figure 6) [152].

Cell cycle progression can be delayed or blocked at several checkpoints due to DNA damage or other cellular insults. p53 is essential for the G1/S checkpoint in the S phase, and stimulates the transcription of different genes including that of *p21* inhibited CDK activity, and *Mdm2* inhibited p53 transcriptional activity and *Bax.* Checkpoint kinase 1 (CHK1) is a key regulatory protein kinase, which is involved in the intra-S phase and G2/M checkpoints. Activation of CHK1 inactivates CDC25, resulting in S or G2 phase arrest via inhibitory activation of CDK. The WEE1 kinase inhibits entry into the mitotic process via inhibitory activation of CDK1, which controls CDK1 and CDK2 activities during the S phase [152-154].

Cell cycle dysregulation occurs in various human cancers. Constitutive and deregulated CDK are frequently characterized by unscheduled proliferation, genomic instability and chromosomal instability in cancer cells. In several malignancies, upregulation of CDKs commonly manifests as over-expression of cyclin or inactivation of CDK inhibitors.

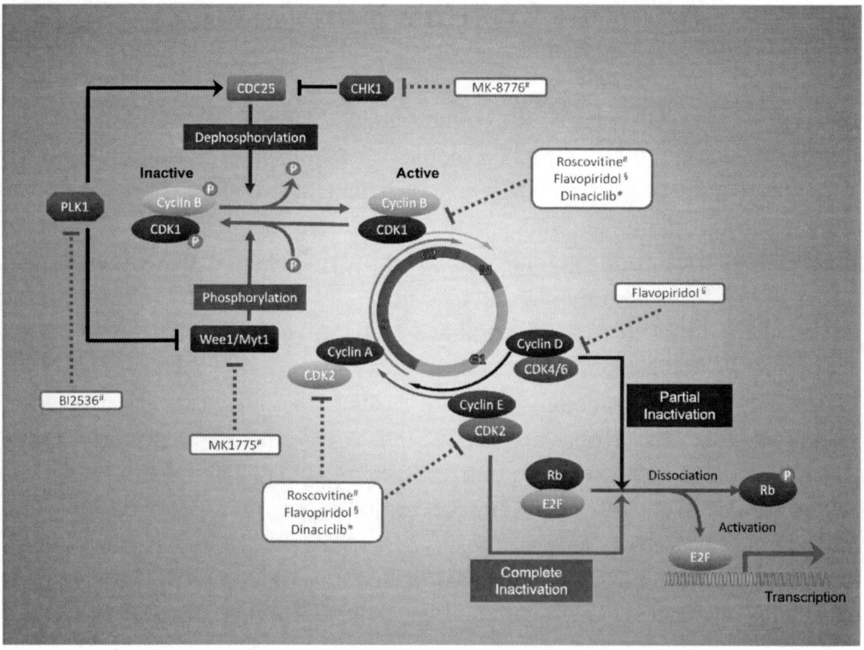

*: Studied in vitro, #: Studied both in vitro and in vivo, §: Developed into clinical trials.

Figure 6. Cell cycle associated kinases and potential target sites in osteosarcoma. The cyclin D-CDK4/6 and cyclin E–CDK2 complex lead to inactivation of Rb, resulting in dissociation and thereby activation of E2F transcription factors, and is essential for promoting entry into the S phase and DNA synthesis. PLK1 phosphorylates CDC25 and inhibits WEE1/ Myt1, thereby promoting the activation of CDK1. Activation of CHK1 inactivates CDC25, resulting in S or G2 phase arrest via inhibitory activation of CDK. The WEE1 kinase inhibits entry into the mitotic process via inhibitory activation of CDK1.

These alterations of mitotic checkpoints and the consequent DNA damage frequently increase the activity of CDK resulting in further driving of tumor cell cycles. Hence, the cell cycle and the checkpoint machinery provide potential targets for cancer therapy [155].

Dysregulation of CDKs is frequently associated with genetic alterations in a wide range of cancers[156]. Recently, selective inhibitors of CDKs and mitotic kinases, such as Staurosporine, Flavonoids, Purine, Indole, Pyrimidine, Indirubin, Pyrazole, and Thiazole, have been developed [157]. Roscovitine (seliciclib) is a selective inhibitor of CDK1, 2, 7 and 9 and Flavopiridol (alvocidib) is multiple inhibitors of cyclin-CDK holoenzymes, including cyclin D-cdk4, cyclin A/E-cdk2, and cyclin B-cdk1. These inhibitor of CDKs have been shown to induce not only cell cycle arrest but also apoptosis in various tumor cells including those of melanoma and prostate carcinoma, head and neck squamous carcinoma, and cervical carcinoma[158-160]. A recent study demonstrated Roscovitine (seliciclib) to have been successfully tested *in vivo* for NSCLC, and multiple myeloma [157]. Another CDK inhibitor, Dinaciclib (SCH 727965) which inhibits the activities of CDK1, CDK2 and CDK9, induced cell cycle arrest and apoptosis in osteosarcoma cells [161]. These findings suggest the potential utility of targeting multiple CDK inhibitors as therapeutic interventions for osteosarcoma.

PLK1 regulates multiple stages of mitosis and maintains genomic stability [162]. Overexpression of PLK1 has been reported, and correlates with both tumor progression and patient survival in several human cancers [162]. Inhibition of PLK1 was revealed to significantly induce growth arrest and apoptosis in osteosarcoma cell lines, and is thus a potential treatment target for osteosarcoma [163]. Moreover, BI 2536, a small-molecule inhibitor of PLK1, was demonstrated to induce mitotic arrest and apoptosis in osteosarcoma both *in vitro* and *in vivo* [164].

Aurora kinases regulate chromosome segregation and cytokinesis in the G2 to M phases of mitosis. The three members of this family are Aurora kinases A, B and C. Aurora kinases A and B are ubiquitously expressed in all tissues, whereas Aurora kinase C accumulates mainly at the centrosome. Overexpression or amplification of Aurora kinases has been reported in various tumor cell lines and is involved tumorigenesis, thereby conferring a poor prognosis [165]. Hence, targeting of these kinases might be a good strategy for molecular therapies. In fact, more than 30 Aurora kinase inhibitors have been developed and have been pre-clinically and clinically evaluated for the treatment of various cancers [166].

Recent study have shown that overexpression of Aurora kinases to correlate with a poor prognosis in canine osteosarcoma, which is high similar to the human disease [167]. The aurora kinase A inhibitor alisertib (MLN8237) inhibited tumor growth both *in vitro* and *in vivo*. Complete responses were maintained in only one of six osteosarcoma xenografts, progressive disease was observed in four, and the other showed stable disease [168]. A phase II study of alisertib is now being conducted, as a clinical trial, by the Children's Oncology Group in children with relapsed/treatment-refractory solid tumors including recurrent osteosarcoma (NCT01154816). Unfortunately, a recent study showed canine osteosarcoma cells to exhibit resistance to Aurora kinase inhibitors [169].

WEE1 and CHK1 are involved in the S and G2/M checkpoints, and are upregulated in various cancers. Recent osteosarcoma studies have demonstrated that the CHK1 inhibitor MK-8776 and the WEE1 inhibitor MK1775 induced osteosarcoma cell death and inhibited tumor growth both *in vitro* and *in vivo* [170, 171]. Notably, WEE1 and CHK1 inhibitors have been tested in early stage clinical trials for the treatment of advanced solid tumors [172].

Further investigation of the potential utility of kinase inhibitors, based on their roles in the cell cycle, is anticipated.

4. Angiogenic Pathway (VEGF Pathway) as a Therapeutic Target in Osteosarcoma

Angiogenesis is an essential biological process for the growth and development of normal as well as cancer cells. Angiogenesis is mainly regulated by vascular endothelial growth factor (VEGF) and its cognate receptor, known as vascular endothelial growth factor receptor (VEGFR). In fact, several cells including fibroblasts, inflammatory cells, and numerous tumor cells, are often stimulated to produce more VEGF in response to increasing tumor hypoxia. Therefore, VEGF contributes mainly to the processes of angiogenesis and lymphangiogenesis [173].

VEGFs consist of five proteins designated A, B, C, D and placental growth factor. VEGFA and B promote angiogenesis by serving as important growth factors for blood vessel endothelial cells, resulting in multifaceted effects, including proliferation, cell migration and tube formation. There are three VEGF receptor isoforms designated VEGFR-1, -2, and -3. VEGF-C and -D bind to VEGFR-3, and are involved in lymphangiogenesis. VEGF-A and VEGF-B bind to VEGFR-1 and -2, and these VEGFRs activate several signal pathways including the PI3K/AKT and MAPK pathways [174]. Therefore, VEGF and VEGFR are both essential for tumor growth and progression, and dysregulation of the pathways involved contributes to cell proliferation, survival, invasion, metastasis and angiogenesis in many cancers including osteosarcoma.

Overexpression of VEGF has been reported in various tumor cell lines and leads to tumorigenesis, with the associated poor prognosis, in various cancers including osteosarcoma. In a meta-analysis of all available studies relating

VEGF with clinical outcomes of osteosarcoma patients, overexpression of VEGF was associated with a poor prognosis [175]. Therefore, inhibition of the VEGF pathway may lead to suppression of both angiogenesis and tumor growth in a broad range of cancers, including osteosarcoma. Recently, inhibition of VEGF, achieved with conventional chemotherapy, exerted significant effects on cancers [176]. Thus, VEGF inhibition is a potentially novel therapeutic strategy for osteosarcoma.

Several therapeutic agents targeting the VEGF pathway have been developed. These agents target either VEGF or VEGFRs. A mAb against VEGF has been investigated as an inhibitor of tumor angiogenesis in preclinical studies and clinical trials for various cancers [177]. Bevacizumab, a humanized mAb targeting the VEGF receptor, was investigated in a phase I study on pediatric patients with treatment-refractory solid tumors by a children's oncology group study [178]. Furthermore, a clinical trial of combination chemotherapy (NCT00667342, NCT01492673) was conducting. A trial of Cediranib (AZD2171), with a specific inhibitor of VEGFRs, is underway to determine whether these agents can inhibit activation of VEGFR1, VEGFR2, VEGFR3 and c-KIT. Cediranib showed high efficacy in four of five osteosarcoma xenograft models [179]. Cediranib in combination with gefitinib is currently being evaluated in patients with advanced tumors including osteosarcoma in a phase I trial, and one osteosarcoma patient was confirmed to have shown a partial response (NCT00502060) [180]. Future research and more clinical trials on VEGF are highly anticipated. Pazopanib is a multi-kinase inhibitor, and targets VEGFR-1, -2, and -3, PDGFR-α, -β and c-KIT. Pazopanib is currently being evaluated for children with treatment-*refractory solid tumors including osteosarcoma* in a phase I trial (NCT01130623) [181].

5. Exploring Other Novel Kinase-Based Therapeutic Targets in Osteosarcoma

To identify therapeutic targets that are responsible for the growth and survival of osteosarcoma cells, previous studies were conducted using small interfering RNA (siRNA) library or lentiviral-based short hairpin RNA (shRNA) library screenings [163, 182]. Recent study identified protein kinases such as PLK1, WEE1, EPHA1, CHEK1 and CSNK2B using the siRNA screening library. Loss of these genes significantly reduced the viability of an osteosarcoma cell line [182]. Using a lentiviral-based shRNA library to screen the osteosarcoma cell line our study identified four kinases including MIRK, PLK1, ROCK1 and CDK11, also known as CDC2L or PITSLRE [163]. This study also revealed the functions of four kinases found in osteosarcoma. MIRK and PLK1 are essential for cell growth and survival in osteosarcoma and knock down of these kinases leads to apoptosis and inhibition of proliferation *in vitro*.

High levels of MIRK and PLK1 expression were associated with poor outcomes [163, 183]. ROCK1 is highly expressed in osteosarcoma. Knockdown of ROCK1 reduced cell proliferation and viability, as well as inducing apoptosis, *in vitro*. Clinically, high levels of ROCK1 expression were already known to be associated with poor outcomes in osteosarcoma patients [184]. Moreover, levels of CDK11 expression in osteosarcoma were high compared with those in normal osteoblasts. High levels of CDK11 expression correlated with poor outcomes. In addition, inhibition of CDK11 reduced tumor volume *in vivo* [185]. Taken together, these findings suggest that MIRK, PLK1, ROCK1 and CDK11 are potentially novel therapeutic targets in osteosarcoma.

Conclusion

In this chapter, we have presented recent advances in the development and emerging roles of novel therapeutic strategies employing protein kinases for osteosarcoma. Protein kinases are involved in virtually every signaling pathways of osteosarcoma cell growth. Moreover, various signaling pathways are overexpressed, mutated, and/or constitutively activated in osteosarcoma. These observations suggest targeting protein kinases have a great potential for improving the survival outcomes of osteosarcoma patients.

Numerous protein kinases inhibitors are now under development. At present, several clinical trials are evaluating for protein kinase targetd therapies in osteosarcoma (Table 3). However, in patients with osteosarcoma, the results from these clinical trials have not appeared to dramatically change the outcome of management as seen in CML with Imatinib, nevertheless, protein kinases have a sufficient potential as a target therapy because their crucial roles in osteosarcoma cell growth. Therefore, more clinical trials are anticipated in the future.

Table 3. Clinical trials using protein kinase targetd therapies in osteosarcoma. Source used; clinicaltrials.gov

ClinicalTrials.gov Identifier	Phase	Protein kinase inhibitors	Primary molecular target	Combination with chemotherapy	Status	Response activity	Refe-rence
NCT00642941	2	RG1507	IGF1R	No	Active, not recruiting	Intermediate activity	[61]
NCT00563680	2	AMG 479	IGF1R	No	Complete		N/A
NCT00831844	2	Cixutumumab	IGF1R	No	Active, not recruiting		N/A
NCT00609141	1	Cixutumumab	IGF1R	No	Complete		N/A
NCT01016015	2	Cixutumumab	IGF1R	Yes	Active, not recruiting	Intermediate activity	[58]
NCT01614795	2	Cixutumumab	IGF1R	Yes	Suspen-ded		N/A
NCT00617890	2	SCH 717454	IGF1R	No	Termi-nated		N/A
NCT00132158	1	Gefitinib	EGFR	Yes	Complete		N/A
NCT00077454	1	Erlotinib	EGFR	Yes	Complete		[100]
NCT00023998	2	Trastuzumab	HER2	Yes	Complete	Low activity	[103]
NCT00005033	2	Trastuzumab	HER2	No	Complete		N/A
NCT00889057	2	Sorafenib	Raf-1, FGFR, VEGFR-2, -3, PDGFR-β, RET, FLT-3,c-KIT	No	Complete	Intermediate activity	[142]
NCT00880542	2	Sorafenib	Raf-1, FGFR, VEGFR-2, -3, PDGFR-β, RET, FLT-3,c-KIT	Yes	Termi-nated		N/A
NCT00330421	2	Sorafenib	Raf-1, FGFR, VEGFR-2, -3, PDGFR-β, RET, FLT-3,c-KIT	No	Complete		N/A
NCT01518413	1	Sorafenib	Raf-1, FGFR, VEGFR-2, -3, PDGFR-β, RET, FLT-3,c-KIT	Yes	Recruting		N/A
NCT01804374	2	Sorafenib Everolimus	Sorafenib: Raf-1, FGFR, VEGFR-2, -3, PDGFR-β, RET, FLT-3,c-KIT Everolims: mTOR	Yes	Recruting		N/A

Table 3. (Continued)

ClinicalTrials. gov Identifier	Phase	Protein kinase inhibitors	Primary molecular target	Combination with chemotherapy	Status	Response activity	Refe- rence
NCT00031915	2	Imatinib mesylate	BCR-ABL, PDGFRs, c-KIT	No	Complete	Intermediate activity	[78]
NCT00030667	2	Imatinib - mesylate	BCR-ABL, PDGFRs, c-KIT	No	Active, not recruiting	Low activity	[43]
NCT00154388	2	Imatinib mesylate	BCR-ABL, PDGFRs, c-KIT	No	Complete		N/A
NCT00752206	2	Saracatinib	Src	No	Recruting		N/A
NCT00464620	2	Dasatinib	Abl/Src, c-Kit, PDGFR, Ephrin	No	Active, not recruiting		N/A
NCT00788125	1/2	Dasatinib	Abl/Src, c-Kit, PDGFR, Ephrin	Yes	Active, not recruiting		N/A
NCT01643278	1	Dasatinib Ipilimumab	Abl/Src, c-Kit, PDGFR, Ephrin	Yes	Recruting		N/A
NCT01353625	1	CC-115	mTOR	No	Recruting		N/A
NCT01154816	3	Ridaforoli- mus	mTOR	No	Recruting		N/A
NCT00538239	3	Ridaforoli- mus	mTOR	No	Complete	Intermediate activity	[128]
NCT00093080	2	Ridaforoli- mus	mTOR	No	Complete	Intermedia- te activity	[127]
NCT01216826	2	Everolimus	mTOR	No	Recruting		N/A
NCT01331135	1	Sirolimus	mTOR	No	Recruting		N/A
NCT00743509	2	Sirolimus	mTOR	No	Active, not recruiting		N/A
NCT01204450	1	Temsiro- limus	mTOR	Yes	Terminat ed		N/A
NCT00949325	1/2	Temsiro- limus	mTOR	Yes	Complete		N/A
NCT01830153	2	Everolimus (RAD001)	mTOR	No	Complete	Intermedia- te activity	[129]
NCT00012181	1	Alvocidib	CDK	No	Complete		N/A
NCT01154816	2	Alisertib	Aurora A kinase	No	Recruting		N/A
NCT00667342	2	Bevaci- zumab	VEGF	Yes	Active, not recruiting		N/A
NCT01492673	2	Bevaci- zumab	VEGF	Yes	Recruting		N/A
NCT00474994	2	Sunitinib	VEGFR	No	Complete		N/A
NCT00502060	1	AZD2171 Gefitinib	AZD2171: VEGFR	Yes	Complete		[179]

ClinicalTrials. gov Identifier	Phase	Protein kinase inhibitors	Primary molecular target	Combination with chemotherapy	Status	Response activity	Reference
			Gefitinib: EGFR				
NCT01130623	1	Pazopanib	VEGFR-1, -2, -3, PDGFR-α, -β, c-KIT	No	Withdrawn		N/A

N/A:not applicable.

REFERENCES

[1] Mohseny, A. B., Szuhai, K., Romeo, S., Buddingh, E. P., Briaire-de Bruijn, I., de Jong, D., van Pel, M., Cleton-Jansen, A. M., & Hogendoorn, P. C. (2009) Osteosarcoma originates from mesenchymal stem cells in consequence of aneuploidization and genomic loss of Cdkn2, *The Journal of pathology 219*, 294-305.

[2] Geller, D. S., & Gorlick, R. (2010) Osteosarcoma: a review of diagnosis, management, and treatment strategies, *Clinical advances in hematology & oncology: H&O 8*, 705-718.

[3] Picci, P., Ferrari, S., Bacci, G., & Gherlinzoni, F. (1994) Treatment recommendations for osteosarcoma and adult soft tissue sarcomas, *Drugs 47*, 82-92.

[4] Bielack, S. S., Kempf-Bielack, B., Delling, G., Exner, G. U., Flege, S., Helmke, K., Kotz, R., Salzer-Kuntschik, M., Werner, M., Winkelmann, W., Zoubek, A., Jurgens, H., & Winkler, K. (2002) Prognostic factors in high-grade osteosarcoma of the extremities or trunk: an analysis of 1,702 patients treated on neoadjuvant cooperative osteosarcoma study group protocols, *Journal of clinical oncology: official journal of the American Society of Clinical Oncology 20*, 776-790.

[5] Chou, A. J., Geller, D. S., & Gorlick, R. (2008) Therapy for osteosarcoma: where do we go from here?, *Paediatric drugs 10*, 315-327.

[6] Schwartz, C. L., Gorlick, R., Teot, L., Krailo, M., Chen, Z., Goorin, A., Grier, H. E., Bernstein, M. L., Meyers, P., & Children's Oncology, G. (2007) Multiple drug resistance in osteogenic sarcoma: INT0133 from the Children's Oncology Group, *Journal of clinical oncology: official journal of the American Society of Clinical Oncology 25*, 2057-2062.

[7] Kempf-Bielack, B., Bielack, S. S., Jurgens, H., Branscheid, D., Berdel, W. E., Exner, G. U., Gobel, U., Helmke, K., Jundt, G., Kabisch, H.,

Kevric, M., Klingebiel, T., Kotz, R., Maas, R., Schwarz, R., Semik, M., Treuner, J., Zoubek, A., & Winkler, K. (2005) Osteosarcoma relapse after combined modality therapy: an analysis of unselected patients in the Cooperative Osteosarcoma Study Group (COSS), *Journal of clinical oncology: official journal of the American Society of Clinical Oncology 23*, 559-568.

[8] Broadhead, M. L., Clark, J. C., Myers, D. E., Dass, C. R., & Choong, P. F. (2011) The molecular pathogenesis of osteosarcoma: a review, *Sarcoma 2011*, 959248.

[9] Johnson, J. R., Bross, P., Cohen, M., Rothmann, M., Chen, G., Zajicek, A., Gobburu, J., Rahman, A., Staten, A., & Pazdur, R. (2003) Approval summary: imatinib mesylate capsules for treatment of adult patients with newly diagnosed philadelphia chromosome-positive chronic myelogenous leukemia in chronic phase, *Clinical cancer research: an official journal of the American Association for Cancer Research 9*, 1972-1979.

[10] Arteaga, C. L. (2003) ErbB-targeted therapeutic approaches in human cancer, *Experimental cell research 284*, 122-130.

[11] Ostman, A., & Heldin, C. H. (2007) PDGF receptors as targets in tumor treatment, *Advances in cancer research 97*, 247-274.

[12] Jiang, Y., Ming, L., Montero, A. J., Kimchi, E., Nikfarjam, M., & Staveley-O'Carroll, K. F. (2008) Optimizing imatinib mesylate treatment in gastrointestinal stromal tumors, *Gastrointestinal cancer research: GCR 2*, 245-250.

[13] Manning, G., Whyte, D. B., Martinez, R., Hunter, T., & Sudarsanam, S. (2002) The protein kinase complement of the human genome, *Science 298*, 1912-1934.

[14] MacKeigan, J. P., Murphy, L. O., & Blenis, J. (2005) Sensitized RNAi screen of human kinases and phosphatases identifies new regulators of apoptosis and chemoresistance, *Nature cell biology 7*, 591-600.

[15] Sebolt-Leopold, J. S., & English, J. M. (2006) Mechanisms of drug inhibition of signalling molecules, *Nature 441*, 457-462.

[16] Du, J., Bernasconi, P., Clauser, K. R., Mani, D. R., Finn, S. P., Beroukhim, R., Burns, M., Julian, B., Peng, X. P., Hieronymus, H., Maglathlin, R. L., Lewis, T. A., Liau, L. M., Nghiemphu, P., Mellinghoff, I. K., Louis, D. N., Loda, M., Carr, S. A., Kung, A. L., & Golub, T. R. (2009) Bead-based profiling of tyrosine kinase phosphorylation identifies SRC as a potential target for glioblastoma therapy, *Nature biotechnology 27*, 77-83.

[17] Casaletto, J. B., & McClatchey, A. I. (2012) Spatial regulation of receptor tyrosine kinases in development and cancer, *Nature reviews. Cancer 12*, 387-400.

[18] Paul, M. K., & Mukhopadhyay, A. K. (2004) Tyrosine kinase - Role and significance in Cancer, *International journal of medical sciences 1*, 101-115.

[19] Hunter, T. (2000) Signaling--2000 and beyond, *Cell 100*, 113-127.

[20] Schlessinger, J. (2000) Cell signaling by receptor tyrosine kinases, *Cell 103*, 211-225.

[21] Andrade, L. F., Nahum, L. A., Avelar, L. G., Silva, L. L., Zerlotini, A., Ruiz, J. C., & Oliveira, G. (2011) Eukaryotic protein kinases (ePKs) of the helminth parasite Schistosoma mansoni, *BMC genomics 12*, 215.

[22] Cheong, J. K., & Virshup, D. M. (2011) Casein kinase 1: Complexity in the family, *The international journal of biochemistry & cell biology 43*, 465-469.

[23] Edelman, A. M., Blumenthal, D. K., & Krebs, E. G. (1987) Protein serine/threonine kinases, *Annual review of biochemistry 56*, 567-613.

[24] Kannan, N., Haste, N., Taylor, S. S., & Neuwald, A. F. (2007) The hallmark of AGC kinase functional divergence is its C-terminal tail, a cis-acting regulatory module, *Proceedings of the National Academy of Sciences of the United States of America 104*, 1272-1277.

[25] Varjosalo, M., Keskitalo, S., Van Drogen, A., Nurkkala, H., Vichalkovski, A., Aebersold, R., & Gstaiger, M. (2013) The protein interaction landscape of the human CMGC kinase group, *Cell reports 3*, 1306-1320.

[26] Park, G., Servin, J. A., Turner, G. E., Altamirano, L., Colot, H. V., Collopy, P., Litvinkova, L., Li, L., Jones, C. A., Diala, F. G., Dunlap, J. C., & Borkovich, K. A. (2011) Global analysis of serine-threonine protein kinase genes in Neurospora crassa, *Eukaryotic cell 10*, 1553-1564.

[27] Cohen, P. (2002) Protein kinases--the major drug targets of the twenty-first century?, *Nature reviews. Drug discovery 1*, 309-315.

[28] Han, E. K., & McGonigal, T. (2007) Role of focal adhesion kinase in human cancer: a potential target for drug discovery, *Anti-cancer agents in medicinal chemistry 7*, 681-684.

[29] Hardie, D. G. (2007) AMP-activated protein kinase as a drug target, *Annual review of pharmacology and toxicology 47*, 185-210.

[30] Cortes, J., & Kantarjian, H. (2012) How I treat newly diagnosed chronic phase CML, *Blood 120*, 1390-1397.

[31] Melo, J. V., & Deininger, M. W. (2004) Biology of chronic myelogenous leukemia--signaling pathways of initiation and transformation, *Hematology/oncology clinics of North America 18*, 545-568, vii-viii.

[32] Bayraktar, U. D., Bayraktar, S., & Rocha-Lima, C. M. (2010) Molecular basis and management of gastrointestinal stromal tumors, *World journal of gastroenterology: WJG 16*, 2726-2734.

[33] Hornick, J. L., & Fletcher, C. D. (2007) The role of KIT in the management of patients with gastrointestinal stromal tumors, *Human pathology 38*, 679-687.

[34] Charpidou, A., Blatza, D., Anagnostou, V., & Syrigos, K. N. (2008) Review. EGFR mutations in non-small cell lung cancer--clinical implications, *In vivo 22*, 529-536.

[35] Ross, J. S., & Fletcher, J. A. (1998) The HER-2/neu oncogene in breast cancer: prognostic factor, predictive factor, and target for therapy, *Stem cells 16*, 413-428.

[36] Berardi, R., Santoni, M., Morgese, F., Ballatore, Z., Savini, A., Onofri, A., Mazzanti, P., Pistelli, M., Pierantoni, C., De Lisa, M., Caramanti, M., Pagliaretta, S., Pellei, C., & Cascinu, S. (2013) Novel small molecule EGFR inhibitors as candidate drugs in non-small cell lung cancer, *OncoTargets and therapy 6*, 563-576.

[37] Herbst, R. S., & Shin, D. M. (2002) Monoclonal antibodies to target epidermal growth factor receptor-positive tumors: a new paradigm for cancer therapy, *Cancer 94*, 1593-1611.

[38] Casaluce, F., Sgambato, A., Maione, P., Rossi, A., Ferrara, C., Napolitano, A., Palazzolo, G., Ciardiello, F., & Gridelli, C. (2013) ALK inhibitors: a new targeted therapy in the treatment of advanced NSCLC, *Targeted oncology 8*, 55-67.

[39] Cao, L., Yu, Y., Darko, I., Currier, D., Mayeenuddin, L. H., Wan, X., Khanna, C., & Helman, L. J. (2008) Addiction to elevated insulin-like growth factor I receptor and initial modulation of the AKT pathway define the responsiveness of rhabdomyosarcoma to the targeting antibody, *Cancer research 68*, 8039-8048.

[40] Scotlandi, K., Picci, P., & Kovar, H. (2009) Targeted therapies in bone sarcomas, *Current cancer drug targets 9*, 843-853.

[41] Taniguchi, E., Nishijo, K., McCleish, A. T., Michalek, J. E., Grayson, M. H., Infante, A. J., Abboud, H. E., Legallo, R. D., Qualman, S. J., Rubin, B. P., & Keller, C. (2008) PDGFR-A is a therapeutic target in alveolar rhabdomyosarcoma, *Oncogene 27*, 6550-6560.

[42] Mita, M. M., & Tolcher, A. W. (2007) The role of mTOR inhibitors for treatment of sarcomas, *Current oncology reports 9*, 316-322.

[43] Wan, X., & Helman, L. J. (2007) The biology behind mTOR inhibition in sarcoma, *The oncologist 12*, 1007-1018.

[44] Bond, M., Bernstein, M. L., Pappo, A., Schultz, K. R., Krailo, M., Blaney, S. M., & Adamson, P. C. (2008) A phase II study of imatinib mesylate in children with refractory or relapsed solid tumors: a Children's Oncology Group study, *Pediatric blood & cancer 50*, 254-258.

[45] Hassan, S. E., Bekarev, M., Kim, M. Y., Lin, J., Piperdi, S., Gorlick, R., & Geller, D. S. (2012) Cell surface receptor expression patterns in osteosarcoma, *Cancer 118*, 740-749.

[46] Boussen, H., Cristofanilli, M., Zaks, T., DeSilvio, M., Salazar, V., & Spector, N. (2010) Phase II study to evaluate the efficacy and safety of neoadjuvant lapatinib plus paclitaxel in patients with inflammatory breast cancer, *Journal of clinical oncology: official journal of the American Society of Clinical Oncology 28*, 3248-3255.

[47] Maemondo, M., Inoue, A., Kobayashi, K., Sugawara, S., Oizumi, S., Isobe, H., Gemma, A., Harada, M., Yoshizawa, H., Kinoshita, I., Fujita, Y., Okinaga, S., Hirano, H., Yoshimori, K., Harada, T., Ogura, T., Ando, M., Miyazawa, H., Tanaka, T., Saijo, Y., Hagiwara, K., Morita, S., Nukiwa, T., & North-East Japan Study, G. (2010) Gefitinib or chemotherapy for non-small-cell lung cancer with mutated EGFR, *The New England journal of medicine 362*, 2380-2388.

[48] Pollak, M. (2008) Insulin, insulin-like growth factors and neoplasia, *Best practice & research. Clinical endocrinology & metabolism 22*, 625-638.

[49] Kuijjer, M. L., Peterse, E. F., van den Akker, B. E., Briaire-de Bruijn, I. H., Serra, M., Meza-Zepeda, L. A., Myklebost, O., Hassan, A. B., Hogendoorn, P. C., & Cleton-Jansen, A. M. (2013) IR/IGF1R signaling as potential target for treatment of high-grade osteosarcoma, *BMC cancer 13*, 245.

[50] Bohula, E. A., Playford, M. P., & Macaulay, V. M. (2003) Targeting the type 1 insulin-like growth factor receptor as anti-cancer treatment, *Anti-cancer drugs 14*, 669-682.

[51] McCarthy, T. L., & Centrella, M. (2001) Local IGF-I expression and bone formation, *Growth hormone & IGF research: official journal of the Growth Hormone Research Society and the International IGF Research Society 11*, 213-219.

[52] Rikhof, B., de Jong, S., Suurmeijer, A. J., Meijer, C., & van der Graaf, W. T. (2009) The insulin-like growth factor system and sarcomas, *The Journal of pathology 217*, 469-482.

[53] Wang, Y. H., Han, X. D., Qiu, Y., Xiong, J., Yu, Y., Wang, B., Zhu, Z. Z., Qian, B. P., Chen, Y. X., Wang, S. F., Shi, H. F., & Sun, X. (2012) Increased expression of insulin-like growth factor-1 receptor is correlated with tumor metastasis and prognosis in patients with osteosarcoma, *Journal of surgical oncology 105*, 235-243.

[54] Wang, Y. H., Wang, Z. X., Qiu, Y., Xiong, J., Chen, Y. X., Miao, D. S., & De, W. (2009) Lentivirus-mediated RNAi knockdown of insulin-like growth factor-1 receptor inhibits growth, reduces invasion, and enhances radiosensitivity in human osteosarcoma cells, *Molecular and cellular biochemistry 327*, 257-266.

[55] Wang, Y. H., Xiong, J., Wang, S. F., Yu, Y., Wang, B., Chen, Y. X., Shi, H. F., & Qiu, Y. (2010) Lentivirus-mediated shRNA targeting insulin-like growth factor-1 receptor (IGF-1R) enhances chemosensitivity of osteosarcoma cells in vitro and in vivo, *Molecular and cellular biochemistry 341*, 225-233.

[56] Mulvihill, M. J., Cooke, A., Rosenfeld-Franklin, M., Buck, E., Foreman, K., Landfair, D., O'Connor, M., Pirritt, C., Sun, Y., Yao, Y., Arnold, L. D., Gibson, N. W., & Ji, Q. S. (2009) Discovery of OSI-906: a selective and orally efficacious dual inhibitor of the IGF-1 receptor and insulin receptor, *Future medicinal chemistry 1*, 1153-1171.

[57] Hashemi, J., Worrall, C., Vasilcanu, D., Fryknas, M., Sulaiman, L., Karimi, M., Weng, W. H., Lui, W. O., Rudduck, C., Axelson, M., Jernberg-Wiklund, H., Girnita, L., Larsson, O., & Larsson, C. (2011) Molecular characterization of acquired tolerance of tumor cells to picropodophyllin (PPP), *PloS one 6*, e14757.

[58] Duan, Z., Choy, E., Harmon, D., Yang, C., Ryu, K., Schwab, J., Mankin, H., & Hornicek, F. J. (2009) Insulin-like growth factor-I receptor tyrosine kinase inhibitor cyclolignan picropodophyllin inhibits proliferation and induces apoptosis in multidrug resistant osteosarcoma cell lines, *Molecular cancer therapeutics 8*, 2122-2130.

[59] Schwartz, G. K., Tap, W. D., Qin, L. X., Livingston, M. B., Undevia, S. D., Chmielowski, B., Agulnik, M., Schuetze, S. M., Reed, D. R., Okuno, S. H., Ludwig, J. A., Keedy, V., Rietschel, P., Kraft, A. S., Adkins, D., Van Tine, B. A., Brockstein, B., Yim, V., Bitas, C., Abdullah, A., Antonescu, C. R., Condy, M., Dickson, M. A., Vasudeva, S. D., Ho, A. L., Doyle, L. A., Chen, H. X., & Maki, R. G. (2013) Cixutumumab and

temsirolimus for patients with bone and soft-tissue sarcoma: a multicentre, open-label, phase 2 trial, *The lancet oncology 14*, 371-382.

[60] Kolb, E. A., Gorlick, R., Houghton, P. J., Morton, C. L., Lock, R., Carol, H., Reynolds, C. P., Maris, J. M., Keir, S. T., Billups, C. A., & Smith, M. A. (2008) Initial testing (stage 1) of a monoclonal antibody (SCH 717454) against the IGF-1 receptor by the pediatric preclinical testing program, *Pediatric blood & cancer 50*, 1190-1197.

[61] Asmane, I., Watkin, E., Alberti, L., Duc, A., Marec-Berard, P., Ray-Coquard, I., Cassier, P., Decouvelaere, A. V., Ranchere, D., Kurtz, J. E., Bergerat, J. P., & Blay, J. Y. (2012) Insulin-like growth factor type 1 receptor (IGF-1R) exclusive nuclear staining: a predictive biomarker for IGF-1R monoclonal antibody (Ab) therapy in sarcomas, *European journal of cancer 48*, 3027-3035.

[62] Kolb, E. A., Kamara, D., Zhang, W., Lin, J., Hingorani, P., Baker, L., Houghton, P., & Gorlick, R. (2010) R1507, a fully human monoclonal antibody targeting IGF-1R, is effective alone and in combination with rapamycin in inhibiting growth of osteosarcoma xenografts, *Pediatric blood & cancer 55*, 67-75.

[63] Kohler, N., & Lipton, A. (1974) Platelets as a source of fibroblast growth-promoting activity, *Experimental cell research 87*, 297-301.

[64] Ross, R., Glomset, J., Kariya, B., & Harker, L. (1974) A platelet-dependent serum factor that stimulates the proliferation of arterial smooth muscle cells in vitro, *Proceedings of the National Academy of Sciences of the United States of America 71*, 1207-1210.

[65] Heldin, C. H., Johnsson, A., Wennergren, S., Wernstedt, C., Betsholtz, C., & Westermark, B. (1986) A human osteosarcoma cell line secretes a growth factor structurally related to a homodimer of PDGF A-chains, *Nature 319*, 511-514.

[66] Li, X., Ponten, A., Aase, K., Karlsson, L., Abramsson, A., Uutela, M., Backstrom, G., Hellstrom, M., Bostrom, H., Li, H., Soriano, P., Betsholtz, C., Heldin, C. H., Alitalo, K., Ostman, A., & Eriksson, U. (2000) PDGF-C is a new protease-activated ligand for the PDGF alpha-receptor, *Nature cell biology 2*, 302-309.

[67] Andrae, J., Gallini, R., & Betsholtz, C. (2008) Role of platelet-derived growth factors in physiology and medicine, *Genes & development 22*, 1276-1312.

[68] Uren, A., Merchant, M. S., Sun, C. J., Vitolo, M. I., Sun, Y., Tsokos, M., Illei, P. B., Ladanyi, M., Passaniti, A., Mackall, C., & Toretsky, J. A.

(2003) Beta-platelet-derived growth factor receptor mediates motility and growth of Ewing's sarcoma cells, *Oncogene 22*, 2334-2342.

[69] Kawai, T., Hiroi, S., & Torikata, C. (1997) Expression in lung carcinomas of platelet-derived growth factor and its receptors, *Laboratory investigation; a journal of technical methods and pathology 77*, 431-436.

[70] Paulsson, J., Sjoblom, T., Micke, P., Ponten, F., Landberg, G., Heldin, C. H., Bergh, J., Brennan, D. J., Jirstrom, K., & Ostman, A. (2009) Prognostic significance of stromal platelet-derived growth factor beta-receptor expression in human breast cancer, *The American journal of pathology 175*, 334-341.

[71] Henriksen, R., Funa, K., Wilander, E., Backstrom, T., Ridderheim, M., & Oberg, K. (1993) Expression and prognostic significance of platelet-derived growth factor and its receptors in epithelial ovarian neoplasms, *Cancer research 53*, 4550-4554.

[72] Sulzbacher, I., Birner, P., Trieb, K., Muhlbauer, M., Lang, S., & Chott, A. (2001) Platelet-derived growth factor-alpha receptor expression supports the growth of conventional chondrosarcoma and is associated with adverse outcome, *The American journal of surgical pathology 25*, 1520-1527.

[73] Kubo, T., Piperdi, S., Rosenblum, J., Antonescu, C. R., Chen, W., Kim, H. S., Huvos, A. G., Sowers, R., Meyers, P. A., Healey, J. H., & Gorlick, R. (2008) Platelet-derived growth factor receptor as a prognostic marker and a therapeutic target for imatinib mesylate therapy in osteosarcoma, *Cancer 112*, 2119-2129.

[74] Zhang, L., Leeman, E., Carnes, D. C., & Graves, D. T. (1991) Human osteoblasts synthesize and respond to platelet-derived growth factor, *The American journal of physiology 261*, C348-354.

[75] Oda, Y., Wehrmann, B., Radig, K., Walter, H., Rose, I., Neumann, W., & Roessner, A. (1995) Expression of growth factors and their receptors in human osteosarcomas. Immunohistochemical detection of epidermal growth factor, platelet-derived growth factor and their receptors: its correlation with proliferating activities and p53 expression, *General & diagnostic pathology 141*, 97-103.

[76] Buchdunger, E., Cioffi, C. L., Law, N., Stover, D., Ohno-Jones, S., Druker, B. J., & Lydon, N. B. (2000) Abl protein-tyrosine kinase inhibitor STI571 inhibits in vitro signal transduction mediated by c-kit and platelet-derived growth factor receptors, *The Journal of pharmacology and experimental therapeutics 295*, 139-145.

[77] Druker, B. J., Tamura, S., Buchdunger, E., Ohno, S., Segal, G. M., Fanning, S., Zimmermann, J., & Lydon, N. B. (1996) Effects of a selective inhibitor of the Abl tyrosine kinase on the growth of Bcr-Abl positive cells, *Nature medicine 2*, 561-566.

[78] McGary, E. C., Weber, K., Mills, L., Doucet, M., Lewis, V., Lev, D. C., Fidler, I. J., & Bar-Eli, M. (2002) Inhibition of platelet-derived growth factor-mediated proliferation of osteosarcoma cells by the novel tyrosine kinase inhibitor STI571, *Clinical cancer research: an official journal of the American Association for Cancer Research 8*, 3584-3591.

[79] Chugh, R., Wathen, J. K., Maki, R. G., Benjamin, R. S., Patel, S. R., Meyers, P. A., Priebat, D. A., Reinke, D. K., Thomas, D. G., Keohan, M. L., Samuels, B. L., & Baker, L. H. (2009) Phase II multicenter trial of imatinib in 10 histologic subtypes of sarcoma using a bayesian hierarchical statistical model, *Journal of clinical oncology: official journal of the American Society of Clinical Oncology 27*, 3148-3153.

[80] Hochhaus, A., & Kantarjian, H. (2013) The development of dasatinib as a treatment for chronic myeloid leukemia (CML): from initial studies to application in newly diagnosed patients, *Journal of cancer research and clinical oncology*.

[81] Kolb, E. A., Gorlick, R., Houghton, P. J., Morton, C. L., Lock, R. B., Tajbakhsh, M., Reynolds, C. P., Maris, J. M., Keir, S. T., Billups, C. A., & Smith, M. A. (2008) Initial testing of dasatinib by the pediatric preclinical testing program, *Pediatric blood & cancer 50*, 1198-1206.

[82] Carpenter, G., Lembach, K. J., Morrison, M. M., & Cohen, S. (1975) Characterization of the binding of 125-I-labeled epidermal growth factor to human fibroblasts, *The Journal of biological chemistry 250*, 4297-4304.

[83] Herbst, R. S. (2004) Review of epidermal growth factor receptor biology, *International journal of radiation oncology, biology, physics 59*, 21-26.

[84] Giroux, V., Dagorn, J. C., & Iovanna, J. L. (2009) A review of kinases implicated in pancreatic cancer, *Pancreatology: official journal of the International Association of Pancreatology 9*, 738-754.

[85] Seshacharyulu, P., Ponnusamy, M. P., Haridas, D., Jain, M., Ganti, A. K., & Batra, S. K. (2012) Targeting the EGFR signaling pathway in cancer therapy, *Expert opinion on therapeutic targets 16*, 15-31.

[86] Ciardiello, F., & Tortora, G. (2008) EGFR antagonists in cancer treatment, *The New England journal of medicine 358*, 1160-1174.

[87] Salomon, D. S., Brandt, R., Ciardiello, F., & Normanno, N. (1995) Epidermal growth factor-related peptides and their receptors in human malignancies, *Critical reviews in oncology/hematology 19*, 183-232.

[88] Baselga, J. (2006) Targeting tyrosine kinases in cancer: the second wave, *Science 312*, 1175-1178.

[89] Lee, J. W., Soung, Y. H., Kim, S. Y., Nam, H. K., Park, W. S., Nam, S. W., Kim, M. S., Sun, D. I., Lee, Y. S., Jang, J. J., Lee, J. Y., Yoo, N. J., & Lee, S. H. (2005) Somatic mutations of EGFR gene in squamous cell carcinoma of the head and neck, *Clinical cancer research: an official journal of the American Association for Cancer Research 11*, 2879-2882.

[90] Moroni, M., Veronese, S., Benvenuti, S., Marrapese, G., Sartore-Bianchi, A., Di Nicolantonio, F., Gambacorta, M., Siena, S., & Bardelli, A. (2005) Gene copy number for epidermal growth factor receptor (EGFR) and clinical response to antiEGFR treatment in colorectal cancer: a cohort study, *The lancet oncology 6*, 279-286.

[91] Pao, W., & Miller, V. A. (2005) Epidermal growth factor receptor mutations, small-molecule kinase inhibitors, and non-small-cell lung cancer: current knowledge and future directions, *Journal of clinical oncology: official journal of the American Society of Clinical Oncology 23*, 2556-2568.

[92] Bunn, P. A., Jr., & Franklin, W. (2002) Epidermal growth factor receptor expression, signal pathway, and inhibitors in non-small cell lung cancer, *Seminars in oncology 29*, 38-44.

[93] Do, S. I., Jung, W. W., Kim, H. S., & Park, Y. K. (2009) The expression of epidermal growth factor receptor and its downstream signaling molecules in osteosarcoma, *International journal of oncology 34*, 797-803.

[94] Dobashi, Y., Suzuki, S., Sugawara, H., & Ooi, A. (2007) Involvement of epidermal growth factor receptor and downstream molecules in bone and soft tissue tumors, *Human pathology 38*, 914-925.

[95] Dobashi, Y., Takei, N., Suzuki, S., Yoneyama, H., Hanawa, M., & Ooi, A. (2004) Aberration of epidermal growth factor receptor expression in bone and soft-tissue tumors: protein overexpression, gene amplification and activation of downstream molecules, *Modern pathology: an official journal of the United States and Canadian Academy of Pathology, Inc 17*, 1497-1505.

[96] Freeman, S. S., Allen, S. W., Ganti, R., Wu, J., Ma, J., Su, X., Neale, G., Dome, J. S., Daw, N. C., & Khoury, J. D. (2008) Copy number gains in

EGFR and copy number losses in PTEN are common events in osteosarcoma tumors, *Cancer 113*, 1453-1461.

[97] Wen, Y. H., Koeppen, H., Garcia, R., Chiriboga, L., Tarlow, B. D., Peters, B. A., Eigenbrot, C., Yee, H., Steiner, G., & Greco, M. A. (2007) Epidermal growth factor receptor in osteosarcoma: expression and mutational analysis, *Human pathology 38*, 1184-1191.

[98] Lee, J. A., Ko, Y., Kim, D. H., Lim, J. S., Kong, C. B., Cho, W. H., Jeon, D. G., Lee, S. Y., & Koh, J. S. (2012) Epidermal growth factor receptor: is it a feasible target for the treatment of osteosarcoma?, *Cancer research and treatment: official journal of Korean Cancer Association 44*, 202-209.

[99] Kersting, C., Gebert, C., Agelopoulos, K., Schmidt, H., van Diest, P. J., Juergens, H., Winkelmann, W., Kevric, M., Gosheger, G., Brandt, B., Bielack, S., & Buerger, H. (2007) Epidermal growth factor receptor expression in high-grade osteosarcomas is associated with a good clinical outcome, *Clinical cancer research: an official journal of the American Association for Cancer Research 13*, 2998-3005.

[100] Ocvirk, J., Heeger, S., McCloud, P., & Hofheinz, R. D. (2013) A review of the treatment options for skin rash induced by EGFR-targeted therapies: Evidence from randomized clinical trials and a meta-analysis, *Radiology and oncology 47*, 166-175.

[101] Jakacki, R. I., Hamilton, M., Gilbertson, R. J., Blaney, S. M., Tersak, J., Krailo, M. D., Ingle, A. M., Voss, S. D., Dancey, J. E., & Adamson, P. C. (2008) Pediatric phase I and pharmacokinetic study of erlotinib followed by the combination of erlotinib and temozolomide: a Children's Oncology Group Phase I Consortium Study, *Journal of clinical oncology: official journal of the American Society of Clinical Oncology 26*, 4921-4927.

[102] Slamon, D. J., Leyland-Jones, B., Shak, S., Fuchs, H., Paton, V., Bajamonde, A., Fleming, T., Eiermann, W., Wolter, J., Pegram, M., Baselga, J., & Norton, L. (2001) Use of chemotherapy plus a monoclonal antibody against HER2 for metastatic breast cancer that overexpresses HER2, *The New England journal of medicine 344*, 783-792.

[103] Onda, M., Matsuda, S., Higaki, S., Iijima, T., Fukushima, J., Yokokura, A., Kojima, T., Horiuchi, H., Kurokawa, T., & Yamamoto, T. (1996) ErbB-2 expression is correlated with poor prognosis for patients with osteosarcoma, *Cancer 77*, 71-78.

[104] Ebb, D., Meyers, P., Grier, H., Bernstein, M., Gorlick, R., Lipshultz, S. E., Krailo, M., Devidas, M., Barkauskas, D. A., Siegal, G. P., Ferguson, W. S., Letson, G. D., Marcus, K., Goorin, A., Beardsley, P., & Marina, N. (2012) Phase II trial of trastuzumab in combination with cytotoxic chemotherapy for treatment of metastatic osteosarcoma with human epidermal growth factor receptor 2 overexpression: a report from the children's oncology group, *Journal of clinical oncology: official journal of the American Society of Clinical Oncology 30*, 2545-2551.

[105] Hubbard, J. M., & Alberts, S. R. (2013) Alternate dosing of cetuximab for patients with metastatic colorectal cancer, *Gastrointestinal cancer research: GCR 6*, 47-55.

[106] Pahl, J. H., Ruslan, S. E., Buddingh, E. P., Santos, S. J., Szuhai, K., Serra, M., Gelderblom, H., Hogendoorn, P. C., Egeler, R. M., Schilham, M. W., & Lankester, A. C. (2012) Anti-EGFR antibody cetuximab enhances the cytolytic activity of natural killer cells toward osteosarcoma, *Clinical cancer research: an official journal of the American Association for Cancer Research 18*, 432-441.

[107] Bose, P., & Ozer, H. (2009) Neratinib: an oral, irreversible dual EGFR/HER2 inhibitor for breast and non-small cell lung cancer, *Expert opinion on investigational drugs 18*, 1735-1751.

[108] Engelman, J. A., Zejnullahu, K., Gale, C. M., Lifshits, E., Gonzales, A. J., Shimamura, T., Zhao, F., Vincent, P. W., Naumov, G. N., Bradner, J. E., Althaus, I. W., Gandhi, L., Shapiro, G. I., Nelson, J. M., Heymach, J. V., Meyerson, M., Wong, K. K., & Janne, P. A. (2007) PF00299804, an irreversible pan-ERBB inhibitor, is effective in lung cancer models with EGFR and ERBB2 mutations that are resistant to gefitinib, *Cancer research 67*, 11924-11932.

[109] Gorlick, R., Kolb, E. A., Houghton, P. J., Morton, C. L., Phelps, D., Schaiquevich, P., Stewart, C., Keir, S. T., Lock, R., Carol, H., Reynolds, C. P., Maris, J. M., Wu, J., & Smith, M. A. (2009) Initial testing (stage 1) of lapatinib by the pediatric preclinical testing program, *Pediatric blood & cancer 53*, 594-598.

[110] Arcaro, A., & Guerreiro, A. S. (2007) The phosphoinositide 3-kinase pathway in human cancer: genetic alterations and therapeutic implications, *Current genomics 8*, 271-306.

[111] Cantley, L. C. (2002) The phosphoinositide 3-kinase pathway, *Science 296*, 1655-1657.

[112] Saini, K. S., Loi, S., de Azambuja, E., Metzger-Filho, O., Saini, M. L., Ignatiadis, M., Dancey, J. E., & Piccart-Gebhart, M. J. (2013) Targeting

the PI3K/AKT/mTOR and Raf/MEK/ERK pathways in the treatment of breast cancer, *Cancer treatment reviews*.

[113] Stambolic, V., Suzuki, A., de la Pompa, J. L., Brothers, G. M., Mirtsos, C., Sasaki, T., Ruland, J., Penninger, J. M., Siderovski, D. P., & Mak, T. W. (1998) Negative regulation of PKB/Akt-dependent cell survival by the tumor suppressor PTEN, *Cell 95*, 29-39.

[114] Gaikwad, S. M., & Ray, P. (2012) Non-invasive imaging of PI3K/Akt/mTOR signalling in cancer, *American journal of nuclear medicine and molecular imaging 2*, 418-431.

[115] Choy, E., Hornicek, F., MacConaill, L., Harmon, D., Tariq, Z., Garraway, L., & Duan, Z. (2012) High-throughput genotyping in osteosarcoma identifies multiple mutations in phosphoinositide-3-kinase and other oncogenes, *Cancer 118*, 2905-2914.

[116] Ji, M., Guan, H., Gao, C., Shi, B., & Hou, P. (2011) Highly frequent promoter methylation and PIK3CA amplification in non-small cell lung cancer (NSCLC), *BMC cancer 11*, 147.

[117] Shi, J., Yao, D., Liu, W., Wang, N., Lv, H., Zhang, G., Ji, M., Xu, L., He, N., Shi, B., & Hou, P. (2012) Highly frequent PIK3CA amplification is associated with poor prognosis in gastric cancer, *BMC cancer 12*, 50.

[118] Yuan, T. L., & Cantley, L. C. (2008) PI3K pathway alterations in cancer: variations on a theme, *Oncogene 27*, 5497-5510.

[119] Gong, C., Liao, H., Wang, J., Lin, Y., Qi, J., Qin, L., Tian, L. Q., & Guo, F. J. (2012) LY294002 induces G0/G1 cell cycle arrest and apoptosis of cancer stem-like cells from human osteosarcoma via down-regulation of PI3K activity, *Asian Pacific journal of cancer prevention: APJCP 13*, 3103-3107.

[120] Khan, K. H., Yap, T. A., Yan, L., & Cunningham, D. (2013) Targeting the PI3K-AKT-mTOR signaling network in cancer, *Chinese journal of cancer 32*, 253-265.

[121] Laplante, M., & Sabatini, D. M. (2012) mTOR signaling in growth control and disease, *Cell 149*, 274-293.

[122] Xu, X., Ye, L., Araki, K., & Ahmed, R. (2012) mTOR, linking metabolism and immunity, *Seminars in immunology 24*, 429-435.

[123] Cornu, M., Albert, V., & Hall, M. N. (2013) mTOR in aging, metabolism, and cancer, *Current opinion in genetics & development 23*, 53-62.

[124] Zhou, Q., Deng, Z., Zhu, Y., Long, H., Zhang, S., & Zhao, J. (2010) mTOR/p70S6K signal transduction pathway contributes to osteosarcoma progression and patients' prognosis, *Medical oncology 27*, 1239-1245.

[125] Hidalgo, M., Buckner, J. C., Erlichman, C., Pollack, M. S., Boni, J. P., Dukart, G., Marshall, B., Speicher, L., Moore, L., & Rowinsky, E. K. (2006) A phase I and pharmacokinetic study of temsirolimus (CCI-779) administered intravenously daily for 5 days every 2 weeks to patients with advanced cancer, *Clinical cancer research: an official journal of the American Association for Cancer Research 12*, 5755-5763.

[126] Mita, M. M., Mita, A. C., Chu, Q. S., Rowinsky, E. K., Fetterly, G. J., Goldston, M., Patnaik, A., Mathews, L., Ricart, A. D., Mays, T., Knowles, H., Rivera, V. M., Kreisberg, J., Bedrosian, C. L., & Tolcher, A. W. (2008) Phase I trial of the novel mammalian target of rapamycin inhibitor deforolimus (AP23573; MK-8669) administered intravenously daily for 5 days every 2 weeks to patients with advanced malignancies, *Journal of clinical oncology: official journal of the American Society of Clinical Oncology 26*, 361-367.

[127] Houghton, P. J., Morton, C. L., Kolb, E. A., Gorlick, R., Lock, R., Carol, H., Reynolds, C. P., Maris, J. M., Keir, S. T., Billups, C. A., & Smith, M. A. (2008) Initial testing (stage 1) of the mTOR inhibitor rapamycin by the pediatric preclinical testing program, *Pediatric blood & cancer 50*, 799-805.

[128] Chawla, S. P., Staddon, A. P., Baker, L. H., Schuetze, S. M., Tolcher, A. W., D'Amato, G. Z., Blay, J. Y., Mita, M. M., Sankhala, K. K., Berk, L., Rivera, V. M., Clackson, T., Loewy, J. W., Haluska, F. G., & Demetri, G. D. (2012) Phase II study of the mammalian target of rapamycin inhibitor ridaforolimus in patients with advanced bone and soft tissue sarcomas, *Journal of clinical oncology: official journal of the American Society of Clinical Oncology 30*, 78-84.

[129] Demetri, G. D., Chawla, S. P., Ray-Coquard, I., Le Cesne, A., Staddon, A. P., Milhem, M. M., Penel, N., Riedel, R. F., Bui-Nguyen, B., Cranmer, L. D., Reichardt, P., Bompas, E., Alcindor, T., Rushing, D., Song, Y., Lee, R. M., Ebbinghaus, S., Eid, J. E., Loewy, J. W., Haluska, F. G., Dodion, P. F., & Blay, J. Y. (2013) Results of an international randomized phase III trial of the mammalian target of rapamycin inhibitor ridaforolimus versus placebo to control metastatic sarcomas in patients after benefit from prior chemotherapy, *Journal of clinical oncology: official journal of the American Society of Clinical Oncology 31*, 2485-2492.

[130] Yoo, C., Lee, J., Rha, S. Y., Park, K. H., Kim, T. M., Kim, Y. J., Lee, H. J., Lee, K. H., & Ahn, J. H. (2013) Multicenter phase II study of everolimus in patients with metastatic or recurrent bone and soft-tissue sarcomas after failure of anthracycline and ifosfamide, *Investigational new drugs*.

[131] Dhillon, A. S., Hagan, S., Rath, O., & Kolch, W. (2007) MAP kinase signalling pathways in cancer, *Oncogene 26*, 3279-3290.

[132] Yoon, S., & Seger, R. (2006) The extracellular signal-regulated kinase: multiple substrates regulate diverse cellular functions, *Growth factors 24*, 21-44.

[133] Rincon, M., & Davis, R. J. (2009) Regulation of the immune response by stress-activated protein kinases, *Immunological reviews 228*, 212-224.

[134] Cuadrado, A., & Nebreda, A. R. (2010) Mechanisms and functions of p38 MAPK signalling, *The Biochemical journal 429*, 403-417.

[135] Yu, Y., Luk, F., Yang, J. L., & Walsh, W. R. (2011) Ras/Raf/MEK/ERK pathway is associated with lung metastasis of osteosarcoma in an orthotopic mouse model, *Anticancer research 31*, 1147-1152.

[136] Malumbres, M., & Barbacid, M. (2003) RAS oncogenes: the first 30 years, *Nature reviews. Cancer 3*, 459-465.

[137] Yokoyama, R., Schneider-Stock, R., Radig, K., Wex, T., & Roessner, A. (1998) Clinicopathologic implications of MDM2, p53 and K-ras gene alterations in osteosarcomas: MDM2 amplification and p53 mutations found in progressive tumors, *Pathology, research and practice 194*, 615-621.

[138] Pompetti, F., Rizzo, P., Simon, R. M., Freidlin, B., Mew, D. J., Pass, H. I., Picci, P., Levine, A. S., & Carbone, M. (1996) Oncogene alterations in primary, recurrent, and metastatic human bone tumors, *Journal of cellular biochemistry 63*, 37-50.

[139] Kawaguchi, K., Oda, Y., Sakamoto, A., Saito, T., Tamiya, S., Iwamoto, Y., & Tsuneyoshi, M. (2002) Molecular analysis of p53, MDM2, and H-ras genes in osteosarcoma and malignant fibrous histiocytoma of bone in patients older than 40 years, *Modern pathology: an official journal of the United States and Canadian Academy of Pathology, Inc 15*, 878-888.

[140] Ikeda, S., Sumii, H., Akiyama, K., Watanabe, S., Ito, S., Inoue, H., Takechi, H., Tanabe, G., & Oda, T. (1989) Amplification of both c-myc and c-raf-1 oncogenes in a human osteosarcoma, *Japanese journal of cancer research: Gann 80*, 6-9.

[141] Pignochino, Y., Grignani, G., Cavalloni, G., Motta, M., Tapparo, M., Bruno, S., Bottos, A., Gammaitoni, L., Migliardi, G., Camussi, G., Alberghini, M., Torchio, B., Ferrari, S., Bussolino, F., Fagioli, F., Picci, P., & Aglietta, M. (2009) Sorafenib blocks tumour growth, angiogenesis and metastatic potential in preclinical models of osteosarcoma through a mechanism potentially involving the inhibition of ERK1/2, MCL-1 and ezrin pathways, *Molecular cancer 8*, 118.

[142] Keir, S. T., Maris, J. M., Lock, R., Kolb, E. A., Gorlick, R., Carol, H., Morton, C. L., Reynolds, C. P., Kang, M. H., Watkins, A., Houghton, P. J., & Smith, M. A. (2010) Initial testing (stage 1) of the multi-targeted kinase inhibitor sorafenib by the pediatric preclinical testing program, *Pediatric blood & cancer 55*, 1126-1133.

[143] Grignani, G., Palmerini, E., Dileo, P., Asaftei, S. D., D'Ambrosio, L., Pignochino, Y., Mercuri, M., Picci, P., Fagioli, F., Casali, P. G., Ferrari, S., & Aglietta, M. (2012) A phase II trial of sorafenib in relapsed and unresectable high-grade osteosarcoma after failure of standard multimodal therapy: an Italian Sarcoma Group study, *Annals of oncology: official journal of the European Society for Medical Oncology / ESMO 23*, 508-516.

[144] Kolb, E. A., Gorlick, R., Houghton, P. J., Morton, C. L., Neale, G., Keir, S. T., Carol, H., Lock, R., Phelps, D., Kang, M. H., Reynolds, C. P., Maris, J. M., Billups, C., & Smith, M. A. (2010) Initial testing (stage 1) of AZD6244 (ARRY-142886) by the Pediatric Preclinical Testing Program, *Pediatric blood & cancer 55*, 668-677.

[145] Susa, M., Hornicek, F., Liu, X., & Duan, Z. (2010) Signal Transducer and Activator of Transcription 3 Signaling Pathway: A Potential Target in Sarcoma Treatment., *Current Enzyme Inhibition 6*, 105-115.

[146] LoPiccolo, J., Blumenthal, G. M., Bernstein, W. B., & Dennis, P. A. (2008) Targeting the PI3K/Akt/mTOR pathway: effective combinations and clinical considerations, *Drug resistance updates: reviews and commentaries in antimicrobial and anticancer chemotherapy 11*, 32-50.

[147] Ryu, K., Choy, E., Yang, C., Susa, M., Hornicek, F. J., Mankin, H., & Duan, Z. (2010) Activation of signal transducer and activator of transcription 3 (Stat3) pathway in osteosarcoma cells and overexpression of phosphorylated-Stat3 correlates with poor prognosis, *Journal of orthopaedic research: official publication of the Orthopaedic Research Society 28*, 971-978.

[148] Liu, Y., Wang, L., Wu, Y., Lv, C., Li, X., Cao, X., Yang, M., Feng, D., & Luo, Z. (2013) Pterostilbene exerts antitumor activity against human

osteosarcoma cells by inhibiting the JAK2/STAT3 signaling pathway, *Toxicology 304*, 120-131.
[149] Fossey, S. L., Liao, A. T., McCleese, J. K., Bear, M. D., Lin, J., Li, P. K., Kisseberth, W. C., & London, C. A. (2009) Characterization of STAT3 activation and expression in canine and human osteosarcoma, *BMC cancer 9*, 81.
[150] Lai, S. Y., & Johnson, F. M. (2010) Defining the role of the JAK-STAT pathway in head and neck and thoracic malignancies: implications for future therapeutic approaches, *Drug resistance updates: reviews and commentaries in antimicrobial and anticancer chemotherapy 13*, 67-78.
[151] Chen, C. L., Loy, A., Cen, L., Chan, C., Hsieh, F. C., Cheng, G., Wu, B., Qualman, S. J., Kunisada, K., Yamauchi-Takihara, K., & Lin, J. (2007) Signal transducer and activator of transcription 3 is involved in cell growth and survival of human rhabdomyosarcoma and osteosarcoma cells, *BMC cancer 7*, 111.
[152] Aarts, M., Linardopoulos, S., & Turner, N. C. (2013) Tumour selective targeting of cell cycle kinases for cancer treatment, *Current opinion in pharmacology 13*, 529-535.
[153] Malumbres, M., & Barbacid, M. (2007) Cell cycle kinases in cancer, *Current opinion in genetics & development 17*, 60-65.
[154] Vermeulen, K., Van Bockstaele, D. R., & Berneman, Z. N. (2003) The cell cycle: a review of regulation, deregulation and therapeutic targets in cancer, *Cell proliferation 36*, 131-149.
[155] Shapiro, G. I. (2006) Cyclin-dependent kinase pathways as targets for cancer treatment, *Journal of clinical oncology: official journal of the American Society of Clinical Oncology 24*, 1770-1783.
[156] Ortega, S., Malumbres, M., & Barbacid, M. (2002) Cyclin D-dependent kinases, INK4 inhibitors and cancer, *Biochimica et biophysica acta 1602*, 73-87.
[157] Canavese, M., Santo, L., & Raje, N. (2012) Cyclin dependent kinases in cancer: potential for therapeutic intervention, *Cancer biology & therapy 13*, 451-457.
[158] Cui, C., Wang, Y., Wang, Y., Zhao, M., & Peng, S. (2013) Exploring the Relationship between the Inhibition Selectivity and the Apoptosis of Roscovitine-Treated Cancer Cells, *Journal of analytical methods in chemistry 2013*, 389390.
[159] Mohapatra, S., Chu, B., Zhao, X., & Pledger, W. J. (2005) Accumulation of p53 and reductions in XIAP abundance promote the apoptosis of prostate cancer cells, *Cancer research 65*, 7717-7723.

[160] Mohapatra, S., Coppola, D., Riker, A. I., & Pledger, W. J. (2007) Roscovitine inhibits differentiation and invasion in a three-dimensional skin reconstruction model of metastatic melanoma, *Molecular cancer research: MCR 5*, 145-151.
[161] Fu, W., Ma, L., Chu, B., Wang, X., Bui, M. M., Gemmer, J., Altiok, S., & Pledger, W. J. (2011) The cyclin-dependent kinase inhibitor SCH 727965 (dinacliclib) induces the apoptosis of osteosarcoma cells, *Molecular cancer therapeutics 10*, 1018-1027.
[162] Strebhardt, K., & Ullrich, A. (2006) Targeting polo-like kinase 1 for cancer therapy, *Nature reviews. Cancer 6*, 321-330.
[163] Duan, Z., Ji, D., Weinstein, E. J., Liu, X., Susa, M., Choy, E., Yang, C., Mankin, H., & Hornicek, F. J. (2010) Lentiviral shRNA screen of human kinases identifies PLK1 as a potential therapeutic target for osteosarcoma, *Cancer letters 293*, 220-229.
[164] Liu, X., Choy, E., Harmon, D., Yang, S., Yang, C., Mankin, H., Hornicek, F. J., & Duan, Z. (2011) Inhibition of polo-like kinase 1 leads to the suppression of osteosarcoma cell growth in vitro and in vivo, *Anti-cancer drugs 22*, 444-453.
[165] Mountzios, G., Terpos, E., & Dimopoulos, M. A. (2008) Aurora kinases as targets for cancer therapy, *Cancer treatment reviews 34*, 175-182.
[166] Kollareddy, M., Zheleva, D., Dzubak, P., Brahmkshatriya, P. S., Lepsik, M., & Hajduch, M. (2012) Aurora kinase inhibitors: progress towards the clinic, *Investigational new drugs 30*, 2411-2432.
[167] Mueller, F., Fuchs, B., & Kaser-Hotz, B. (2007) Comparative biology of human and canine osteosarcoma, *Anticancer research 27*, 155-164.
[168] Maris, J. M., Morton, C. L., Gorlick, R., Kolb, E. A., Lock, R., Carol, H., Keir, S. T., Reynolds, C. P., Kang, M. H., Wu, J., Smith, M. A., & Houghton, P. J. (2010) Initial testing of the aurora kinase A inhibitor MLN8237 by the Pediatric Preclinical Testing Program (PPTP), *Pediatric blood & cancer 55*, 26-34.
[169] Cannon, C. M., Pozniak, J., Scott, M. C., Ito, D., Gorden, B. H., Graef, A. J., & Modiano, J. F. (2013) Canine osteosarcoma cells exhibit resistance to aurora kinase inhibitors, *Veterinary and comparative oncology*.
[170] Kreahling, J. M., Foroutan, P., Reed, D., Martinez, G., Razabdouski, T., Bui, M. M., Raghavan, M., Letson, D., Gillies, R. J., & Altiok, S. (2013) Wee1 inhibition by MK-1775 leads to tumor inhibition and enhances efficacy of gemcitabine in human sarcomas, *PloS one 8*, e57523.

[171] Thompson, R., Montano, R., & Eastman, A. (2012) The Mre11 nuclease is critical for the sensitivity of cells to Chk1 inhibition, *PloS one 7*, e44021.

[172] Guertin, A. D., Martin, M. M., Roberts, B., Hurd, M., Qu, X., Miselis, N. R., Liu, Y., Li, J., Feldman, I., Benita, Y., Bloecher, A., Toniatti, C., & Shumway, S. D. (2012) Unique functions of CHK1 and WEE1 underlie synergistic anti-tumor activity upon pharmacologic inhibition, *Cancer cell international 12*, 45.

[173] Kieran, M. W., Kalluri, R., & Cho, Y. J. (2012) The VEGF pathway in cancer and disease: responses, resistance, and the path forward, *Cold Spring Harbor perspectives in medicine 2*, a006593.

[174] Aldebasi, Y. H., Rahmani, A. H., Khan, A. A., & Aly, S. M. (2013) The effect of vascular endothelial growth factor in the progression of bladder cancer and diabetic retinopathy, *International journal of clinical and experimental medicine 6*, 239-251.

[175] Yu, X. W., Wu, T. Y., Yi, X., Ren, W. P., Zhou, Z. B., Sun, Y. Q., & Zhang, C. Q. (2013) Prognostic significance of VEGF expression in osteosarcoma: a meta-analysis, *Tumour biology: the journal of the International Society for Oncodevelopmental Biology and Medicine*.

[176] Kerbel, R. S. (2006) Antiangiogenic therapy: a universal chemosensitization strategy for cancer?, *Science 312*, 1171-1175.

[177] Glade-Bender, J., Kandel, J. J., & Yamashiro, D. J. (2003) VEGF blocking therapy in the treatment of cancer, *Expert opinion on biological therapy 3*, 263-276.

[178] Glade Bender, J. L., Adamson, P. C., Reid, J. M., Xu, L., Baruchel, S., Shaked, Y., Kerbel, R. S., Cooney-Qualter, E. M., Stempak, D., Chen, H. X., Nelson, M. D., Krailo, M. D., Ingle, A. M., Blaney, S. M., Kandel, J. J., Yamashiro, D. J., & Children's Oncology Group, S. (2008) Phase I trial and pharmacokinetic study of bevacizumab in pediatric patients with refractory solid tumors: a Children's Oncology Group Study, *Journal of clinical oncology: official journal of the American Society of Clinical Oncology 26*, 399-405.

[179] Maris, J. M., Courtright, J., Houghton, P. J., Morton, C. L., Gorlick, R., Kolb, E. A., Lock, R., Tajbakhsh, M., Reynolds, C. P., Keir, S. T., Wu, J., & Smith, M. A. (2008) Initial testing of the VEGFR inhibitor AZD2171 by the pediatric preclinical testing program, *Pediatric blood & cancer 50*, 581-587.

[180] van Cruijsen, H., Voest, E. E., Punt, C. J., Hoekman, K., Witteveen, P. O., Meijerink, M. R., Puchalski, T. A., Robertson, J., Saunders, O.,

Jurgensmeier, J. M., van Herpen, C. M., & Giaccone, G. (2010) Phase I evaluation of cediranib, a selective VEGFR signalling inhibitor, in combination with gefitinib in patients with advanced tumours, *European journal of cancer 46*, 901-911.
[181] Keir, S. T., Morton, C. L., Wu, J., Kurmasheva, R. T., Houghton, P. J., & Smith, M. A. (2012) Initial testing of the multitargeted kinase inhibitor pazopanib by the Pediatric Preclinical Testing Program, *Pediatric blood & cancer 59*, 586-588.
[182] Yamaguchi, U., Honda, K., Satow, R., Kobayashi, E., Nakayama, R., Ichikawa, H., Shoji, A., Shitashige, M., Masuda, M., Kawai, A., Chuman, H., Iwamoto, Y., Hirohashi, S., & Yamada, T. (2009) Functional genome screen for therapeutic targets of osteosarcoma, *Cancer science 100*, 2268-2274.
[183] Yang, C., Ji, D., Weinstein, E. J., Choy, E., Hornicek, F. J., Wood, K. B., Liu, X., Mankin, H., & Duan, Z. (2010) The kinase Mirk is a potential therapeutic target in osteosarcoma, *Carcinogenesis 31*, 552-558.
[184] Liu, X., Choy, E., Hornicek, F. J., Yang, S., Yang, C., Harmon, D., Mankin, H., & Duan, Z. (2011) ROCK1 as a potential therapeutic target in osteosarcoma, *Journal of orthopaedic research: official publication of the Orthopaedic Research Society 29*, 1259-1266.
[185] Duan, Z., Zhang, J., Choy, E., Harmon, D., Liu, X., Nielsen, P., Mankin, H., Gray, N. S., & Hornicek, F. J. (2012) Systematic kinome shRNA screening identifies CDK11 (PITSLRE) kinase expression is critical for osteosarcoma cell growth and proliferation, *Clinical cancer research: an official journal of the American Association for Cancer Research 18*, 4580-4588.

In: Osteosarcoma
Editors: Edwin Choy

ISBN: 978-1-63321-052-3

Chapter 9

CLINICAL TRIALS FOR OSTEOSARCOMA

Jacson K. Shen and Edwin Choy
Center for Sarcoma and Connective Tissue Oncology,
Massachusetts General Hospital, Boston, MA, US

ABSTRACT

Osteosarcoma is the most common form of primary bone malignancy. Proper diagnosis and surgical resection plays a critical role in the treatment of osteosarcoma, and the introduction of chemotherapy has improved patient survival. However, surviving patients endure potential for late adverse effects and secondary malignancies. Advances in our understanding of the biology of osteosarcoma will lead to better patient outcomes in the future. Development of imaging tools for diagnosis and prognosis will provide patients with the proper information for their treatment decisions. Genomic studies allow for both observational and interventional approaches for patients. Various treatment strategies for osteosarcoma utilize other combination chemotherapies; radiation therapies; targeted therapies, including tumor-associated biomarkers and pathways; and immunotherapies, including immunostimulants and vaccine therapy. Supportive care therapies also improve patient quality of life from the exhaustive nature of these treatments. This review surveys current clinical research strategies and recent innovations in the care of patients with osteosarcoma.

INTRODUCTION

Osteosarcoma is the most commonly diagnosed form of primary bone malignancy [1]. Untreated osteosarcoma is aggressively systemic and leads to death within months [2]. Improper diagnostics and unsuitable therapy can drastically undermine the chances of being cured. Traditionally, radical en bloc surgical resection is a critical part of the recommended treatment. Wide negative margins attempt to ensure local tumor control. While patients who present with non-metastatic disease can be cured, fewer than 20 percent of patients remain relapse-free without adjuvant chemotherapy. With effective adjuvant chemotherapy, the five-year survival rate has increased to 70 percent [3]. Studies have hypothesized and demonstrated that clinically immeasurable metastatic disease may be present at the time of diagnosis, emphasizing the importance of a multidisciplinary approach [4, 5].

Unfortunately, osteosarcoma patients face one of the most difficult chemotherapy treatments of any of the solid tumors, and progress has slowed over the past twenty years [6, 7]. Of the two-thirds of the long-term surviving patients with non-metastatic extremity osteosarcomas, up to 50 percent of those with limited lung metastases can be cured, and approximately 25 percent of patients with greater metastases can expect long-term relapse-free survival [6]. Furthermore, there is no standard, second line therapy for patients who relapse, and dose intensification shows limited improvement and increased complications [4, 8-10]. Current advancements in cancer treatment have seen the development of novel strategies and genomic studies. As a result, these new biological insights and investigational strategies hold the potential to improve the outcome and quality of life for patients treated for osteosarcoma.

Along with the specialized multi-modal treatments, it has become standard practice to provide patients with the option of prospective clinical trials. This chapter provides an overview of osteosarcoma observational studies and interventional diagnostic and treatment options, describing recent innovations in the care of patients with osteosarcoma through a survey of current clinical research strategies in the United States through ClinicalTrials.gov.

IMAGING

Diagnostic

Typically, clinical presentation of osteosarcoma is localized pain and/or mass over several months, which is then imaged by plain radiograph [4]. X-ray characteristics of osteosarcoma include destruction of the normal trabecular bone pattern, obscure margins between lytic and/or sclerotic lesions and normal bone, and absence of endosteal bone response [4]. Involved bone is visualized as indistinct radiodense and radiolucent areas, including new periosteal bone formation, and formation of Codman's triangle. Affected soft tissue mass is sometimes ossified in a radial pattern [11].

While a correct diagnosis can be predicted from radiographic appearance in a majority of cases, a necessary biopsy is performed in the suspected osteosarcoma case for a definitive differential diagnosis. An experienced orthopaedic surgeon is required to carefully plan and perform the biopsy in consideration with the later treatment plan, especially in limb-sparing procedures. Histologically, osteosarcoma is characterized by osteoid formation in the malignant tumor, which is visible by microscopy. Because it is thought to originate from mesenchymal stem cells, osteosarcoma may appear similar to other sarcomas of bone, such as chondrosarcoma and fibrosarcoma, with the fundamental difference being the woven bone matrix in osteosarcoma diagnoses. Some osteosarcomas display variable histomorphologies, which require additional immunohistochemistry to confirm the diagnosis. Laboratory reports show elevated levels of lactate dehydrogenase (LDH) and alkaline phosphatase [4]. Osteosarcomas are not characterized by chromosomal translocations [12].

Following diagnosis, staging work-up is performed via imaging studies, in which cross-sectional imaging is important for surgical planning, prognosis, and treatment. Magnetic Resonance Imaging (MRI) of the entire afflicted bone is the preferred method of assessment because of its precise imaging of soft tissue extension. To determine the presence of pulmonary metastases, computer tomography (CT) of the chest is necessary, as approximately 80 percent of metastases travel to the lung [13]. Radionuclide bone scanning or positron emission tomography (PET) is recommended to detect metastases throughout the entire skeleton, according to the National Comprehensive Cancer Network (NCCN) guidelines.

With the development of innovative imaging techniques, investigators aim for more accurate and non-invasive approaches to diagnosis. Using carbon-11

(C-11), Shulkin et al. are able to exploit its integration into methionine, which is highly valuable in monitoring neoplasms, and detect tumors using PET/CT (NCT00840047). Quon et al. propose fluorine F-18 sodium fluoride PET/CT as a more sensitive approach to detecting and characterizing skeletal lesions and malignancies (NCT01541358). While some conventional scans may misdiagnosis certain lesions resulting in treatments that lead to unintentional tumor progression or improper biopsies leading to limb amputation, Marina et al. propose to establish a clinically applicable imaging test for the differentiation of bone sarcomas and osteomyelitis with ferumoxytol-enhanced MRI (NCT01336803). Using FDA-approved ultra small superparamagnetic iron oxide (USPIO) Ferumoxytol nanoparticles, they propose to exploit the differences in cellular composition and uptake of sarcomas and inflammations. Phagocytosis of USPIOs by macrophages in an inflammatory event such as osteomyletis, but not in malignant tumors, allows for high soft tissue contrast, three-dimensional information, and sub-millimeter detection via MRI. Such an immediate, non-invasive diagnostic technique will enable more efficient and appropriate patient referrals for proper treatment.

Prognostic

The Muscoloskeletal Tumor Society (MSTS) as a surgical staging system developed by Enneking is a strong pretreatment indicator of prognosis. Pretreatment prognosis is dependent upon site and size, and primary metastases [14, 15]. The MSTS staging system describes the size and site of the non-metastatic primary tumor (low grade, stage I versus high grade, stage II; intracompartmental, A versus extracompartmental, B) or the presence of clinically detectable metastatic disease (stage III). However for clinically undetectable metastatic disease, the greatest predictors of outcome are treatment-related prognostic indicators, such as extent of surgery and response to chemotherapy [4, 14, 16, 17]. Histologic evaluation of pre-operative chemotherapy response can only be determined post-operatively. Good responders are considered patients with greater than 90 percent tumor necrosis and have a disease-free survival rate of 80 percent, while poor responders exhibit less than 90 percent necrosis and have a disease-free survival rate of 40 to 50 percent [9, 18, 19]. Meyers et al. state that this is not a true prognostic tool, as assessment cannot be made at the time of initial diagnosis. There is a lack of clinically useful prognostic indicators; thus, more efficient tools and techniques are in development to determine pre-operative chemotherapy response in patients.

Current areas of interest include imaging techniques to determine if a chemotherapy regimen is working by evaluating percent necrosis. With a less invasive approach, it is possible to make evidence-based changes to treatment strategies in patients who do not show response, and repeat such analysis until an effective therapy is determined. Previous studies have reported strong correlation of nuclear imaging techniques with histologic response using isotopic thallium and gadolinium [20, 21]. Fluorine-18 fluoro-L-thymidine (18F-FLT) and fludeoxyglucose (FDG) have emerged as novel radioisotope markers to evaluate tumor cell proliferation in sarcomas via PET studies [22]. Keedy et al. propose a quantitative imaging technique using 18F-FLT-PET/CT to determine osteosarcoma tumor response after one cycle of neoadjuvant chemotherapy, with the hypothesis that a significant decrease in 18F-FLT uptake after two cycles will correlate with decreased tumor volume and slowed tumor growth (NCT01882231). Czernin et al. aim to employ FDG-PET/CT to monitor changes in glucose metabolic activity, and therefore propose to accurately locate and determine the extent of disease in osteosarcoma patients undergoing treatment (NCT00335751). Diffuse Optical Spectroscopic Imaging (DOSI) is another useful technique in monitoring the metabolic tissue function of tumors, enabling evaluation of chemotherapy response. Tromberg et al. propose to monitor patient response to pre-operative chemotherapy by determining if measurable analogous biomarkers of response exist for osteosarcoma patients, comparable to clinical MRI or PET/CT (NCT01263405).

Careful delineation of target volume allows for clearer surgical planning and prevention of marginal recurrence. Koutcher et al. currently propose the use of Dynamic Contrast Enhanced MRI (DCE-MRI) as a reliable a priori or early prognostic marker of osteosarcoma tumor response pre-operatively, as well as to predict percent necrosis at the time of surgery and evaluate disease-free survival (NCT00598741). This study aims to establish DCE-MRI as an independent marker of tumor response, similar to currently established markers of disease size, site, stage, and levels of LDH and alkaline phosphatase. To solidify their findings, the study also looks at the potential for the DCE-MRI results to correlate with key molecular markers and pathways of osteosarcoma including expression of HER-2, platelet derived growth factor, reduced folate carrier, and p-glycoprotein.

PREDICTIVE BIOMARKERS

The need for alternative treatment for patients who do not respond to standard therapy and the search for chemotherapy alternatives and/or targeted adjuvants have brought light to research on biomarkers that may predict outcome in osteosarcoma. Biomarkers to determine outcome in osteosarcoma have been examined in two distinct manners: determining the role of individual genetic alterations in osteosarcoma, and utilizing high-throughput arrays to identify predictors of prognosis.

Single gene alterations can provide information on how they affect osteosarcoma tumorigenesis and/or predict outcome, and can be effective in identifying possible targets for therapy as well. Both the Retinoblastoma Susceptibility gene (RB1) and the TP53 pathway have been shown to play a crucial role in osteosarcoma tumorigenesis, but have not been correlated with survival outcome [6, 23, 24]. The role of RB1 is notable in many regulatory cellular functions such as proliferation, differentiation, and apoptosis. RB1 is a tumor suppressor gene located on human chromosome 13q14 and is a shared mutation with retinoblastoma tumors [25]. The mutation is usually inherited as a heterozygous mutation, in which a loss of heterozygosity (LoH) of the remaining wildtype allele drives tumorigenesis by being unable to bind transcription factor proteins and inappropriately activating transcription in the G1 growth stage and S phase [26]. TP53 has been suggested to act as a tumor suppressor gene, as inherited loss of heterozygosity mutations are also commonly observed in osteosarcoma and many other human cancers [27]. The p53 protein plays a critical role as a checkpoint for DNA damage and regulator of apoptosis [28]. Some biomarkers for tumorigenesis in osteosarcoma have been controversial. The role of HER-2/neu (ERBB2) is more established in tumorigenesis and targeted therapeutics for breast cancer than for osteosarcoma [6]. One study has demonstrated that ERBB2 in osteosarcoma becomes internalized, and therefore does not respond to ERBB2-targeted therapy [29, 30]. Thus, investigators are looking into other possible predictors of tumorigenesis.

Biomarkers of tumorigenesis by inheritance and loss of heterozygosity or other genetic aberrations are currently being uncovered through observational studies by tissue sample collection and gene expression analysis. Previous studies have described a loss of heterozygosity in chromosome 18q for osteosarcoma tumorigenesis in relation to Paget's disease. Damron et al. aim to delineate the inheritance of a proposed tumor suppressor gene from the father as seen in the son (NCT00615628). High-throughput array-based gene expression assays are being employed for genomic analysis by several groups to investigate, classify, and map genetic alterations to predict tumorigenesis (NCT01807143, NCT01050296, NCT00615329, NCT00003793). In some studies, these expression profiles also allow researchers to determine and investigate biomarkers associated with patient outcome and chemotherapy response prognosis.

Treatment response and chemotherapy resistance are strong indicators of patient survival. Glutathione S-transferase P1 (GSTP1) plays a role in cell detoxification. The upregulation of GSTP1 expression in osteosarcoma cells induced increased cell detoxification after treatment with doxorubicin and cisplatin, and the cells became more resistant to these chemotherapeutic agents [31]. Therefore, increased expression of GSTP1 has been shown to significantly correlate with higher relapse rate and poorer prognosis. Transmembrane protein p-glycoprotein may also play a role in chemotherapy response and drug resistance, as it facilitates the efflux of chemotherapeutic agents. Some studies have shown results associating higher p-glycoprotein expression with chemotherapy resistance and poorer prognosis in osteosarcoma. However, others have demonstrated through histologic analysis that higher expression of p-glycoprotein does not correlate with prognosis. Thus, groups have begun to look for other biomarkers that may be stronger indicators of acquired or intrinsic resistance to pre-operative chemotherapy, and correlate their findings with clinical outcome (NCT00898755, NCT00580385). By collecting, culturing, and analyzing chemotherapy-resistant tissue samples, investigators will be able to study molecular markers associated with drug sensitivity and cytotoxicity. Investigators also aim to identify and validate novel therapeutic targets for metastatic osteosarcoma by understanding the genetic alterations through patient tissue samples and peripheral blood DNA (NCT00579930, NCT01190943), as well as novel detection methods (NCT00588510, NCT00899496). Other repositories for osteosarcoma tissue samples are also being established for storage and study linking patients' clinical data, percent necrosis, and overall survival and event-free survival (NCT00899275, NCT01807052, NCT01047878).

CURRENT STANDARD OF CARE FOR OSTEOSARCOMA

Neoadjuvant Chemotherapy, Surgical Resection, Adjuvant Chemotherapy

Localized, non-metastatic osteosarcoma was treated solely by surgical resection prior to the 1970s. While surgery maintained high rates of local control, the majority of patients would very quickly succumb to pulmonary metastases. Since the introduction of chemotherapy in the late 1970s, prognosis for high-grade osteosarcoma has improved dramatically allowing long-term, disease-free survival in 60 to 70 percent of patients [2, 9, 32]. Today, the standard of care for curable, non-metastatic resectable osteosarcoma consists of ten weeks of pre-operative chemotherapy, local surgical resection, followed by 20 weeks of post-operative chemotherapy. Neither surgery alone nor chemotherapy alone is a curative method of treatment for osteosarcoma. The goal of limb-sparing "wide" surgical resection is to remove the primary tumor as well as all clinically detectable metastases to allow for local control.

A majority of patients with osteosarcoma have micrometastases [32], but for those who present with clinically detectable metastatic disease, their probability of being disease-free after five years is 11 percent, drastically lower than the 69 percent probability of disease-free survival for those without [33]. Chemotherapy acts to systemically eradicate these micrometastases. For patients who present with clinical metastases or recurrent tumors, treatment is directed towards all tumor masses, as chemotherapy alone is not enough to eradicate the tumors.

Though multiple groups have studied the effect of chemotherapy only after definitive surgery or including pre-operative chemotherapy, no difference was seen between the two groups on patient survival in non-metastatic disease (NCT00001217) [34-36]. Pre-operative chemotherapy remains to be the standard of care as it provides other advantages to patient care and treatment planning, including: allowing a wider timeframe in preparation for the surgical procedure; delineation of tumor volume allowing for better quality surgical margins, therefore reducing the probability of local recurrence; and histological evaluation of percent necrosis of tumor, indicating response to treatment and defining good responders from poor responders.

The most common components of the standard chemotherapy regimen for non-metastatic and resectable osteosarcoma are doxorubicin, cisplatin, and high-dose methotrexate (MAP). The addition of ifosamide as a fourth chemotherapy agents has not yet been confirmed, as some groups have shown its benefit in the prevention of recurrent osteosarcoma, while others have seen no additional benefit [37, 38]. For metastatic or non-resectable tumors, patients undergo a chemotherapy regimen of doxorubicin, cisplatin, high-dose methotrexate, ifosfamide, and etoposide. If the tumor is resectable, surgery is usually performed after ten weeks of chemotherapy, and additional chemotherapy is given.

COMBINATION CHEMOTHERAPY

Although the aforementioned chemotherapy regimen has been established as the standard of care for osteosarcoma, challenges still remain to optimize treatment and prevent chemotherapy resistance. Chemotherapy agents each work in different ways to stop the growth of tumor cells by killing the cells or preventing cell division, and the combination of more than one drug may therefore kill a greater number of tumor cells; however, clones may escape one treatment approach resulting in multidrug resistant tumors. Currently, investigators are looking for additional agents that may be more effective as a monotherapy or in combination with the standard chemotherapy treatments.

Previous studies have demonstrated in adults that adjuvant high-dose methotrexate did not show a statistically significant survival benefit versus doxorubicin and cisplatin alone [39]. Thus, investigators have examined the efficacy of ifosfamide and carboplatin with or without doxorubicin neoadjuvant and post-operative chemotherapy in adolescents with non-metastatic resectable osteosarcomas (NCT00145639). Liposomal doxorubicin has been shown to allow for the prolonged release of the drug for treatment of refractory osteosarcoma in children (NCT00019630). A current clinical trial is studying the use of the anti-cancer drug trabectedin as a monotherapy for metastatic and refractory osteosarcoma for children (NCT00070109), as efficacy has been shown in adult trials (NCT00005625). Combination chemotherapy of trabectedin and doxorubicin is also in clinical trials for metastatic osteosarcoma (NCT01189253).

For children with recurrent or refractory osteosarcoma, there are several chemotherapeutic agents being investigated as immunotherapy that have been shown to be effective in other types of cancers. These hold the potential to overcome certain mechanisms of resistance without dose-intensification and the related toxicities. In a retrospective study of adults with osteosarcoma, combination therapy of gemcitabine followed by docetaxel showed a synergistic response and an overall response rate of 43 percent [40]. Another review of children and adolescents with the same regimen showed similar efficacy in osteosarcoma patients [41]. Zwerdling et al. have examined the response rates of children to docetaxel alone (NCT00002825), however found it to be ineffective in recurrent solid tumors other than Ewing sarcoma [42]. Topotecan clinical trials in pediatric osteosarcoma was shown to be tolerable, but ineffective (NCT00003745) [43]. The study of becatecarin in monotherapy has been conducted (NCT00006102), but ineffective [44]. Other chemotherapeutic agents in monotherapy clinical trials include ixabepilone (NCT00030108) and ABT-751 (NCT00036959). Previous studies have examined irinotecan (NCT00004078) and oxaliplatin (NCT00091182) as monotherapies for osteosarcoma, as they have each been approved for the treatment of colorectal cancer. McGregor et al. investigated the efficacy and toxicity of both irinotecan and oxaliplatin together for the treatment of recurrent or refractory osteosarcoma in children (NCT00101270); however, found greater toxicity than evidence of antitumor activity [45]. Several other groups are investigating combination chemotherapies for the treatment of refractory osteosarcoma in children in hopes of increasing potency and efficacy. Chemotherapy regimens of talabostat and temozolomide or carboplatin (NCT00303940) are being investigated for treatment in children with refractory osteosarcoma. Temozolomide and O6-benzylguanine were studied (NCT00020150) and evidence of activity was observed with mild toxcities [46].

Other alkylating chemotherapeutic agents have been studied for potential therapy in sarcomas. Palifosfamide is the active metabolite of ifosfamide, and acts by alkylating DNA, preventing tumor proliferation. Studies in soft tissue sarcoma of palifosfamide monotherapy or in combination with doxorubicin failed to show efficacy. A current clinical trial proposes the use of etoposide and carboplatin with palifosfamide for osteosarcoma (NCT01242072). Another alkylating agent that has been controversial is dacarbazine for metastatic osteosarcoma, as some studies have shown it to be less effective and it has greater toxicity. However, Van Tine et al. aim to reexamine the tumor anatomic response rate and determine the risk of emesis and neutropenia when given supportive care of anti-emetic drugs and pegfilgrastim (NCT00802880).

Novel antifolates have been of interest in developing compounds to overcome chemotherapy resistance in the treatment of osteosarcoma. Methotrexate is the standard antifolate compound used against osteosarcoma by inhibiting dihydrofolate reductase (DHFR). However, mechanisms of methotrexate resistance include the upregulation of DHFR expression by gene amplification, aberrant transport by lower levels of reduced folate carrier, and defective intracellular retention of the drug [47]. Trimetrexate is a methotrexate analog and DHFR inhibitor. The mechanism of action of trimetrexate does not involve the reduced folate carrier, and therefore may still be effective in drug transportation into cells. Several studies have examined the efficacy of trimetrexate for treatment of osteosarcoma with leucovorin support for bone marrow recovery. Trimetrexate has been previously studied as a monotherapy in children with recurrent osteosarcoma (NCT00002738), in combination with methotrexate in recurrent osteosarcoma in adults (NCT00119301), and with conventional chemotherapy in metastatic osteosarcoma (NCT00003776). Pemetrexed is another alkylating agent that inhibits DHFR, as well as other folate-metabolic enzymes including thymidylate synthase, glycinamide ribonucleotide formyltransferase, and aminoimidazole carboxamide ribonucleotide formyltransferase [48]. These other mechanisms of action may allow pemetrexed to overcome osteosarcoma resistance to methotrexate working around DHFR overexpression, and is currently being studied for monotherapy treatment of recurrent osteosarcoma in children (NCT00520936).

Bisphosphonates are a type of drug used for the treatment of osteolytic bone diseases by inhibiting osteoclast activity, causing osteoclasts to undergo apoptosis, and therefore slowing bone degradation. This has led to the recent interest towards the application of bisphosphonates for the treatment of osteosarcoma. It has been suggested that osteosarcomas and bone malignacies may potentially arise from a positive-feedback loop, in which activated osteoclasts release growth factors that bind to receptors on tumor cells, which promotes proliferation and further release of growth factors [49]. The inhibition of osteoclasts may therefore prevent this tumor-growth mechanism. Several *in vitro* and *in vivo* animal studies have shown bisphosphonates to have a direct effect as an anti-neoplastic agent in osteosarcoma [50-52]. Additionally, bisphosphonates may have an added benefit of aiding in the prevention of osteoporosis due to chemotherapy treatment. Adjuvant administration of bisphosphonate pamidronate treatment for newly diagnosed high-grade osteosarcoma has been suggested to improve limb reconstruction and does not interfere with efficacy of chemotherapy in clinical trials (NCT00586846) [53]. This has led to further investigational studies of bisphosphonates. For patients with metastatic osteosarcoma, clinical trials for zoledronic acid with conventional chemotherapy (NCT00742924), as well as zoledronic acid as a monotherapy (NCT00320710) are currently being conducted.

Therapeutic strategies for pulmonary metastases are challenging due to the limited improvement and increased toxicity seen with dose intensification of chemotherapy. After surgical removal of lung masses, new pulmonary metastases are likely to develop, which suggests the presence of further micrometastases resistant to systemic chemotherapy. Researchers are investigating a more site-concentrated method of treatment with low systemic exposure. Because osteosarcoma preferentially metastasizes to the lung, aerosols and inhalation treatment methods are of interest. Clinical trials have been proposed for evaluating whether inhaled lipid-complexed cisplatin is effective in preventing pulmonary relapse of osteosarcoma patients with previous pulmonary relapses (NCT01650090). The goal of this trial is to increase local cisplatin concentration over a sustained period of time and reduce systemic exposure of the chemotherapy, and to determine event-free survival of patients.

RADIATION THERAPY

Generally, osteosarcomas are insensitive to radiation therapy alone; however, in combination with chemotherapy, radiation therapy may be useful in controlling a site of local or unresectable tumor [4]. Dosing of radiation treatment is determined and modified according to the radiation oncologist based on surround tissue tolerance. Giving radiation therapy before surgery, similar to or in conjuction with neoadjuvant chemotherapy, may delineate tumor volume to further reduce the amount of normal tissue to that needs to be surgically resected.

Further studies are needed in examining the effectiveness of radiation therapy in combination with chemotherapy and/or surgery. Some studies aim to optimize a regimen for treating osteosarcoma, as some patients after surgery may not need maintenance treatment until there is clinical progression of disease (NCT00346164). Examining the various permutations of neoadjuvant and/or maintenance chemoradiotherapy or observation alone, the goal of these studies is to optimize the survival rates for low-risk patients while monitoring toxicity. Several other groups are focusing on combination chemoradiotherapy post-operatively to reduce radiation exposure especially in pediatric patients, while maintaining the standard neoadjuvant chemotherapy treatment to kill remaining tumor cells that may have become chemotherapy resistant (NCT00592293).

Because it has been suggested that osteosarcoma may arise from previous irradiation sites, more effective ways to deliver radiation therapy are needed especially in pediatric patients. Using image-guided radiation therapy (IGRT) in combination with CT, MRI, and PET scan, investigators aim to more precisely define tumor location and treatment planning to minimize radiation side effects without affecting nearby normal tissues (NCT00186992). Intensity-Modulated Radiation Therapy (IMRT) also allows for a highly conformal dose delivery method as each radiation beam shape and intensity may be modified and directed towards the tumor for pre-operative therapy as previously studied (NCT00740597).

For metastatic disease, radiation therapy may be effective in treating unresectable metastases or eradicating the presence of possible chemotherapy resistant clones. Several groups are studying stereotactic methods of radiation delivery to metastases of difficult areas such as the brain and lungs to reduce exposure of normal tissues (NCT01586104). Intravenous radiation therapy may be able to target and kill tumor cells that are actively forming bone. Some radiocompounds are administered by infusion method to seek out bone. A novel compound radium-223 dichloride is being investigated for its effectiveness against metastatic osteosarcoma (NCT01833520). For unresectable metastatic osteosarcoma, 153Sm-EDTMP is used to target cancer that has invaded into the bone and kills the cells in combination with external beam radiotherapy (NCT01886105). 153Sm-EDTMP is also used in the palliation of pain.

Ultrasound therapy may also be used for the palliation of pain in metastatic osteosarcomas where the patient has not responded to radiation therapy. ExAblate is a MR-guided focused ultrasound surgery in clinical trials (NCT00981578, NCT00656305, NCT00350233).

Targeted Therapy

A greater understanding of molecular mechanisms and signal transduction pathways underlying the pathogenesis of osteosarcoma and the tumor microenvironment have led to the development of novel targeted therapies. By specifically targeting tumor cells and/or their microenvironment, toxicity to normal cells can be minimized. Targeted therapy for osteosarcoma has not yet been extensively studied, but developing effective agents is promising for patient outcomes in the future. Current areas of interest include receptor tyrosine kinases (RTKs), signal-transduction pathways, the tumor microenvironment, and immunomodulators. Monoclonal antibodies and small molecule inhibitors are effective in the targeting and inhibition of these mechanisms that have been linked to poorer prognosis in cancer.

Receptor Tyrosine Kinases

The study of RTKs for signal transduction towards cell growth or apoptosis in cancer has led to the development of monoclonal antibodies and small molecule inhibitors. Elucidating these pathways in osteosarcoma may also lead to their application as potential novel targeted therapies for osteosarcoma.

Insulin-like Growth Factor-1 Receptor

IGF-1R plays an important role in cell proliferation and suppression of apoptosis, and has been linked to the development of the malignant phenotype of cancer. Studies have linked high serum levels of IGF-1 to increased risk of colon, prostate, breast, and lung cancer [54-57]. High expression of IGF-1R has also been shown in primary sarcomas [58]. Thus, the development of therapeutic agents towards the inhibition of IGF-1 binding to IGF-1R and subsequent pathway activation has been of recent interest. Studies have examined the use of small molecule inhibitors, which bind to the ATP-binding or substrate-binding site of the receptor, and monoclonal antibodies. Due to the homology of IGF-1R and insulin receptor, small molecule inhibitors may not be ideal candidates due to possible cross-reactivity and interference with glucose metabolism. Monoclonal antibodies that target the receptor, however, may be able to downregulate the cell surface expression of IGF-1R.

Currently, several clinical trials utilizing monoclonal antibodies against IGF-1R have been in development for advanced osteosarcomas. Clinical trials are looking at the effectiveness of cixutumumab (IMC-A12) monotherapy for recurrent osteosarcoma (NCT00831844). Another monotherapy employing recombinant human monoclonal antibody R1507 is also being studied (NCT00642941). Chugh et al. is studying the combination treatment of cixutumumab given together with doxorubicin for patients with unresectable, locally advanced, or metastatic osteosarcoma (NCT00720174).

The binding of growth factors to IGF-1R activates the IGF pathway, leading to downstream signaling of the mitogen-activated protein kinase

(MAPK), phosphatidylinsolitol 3'-kinase (PI3K), and mammalian target of rapamycin (mTOR) kinase pathways. MAPK promotes cell proliferation, and PI3K and mTOR are regulators of the cell cycle and apoptosis, but their pathways are closely connected and are able to signal each other. In osteosarcoma, targeting the growth factors that bind to their receptors within these pathways is of interest. Therapeutic agents have also been shown to be effective in targeting these signalling-transduction pathways.

PI3K/Akt and mTOR Pathway

The PI3K/Akt and mTOR pathway is activated by IGF-1R, and plays an important role in cell proliferation and apoptosis. This pathway is aberrant in many cancers including sarcomas, causing tumor growth [59-61]. mTOR integrates growth factors such as amino acids and energy sources, inducing the G1 to S progression of the cell cycle [60, 62]. Rapamycin is an antibiotic that targets and arrests the G1 to S progression, and is currently in clinical use for immunosuppressive indications to prevent transplant rejection. More recently, rapamycin (sirolimus) and similar analogs (temsirolimus) have been investigated as potential anti-cancer agents.

Some studies suggest that sirolimus may be effective in combination with conventional chemotherapy drugs to treat patients with recurrent or refractory osteosarcoma. Monotherapy of sirolimus has been demonstrated to be an effective anti-cancer agent in pediatric patients with solid tumors xenografts in previous studies. Current clinical trials propose that administration of sirolimus in combination with chemotherapy may be a viable treatment option for patients in need of novel approaches. Several groups are investigating the efficacy of oral sirolimus and alternating etoposide and cyclophosphamide in children with refractory osteosarcoma (NCT01331135), and oral sirolimus and cyclophosphamide in adults with advanced osteosarcoma (NCT00743509). Another approach being studied for recurrent or refractory osteosarcomas is treatment with temsirolimus and liposomal doxorubicin for prolonged drug release (NCT00949325).

Though mTOR is downstream from PI3K/Akt, mTOR inhibition induces upstream activation of Akt. Studies have shown, however, that blocking IGF-1R prevents the activation of Akt by mTOR [63]. This indicates that targets further upstream of mTOR are also critical in the inhibition of the IGF-1R and PI3K/Akt/mTOR pathway to arrest cell cycle progression. Temsirolimus, targeting mTOR, and cixutumumab, targeting IGF-1R, are in clinical trials for the treatment of metastatic (NCT01016015) and relapsed (NCT01614795) osteosarcomas. CC-115 is a novel mTOR inhibitor that also acts as a dual inhibitor of DNA-dependent protein kinase (DNA-PK), related to the PI3K kinases. Clinical trials are underway to study the safety, action, and efficacy of oral administration of CC-115 in patients with advanced and refractory osteosarcoma (NCT01353625).

MAPK/ERK

The MAPK signalling pathway plays a critical role in gene expression, cell proliferation, and apoptosis. The MAPK pathway is a three-tiered cascade from which MAPK is activated by the phosphorylation of MAPKK, which is activated by the phosphorylation of MAPKKK. There are several classes of MAPKs, with ERK being the most widely studied in cancer, as it is demonstrated to be mutated in nearly one-third of cancers [64]. ERK signalling is activated by MEK phosphorylation, which is activated by Raf phosphorylation. Activated ERKs subsequently phosphorylate many cytoplasmic kinases, phosphotases, transcription factors, and cytoskeleton proteins, in which overactivation leads to deregulated cell proliferation, differentiation, survival, migration, angiogenesis, and chromatin remodelling [65], as well as overexpression of genes that limit proliferation [66]. In many cases, overactivation of ERK is due to the overexpression of upstream tyrosine receptor kinases, activating mutations of these tyrosine receptor kinases, or ubiquitous release of activating ligands.

Because of the network cascade of these pathways, downstream target specificity is an important factor in ensuring that only certain functions may be inhibited. With its downstream location and multiple effectors in cell proliferation, differentiation, survival, migration, angiogenesis, and chromatin remodelling, the ERK pathway is an attractive target. For similar reasons, another target of interest is heat shock protein 90 (Hsp90). Hsp90 is a critical chaperone for many signalling proteins, such as Raf, Akt, and epidermal growth factor receptors (EGFR). Targeting and inhibition of Hsp90 result in the degradation of these proteins. Studies using tanespimycin monotherapy to target Hsp90 in advanced or refractory osteosarcoma in children (NCT00093821) and adults (NCT00004241) have been examined, but need further investigation [67].

One drug that has been approved for use in renal and liver cancer that targets a similar pathway is sorafenib. Studies have also shown strong evidence that sorafenib acts through platelet-derived growth factor (PDGF) and vascular endothelial growth factor receptor (VEGF). Several groups are investigating sorafenib for the treatment of osteosarcoma. Tap et al. aim to examine the efficacy of neoadjuvant and post-operative sorafenib treatment in combination with ifosfamide in resectable osteosarcomas (NCT00880542). Oral sorafenib monotherapy and surgery has been studied for treatment of metastatic and inoperable osteosarcoma, as well as evaluated for its effect on VEGF and PDGF (NCT00330421); however, it showed little efficacy in sarcomas other than angiosarcoma [68]. For pediatric patients with refractory osteosarcomas, a different chemotherapy from the standard regimen may help to overcome possible drug resistance. Oral sorafenib and irinotecan have been shown to be effective in adults, and each exhibit different mechanisms of action from previous studies. This strategy is being studied for its efficacy and tolerability in pediatric patients with refractory osteosarcoma (NCT01518413).

Vascular Endothelial Growth Factor

VEGF is an essential signalling molecule for the induction of vasculogenesis and angiogenesis. Solid tumors that express VEGF are more likely to grow, as the formation of blood vessels provides a greater surface area and permeability for the tumor cells to exchange blood supply and nutrients, as well as metastasize [69]. Several studies have shown a correlation of VEGF expression, metastasis rate, and prognostic outcome [70-72]. In cases of osteosarcoma, one study examined the expression of VEGF in untreated disease, and found a correlation with increased microvessel density, pulmonary metastases (82 percent in VEGF+, while only 10 percent in VEGF- tumors), and lower overall survival [73]. Similar results were found in a study with pre-operative chemotherapy treatment, in that VEGF expression correlated with lower disease-free and overall survival [74]. These findings show promise in targeting VEGF for the treatment of patients with osteosarcoma.

Bevacizumab is a monoclonal antibody that has been demonstrated in the clinic to successfully inhibit angiogenesis and has been approved for the treatment of metastatic colorectal cancer in combination with chemotherapy. Current clinical trials aim to adopt this strategy as a novel approach to first-line treatment of osteosarcoma. For patients with localized and resectable tumors, bevacizumab in combination with the conventional regimen of high-dose methotrexate, doxorubicin, and cisplatin will be administered to determine the rate of event-free survival. For unresectable and metastatic tumors, the regimen additionally includes ifosfamide and etoposide (NCT00667342).

Pazopanib is a small molecule inhibitor that acts to prevent angiogenesis by blocking the VEGFR-1, VEGFR-2, VEGFR-3, and platelet-derived growth factor (PDGF) receptors. Pazopanib has been approved for the treatment of renal cell carcinoma and soft tissue sarcomas. Thus, investigators propose a pazopanib monotherapy for osteosarcoma that has metastasized to the lung (NCT01759303), as well as examining its efficacy in children with refractory osteosarcoma (NCT01130623).

Other signalling pathways that influence angiogenesis include the Notch signalling pathway and the Hedgehog signalling pathway. In angiogenesis, endothelial cells use the Notch signalling pathway to communicate and coordinate the development and migration of blood vessels between cells. RO4929097, a novel inhibitor of gamma secretase, which is a necessary enzyme in the activation of Notch, was recently examined in *in vitro* and *in vivo* melanoma xenograft models. Expression of genes within the Notch signalling pathway were seen to be upregulated and correlated with disease outcome in melanoma. RO4929097 successfully demonstrated inhibition of primary and metastatic melanoma growth and invasion [75].

The Hedgehog signalling pathway is required for proper embryonic development, and has also been shown to be involved in regulating adult stem cells for maintenance and tissue repair. However, dysregulation of this pathway in adults has been associated with cancer. Studies have suggested that Hedgehog signalling also plays an important role in angiogenesis [76]. Therefore, targeting the Hedgehog pathway with specific inhibitors may provide an effective treatment option. Vismodegib is a small molecule inhibitor specifically targeted to the Hedgehog pathway, and is the first approved drug for the treatment of basal cell carcinomas. Investigators propose to exploit these two pathways in the treatment of metastatic or advanced osteosarcoma. A current clinical trial is studying the efficacy of gamma secretase/Notch inhibitor RO4929097 together with Hedgehog inhibitor vismodegib in treating patients by oral administration (NCT01154452).

Activation of the Hedgehog pathway also leads to an increase in angiogenic factors, including angiopoietin-1 (Ang I) and angiopoietin-2 (Ang II). Ang I is converted to Ang II by angotensin-converting enzyme (ACE), and Ang II mediates a MAPK pathway promoting cell growth and angiogenesis. ACE2 converts Ang II into its metabolite Angiotensin-(1-7) (Ang-(1-7)), which inhibits the Ang II-mediated MAPK pathway [77]. However, Ang-(1-7) is quickly metabolized into inactive Ang-(1-5) [78, 79]. Petty et al. propose an antiangiogenic treatment using therapeutic Ang-(1-7) for second- or third-line treatment of metastatic and unresectable osteosarcoma (NCT01553539). Therapeutic Ang-(1-7) may prevent the growth of the tumor by blocking blood vessel formation and blood flow.

Epidermal Growth Factor Receptor

EGFR is tyrosine kinase receptor for the family of epidermal growth factors. There are a number of receptor tyrosine kinases that are closely related to EGFR (ErbB-1), including HER2/neu (ErbB-2), Her 3 (ErbB-3), and Her 4 (ErbB-4). These receptors bind a number of epidermal growth factors and transforming growth factor α (TGFα), which induces dimerization and activation of downstream signalling cascades such as MAPKs and PI3K/Akt/mTOR leading to DNA synthesis and cell proliferation [80]. The EGFR kinase domain can cross-phosphorylate other receptors that it may be dimerized with, and vice versa, as well as activate itself in a feedback loop. Overexpression of EGFR has been observed in a number of cancers, including breast, ovarian, endometrial, and lung, and has been correlated with poor prognosis [81], making this oncogene an attractive target for novel anti-cancer therapies. The expression of HER2/neu in osteosarcoma has been studied by several groups with controversial results. While some groups have shown correlation of HER2/neu expression with pulmonary metastasis and poor prognosis in osteosarcoma [82, 83], a number of groups demonstrated that HER2/neu is not a prognostic factor or overexpressed [84, 85]. Nonetheless, this target remains an important tool in understanding the intracellular signalling that promotes tumor growth.

Trastuzumab is a monoclonal antibody blocking the extraceullular ligand binding domain that has been approved for the treatment of breast cancer with HER2/neu overexpression. For patients with recurrent osteosarcoma with confirmed overexpression of HER2/neu, monotherapy treatment with trastuzumab may be effective in targeting tumor cells that have become resistant to doxorubicin after initial systemic chemotherapy (NCT00005033). Maintenance therapy with trastuzumab in combination with standard treatment has also been studied. For newly diagnosed, metastatic disease, Ebb et al. studied the efficacy of the conventional chemotherapy regimen of doxorubicin, cisplatin, and methotrexate with immunostimulatory support, followed by surgical resection or radiation if inoperable, and then addition of trastuzumab in the adjuvant therapy regimen (NCT00023998), but was unable to determine its therapeutic benefits [86].

Small molecule inhibitors are another approach to specifically targeting and inhibiting EGFR tyrosine kinases, but within the cytoplasm. By blocking the EGFR signalling cascade, the kinase is unable to activate itself. Gefitinib and erlotinib are small molecule inhibitors that have been developed for the treatment of lung cancer, which target the EGFR cascade. Clinical trials for the treatment of children with refractory osteosarcomas are employing combination therapies by oral administration of these inhibitors and chemotherapy, including gefitinib with irinotecan (NCT00132158). Phase I trials for erlotinib with temozolomide showed efficacy in recurrent pediatric solid tumors (NCT00077454) [87].

Platelet-derived Growth Factor

PDGF is another important growth factor for cell proliferation and angiogenesis, which acts through receptor tyrosine kinases, such as PDGFR-α and PDGFR-β. There are several dimeric isoforms of PDGF that bind to these two receptors: PDGF-AA, PDGF-BB, PDGF-AB, PDGF-CC, and PDGF-DD. When the PDGF pathway is activated, the receptors dimerize and subsequently induce several signal transduction pathways, including PI3K/Akt, which inhibits BCL, an activator of apoptosis [88]. Previous studies have shown that PDGF may act as a mitogen to drive proliferation of mesenchymal cells, as well as osteosarcoma cell lines [88]. It has also been suggested that coexpression of PDGF-AA and PDGFR-α in osteosarcoma cell lines and human osteosarcoma samples demonstrates an autocrine and/or paracrine activation loop [89]. More recently, a study demonstrated a correlation between coexpression of PDGF-AA and PDGFR-α and poor prognosis, showing PDGFR as a potential therapeutic target [90].

Imatinib is a small molecule inhibitor developed to inhibit the Bcr-Abl tyrosine kinase, and has been shown *in vitro* to also act through c-kit and PDGFR [91]. Other *in vitro* studies have demonstrated efficacy of imatinib to inhibit PDGF-mediated cell proliferation in osteosarcoma cell lines. Several groups are investigating imatinib as a monotherapy for advanced, metastatic, or refractory osteosarcomas (NCT00030667).

Dasatinib was developed as a second-generation Bcr-Abl tyrosine kinase inhibitor for patients who were resistant to imatinib. Dasatinib also targets Src, c-kit, and several other tyrosine receptor kinases. Previous studies have shown *in vitro* that dasatinib inhibition of Src phosphorylation effectively altered the metastatic potential of osteosarcoma cells lines, however were unable to demonstrate similar results *in vivo*, suggesting that other pathways may be involved in the metastasis of osteosarcoma [92]. Thus, groups have proposed to use a combination therapy of dasatinib with ifosfamide, carboplatin, and etoposide chemotherapy in young patients with metastatic or recurrent osteosarcoma (NCT00788125). Another potential target in combination with dasatinib Src inhibition that investigators are pursuing is CTLA-4, which inhibits activation of cytotoxic T lymphocytes (CTLs). Ipilimumab binds to CTLA-4, allowing the CTLs to recognize and destroy cancer cells. Dasatinib in combination with ipilimumab are being studied for their efficacy in treating patients with metastatic or unresectable osteosarcomas (NCT01643278).

Saracatinib is also a dual-specific inhibitor of Src and Abl, as well as an inhibitor of osteoclast bone reasborption. In a double-blind study, investigators aim to evaluate the efficacy of post-operative saracatinib versus placebo for treatment of osteosarcomas that have metastasized to the lung (NCT00752206).

Sunitinib is a small molecule inhibitor of several receptor tyrosine kinases including PDGFR and VEGFR, and was also approved for treatment of imatinib-resistant metastatic melanoma. By targeting PDGFR and preventing angiogenesis, investigators propose sunitinib as a monotherapy for metastatic osteosarcomas (NCT00474994).

Targeting Tumor-Specific/Tumor-Associated Antigens

HDAC

Histone deacetylase (HDAC) inhibitors have recently emerged as potential therapeutic compounds for cancer treatment. Histone deacetylases regulate chromatin structure and gene expression, which have become dysregulated in cancer. HDAC inhibitors play a role in epigenetic processes by modifying acetylation states of genes involved in tumor proliferation, thus inducing an apoptotic effect [93, 94]. Though the exact mechanism of action of HDAC inhibitors and which patient characteristics would most benefit are still to be determined, a number of anti-cancer agents are currently in development. The specificity and potency of HDAC inhibitors towards tumor specific cells *in vivo* and *in vitro* show promise as either a monotherapy or part of combination therapies [94-96].

Several HDAC inhibitor monotherapy clinical trials are being investigated in metastatic osteosarcoma. Savage et al. are studying the efficacy of monotherapy with romidepsin for metastatic osteosarcoma, which has previously been approved for treatment of cutaneous T-cell lymphoma (NCT00112463). PXD101 is being investigated as a monotherapy (NCT00413075), as it has been shown to synergize in combination with chemotherapeutic 5-Fluorouracil in advanced solid tumors (NCT00413322) [97]. Valproic acid acts as a HDAC inhibitor and may also block blood flow to solid tumors. In combination with temsirolimus, an mTOR inhibitor, Blatt et al. propose a study to inhibit growth of relapsed osteosarcomas (NCT01204450).

PARP

Poly ADP ribose polymerase (PARP) play a critical role in DNA repair. PARP1 and PARP2 act to repair single-strand breaks in DNA prior to the DNA replication step in cell division, preventing the formation of double-strand breaks [98]. Several studies have shown that PARP has a greater role within cancer cell regulation than in normal cells, implicating PARP as a potential target for cancer therapy [99]. PARP inhibitors block PARP enzyme activity, thus preventing the repair of DNA damage and subsequently causing cell death. Recent studies have shown that PARP inhibitors have a synergistic and more toxic effect, in that they localize and lock PARP proteins to the sites of DNA damage. The aggregated PARP protein-DNA complex blocks DNA replication, as PARP is unable to be released to allow recruited DNA repair proteins such as BRCA1, BRCA2, and PALB2 into the site to initiate repair [100, 101].

BMN 673 has been developed as a novel highly potent and highly specific PARP inhibitor for anti-cancer treatment [102]. *In vitro*, BMN 673 targeted tumor cells with BRCA1, BCRA2, or PTEN mutations at a higher rate than previous PARP inhibitors, and did not have significant interactions with other enzymes. *In vivo* mouse models showed BMN 673 had anti-tumor activity, as well as synergistic effects with chemotherapy drugs. Clinical trials for first in human studies are being investigated for BMN 673 monotherapy treatment of unresectable or recurrent osteosarcoma (NCT01286987).

Proteasome Inhibitors

Proteasomes hold an important role in the regulation of protein expression by breaking down proteins through the ubiquitin-proteasome pathway [103]. Dysregulation of the proteasome may induce the degradation of pro-apoptotic factors, allowing damaged cells to continue proliferating. Proteasome inhibitors have become an interesting new target for cancer therapy in that proteasome inhibition may prevent malignant cells from proliferating and eliciting a stress response. Studies have shown that treatment with a proteasome inhibitor in combination with radiation or chemotherapy may enhance tumor-killing ability [103].

Bortezomib is a proteasome inhibitor developed for the treatment of multiple myeloma. Recently, groups have proposed bortezomib treatment as a monotherapy for osteosarcoma (NCT00027716), as Phase I trials of bortezomib in combination with gemcitabine (NCT00620295) for metastatic or advanced solid tumors have demonstrated efficacy [104].

AURKA

Aurora A kinase (AURKA) is an important enzyme during mitosis and meiosis, between G2 and M phases of the cell cycle, and cytokinesis for healthy proliferation of the cell. Aurora A dysregulation has been linked to a high occurrence of cancer. Aurora A is usually regulated by p53, however, if a cell becomes unable to complete mitosis via cytokinesis, the resulting cell becomes aneuploidy, which has been implicated in a number of cancers [105]. Studies have demonstrated higher AURKA expression associated with poorer prognosis and metastasis of breast cancer [106]. Alisertib is a small molecule inhibitor of AURKA being studied in oncology clinical trials. For young patients with relapsed or refractory osteosarcoma, Mosse et al. propose an alisertib monotherapy treatment (NCT01154816).

GD2

Disialoganglioside GD2 is a cell surface antigen that is expressed on a number of tumors, but less so on normal tissues. GD2 has been demonstrated to be expressed in approximately 50 percent of osteosarcoma and soft-tissue sarcoma samples, as well as other high-risk tumors such as melanoma and neuroectodermal tumors [107, 108]. Anti-cancer monoclonal antibody development has been of recent interest. Though the exact function of GD2 has not been fully elucidated, it has been suggested that this surface antigen is involved in the attachment of tumor cells to extracellular matrix proteins [109]. GD2 is an attractive target for novel immunotherapies because of its tumor-selective expression. A humanized monoclonal anti-GD-2 antibody hu14.18K322A is being investigated for monotherapy treatment of relapsed or refractory osteosarcoma in children (NCT00743496).

TNFRSF10B

Tumor necrosis factor receptor superfamily, member 10b (TRAIL-R2) contains an intercellular death domain. When this receptor becomes activated by tumor necrosis factor-related apoptosis inducing ligand (TRAIL), apoptosis signalling is tranduced. Lexatumumab is a monoclonal antibody that targets TRAIL-R2 and induces cell death. Mackall et al. are examining the efficacy of lexatumumab for the treatment of metastatic osteosarcoma in children (NCT00428272).

Retroviral Vector Gene Therapy

The recent focus of vector gene therapy in cancer treatment has been on strategies that enhance the effects of immunotherapeutic and chemotherapeutic agents. Vector gene therapeutics allows for the targeting of tumor-specific cells, and in some cases is targeted towards inactivation of oncogenes and gene replacement of tumor suppressor genes [110]. A retrovirus incorporates into DNA to replicate within and destroy tumor cells, and subsequently is able to travel through the bloodstream to other possible tumor sites. Several studies have developed oncolytic therapeutics with immunostimulatory genes to specifically target overactive Ras pathways allowing for use in many cancers, including sarcoma [111]. JX-594 was developed with attenuated vaccinia virus with GM-CSF vector incorporated, and is currently being investigated in clinical trials for pediatric patients with advanced or refractory osteosarcoma (NCT01169584). Reovirus targets the activated Ras signalling pathway and is being evaluated for treatment of patients with osteosarcoma metastatic to the lungs (NCT00503295). Rexin-G is a retroviral vector that encodes mutant human cyclic G1 to inhibit cell proliferation, and is in clinical trials for metastatic osteosarcoma (NCT00572130).

IMMUNOSTIMULANTS

Previously, immunostimulatory agents had mainly been used to enhance neutrophil rescue after chemotherapy. Recent studies have begun to investigate the immunomodulatory potential of these agents. Inhalation of immunostimulants such as IL-2 and Sargramostim are also being studied for pulmonary metastases of osteosarcoma, in which the patient's own immune cells will be stimulated to recover from intensive systemic chemotherapy and attack remaining tumor cells after surgical resection of the large masses (NCT01590069, NCT00066365). PEG-interferon alfa-2b in combination with chemotherapy is also a potential post-surgical maintenance therapy treatment for osteosarcoma (NCT00134030).

In cases of chemorefractory tumors, immune tolerance arises from the suppression of antigen presenting cells (APCs) that activate CD4 T cells, which are subsequently required to stimulate the CD8 T cells directed against the tumors [112, 113]. Previous studies have demonstrated that donor mononuclear cells are able to overcome this tolerance [114]. Furthermore, irradiated donor mononuclear cells may prevent possible graft-versus-host disease [115]. Thus, clinical trials for the treatment of refractory and unresectable osteosarcoma using irradiated donor lymphocytes have been proposed (NCT00161187).

Muramyl tripeptide phosphatidyl-ethanolamine (MTP-PE) is a liposomally encapsulated drug delivery vehicle that activates immune cells such as monocytes and macrophages against osteosarcoma cells [116]. Previous studies on non-metastatic osteosarcoma in pediatric patients demonstrated that MTP-PE in addition to standard chemotherapy significantly increased overall and event free survival [117]. This has prompted a clinical trial to investigate the efficacy of MTP-PE for metastatic osteosarcoma (NCT00631631).

Stem Cell Therapy

Stem cell transplantation may allow for higher-dose chemotherapy by recovering patients' immune systems. Current clinical trials are examining the effectiveness of giving autologous stem cell transplants followed by high-dose combination chemotherapy (NCT00002854, NCT00002601), or cyclophosphamide or thalidomide to prevent new blood vessel growth (NCT01661400). Symons et al. exploit the graft versus tumor mechanism by treatment with reduced intensity chemotherapy followed by haploidentical bone marrow transplant and mTOR inhibitor sirolimus (NCT01804634).

Vaccine Therapy

The development of cancer vaccines to stimulate memory immune cells against tumor-associated antigens may aid in the treatment of osteosarcoma. Multiple treatment vaccines are currently in clinical trials. Goldberg et al. propose exposure of autologous dendritic cells (DCs) with or without gemcitabine *in situ* to refractory osteosarcoma tumor lysate to evaluate patient immune response (NCT01803152). More specific target peptides have previously been tested on tumors that express these antigens, and are currently being examined for their efficacy in stimulating the immune system for osteosarcoma, including NY-ESO-1, MAGE-A1, MAGE-A3 (NCT01241162), and NY-ESO-1 with immunostimulant sirolimus (NCT01522820).

FANG is a bifunctional vaccine that expresses rhGM-CSF to recruit and activate APCs, as well as shRNAfurin, which blocks furin protein production and subsquently inhibits the immunosuppressive TGFβ mechanism. Together the GM-CSF and TGFβ suppression are proposed to enhance the immune system in the treatment of osteosarcoma (NCT01061840).

SUPPORTIVE CARE

The exhaustive nature of chemotherapy and radiation therapy results in systemic complications. The most common complications include infection associated with myelosuppression, mucositis, nephrotoxicity (tubular damage due to ifosfomide and glomerular dysfuction due to cisplatin), hypomagnesaemia, ototoxicity, gonadal dysfunction, anthracycline-induced cardiac dysfunction, fatigue, and cachexia [2]. Clinical trials for supportive care of the multiple effects of chemotherapy have been proposed. Prevention of alopecia due to taxane-based chemotherapy is being tested with topical calcitriol in adults with relapsed disease (NCT01588522). Autologous stem cell transplantation after high-dose chemotherapy may rescue osteosarcoma patients from myelosuppression (NCT00638898). Chemotherapy-induced thrombocytopenia from gemcitabine and docetaxel for bone sarcomas may also be prevented by treatment with eltrombopag (NCT01491594). Other bleeding complications and deep vein thrombosis at the surgical site of lower extremity osteosarcomas are being evaluated with prophylactic treatment of dalteparin (NCT00525057). Pre-operative physical therapy of the lower extremities may strengthen, as well as promote overall healing for osteosarcomas (NCT01674101). Prevention of cancer- or treatment-related weight loss may be alleviated with cyproheptadine in children at high nutritional risk who are receiving moderate to high emetic chemotherapy (NCT01132547). Electroacupuncture is being evaluated for the prevention of nausea and vomiting (NCT00040911). Ototoxicity is a common complication of cisplatin treatment for patients with osteosarcoma, and sodium thiosulfate may prevent this hearing loss (NCT00716976). Pantoprazole may also provide a new approach to prevent hearing loss, as well as nephrotoxcity in osteosarcoma patients treated with high-dose methotrexate (NCT01848457). Dexrazoxane as a chemoprotective agent may provide cardioprotection during the induction of chemotherapy (NCT00003937). Additionally, there are studies that aim to determine the importance of certain genes in B-receptor signalling associated with anthracycline-induced cardiomyopathy by genotyping patients treated with doxorubicin (NCT01135849).

CONCLUSION

While the current standard of care for osteosarcoma can be curative in 70 percent of patients in non-metastatic disease, further progress has slowed in the last twenty years. Diagnostic and prognostic tools are limited in that assessment cannot be made at the time of initial diagnosis. Furthermore, it is suggested that many osteosarcoma patients have micrometastases for which there are no current clinical detection tools. For patients with metastatic or refractory disease, dose-intensification of current chemotherapy regimens is limited by lack of response and greater toxicity. There are numerous clinical trials underway for osteosarcoma patients targeted towards finding more powerful prognostic tools, effective treatments, and supportive care to increase patient survival and quality of life. The next goals for these trials include determining the patient population that would most benefit from these efforts, as well as the timing of these interventions in the course of treatment, especially to improve the outcome of those patients with refractory or clinically detectable metastatic disease at diagnosis. By understanding the molecular mechanisms critical to osteosarcoma and establishing translatable preclinical models, therapeutic or diagnostic agents may improve the outcome for patients with osteosarcoma. With genomic studies, and the development of single agent monotherapies and rational combinations of diagnostic and therapeutic agents, the future outlook for the outcome of osteosarcoma patients is promising.

REFERENCES

[1] Mirabello L, Troisi RJ, Savage SA. Osteosarcoma incidence and survival rates from 1973 to 2004: data from the Surveillance, Epidemiology, and End Results Program. *Cancer* 2009;115:1531-43.

[2] Carrle D, Bielack SS. Current strategies of chemotherapy in osteosarcoma. *International orthopaedics* 2006;30:445-51.

[3] Marina N, Gebhardt M, Teot L, Gorlick R. Biology and therapeutic advances for pediatric osteosarcoma. *The oncologist* 2004;9:422-41.

[4] Meyers PA, Gorlick R. Osteosarcoma. *Pediatric clinics of North America* 1997;44:973-89.

[5] Huvos AG. Osteogenic sarcoma of bones and soft tissues in older persons. A clinicopathologic analysis of 117 patients older than 60 years. *Cancer* 1986;57:1442-9.

[6] Kong C, Hansen MF. *Biomarkers in osteosarcoma*. 2009.

[7] Whelan J, Seddon B, Perisoglou M. Management of osteosarcoma. *Current treatment options in oncology* 2006;7:444-55.

[8] Lewis IJ, Nooij MA, Whelan J, et al. Improvement in histologic response but not survival in osteosarcoma patients treated with intensified chemotherapy: a randomized phase III trial of the European Osteosarcoma Intergroup. *Journal of the National Cancer Institute* 2007;99:112-28.

[9] O'Day K, Gorlick R. Novel therapeutic agents for osteosarcoma. *Expert review of anticancer therapy* 2009;9:511-23.

[10] Meyers PA, Gorlick R, Heller G, et al. Intensification of preoperative chemotherapy for osteogenic sarcoma: results of the Memorial Sloan-Kettering (T12) protocol. *Journal of clinical oncology: official journal of the American Society of Clinical Oncology* 1998;16:2452-8.

[11] Wang LL, Chintagumpala M, Gebhardt MC. Osteosarcoma: Epidemiology, pathogenesis, clinical presentation, diagnosis, and histology. In: Basow DS, ed. UpToDate. Waltham, MA: UpToDate; 2013.

[12] Fletcher JA, Gebhardt MC, Kozakewich HP. Cytogenetic aberrations in osteosarcomas. Nonrandom deletions, rings, and double-minute chromosomes. *Cancer genetics and cytogenetics* 1994;77:81-8.

[13] Jeffree GM, Price CH, Sissons HA. The metastatic patterns of osteosarcoma. *British journal of cancer* 1975;32:87-107.

[14] Bielack SS, Kempf-Bielack B, Delling G, et al. Prognostic factors in high-grade osteosarcoma of the extremities or trunk: an analysis of 1,702 patients treated on neoadjuvant cooperative osteosarcoma study group protocols. *Journal of clinical oncology: official journal of the American Society of Clinical Oncology* 2002;20:776-90.

[15] Pakos EE, Nearchou AD, Grimer RJ, et al. Prognostic factors and outcomes for osteosarcoma: an international collaboration. *Eur. J. Cancer* 2009;45:2367-75.

[16] Glasser DB, Lane JM, Huvos AG, Marcove RC, Rosen G. Survival, prognosis, and therapeutic response in osteogenic sarcoma. The Memorial Hospital experience. *Cancer* 1992;69:698-708.

[17] Provisor AJ, Ettinger LJ, Nachman JB, et al. Treatment of nonmetastatic osteosarcoma of the extremity with preoperative and postoperative

chemotherapy: a report from the Children's Cancer Group. *Journal of clinical oncology: official journal of the American Society of Clinical Oncology* 1997;15:76-84.

[18] Bacci G, Ferrari S, Bertoni F, et al. Long-term outcome for patients with nonmetastatic osteosarcoma of the extremity treated at the istituto ortopedico rizzoli according to the istituto ortopedico rizzoli/osteosarcoma-2 protocol: an updated report. *Journal of clinical oncology: official journal of the American Society of Clinical Oncology* 2000;18:4016-27.

[19] Kim MS, Cho WH, Song WS, Lee SY, Jeon DG. time dependency of prognostic factors in patients with stage II osteosarcomas. *Clinical orthopaedics and related research* 2007;463:157-65.

[20] Caluser CI, Abdel-Dayem HM, Macapinlac HA, et al. The value of thallium and three-phase bone scans in the evaluation of bone and soft tissue sarcomas. *European journal of nuclear medicine* 1994;21:1198-205.

[21] Holscher HC, Bloem JL, van der Woude HJ, et al. Can MRI predict the histopathological response in patients with osteosarcoma after the first cycle of chemotherapy? *Clinical radiology* 1995;50:384-90.

[22] Toner GC, Hicks RJ. PET for sarcomas other than gastrointestinal stromal tumors. *The oncologist* 2008;13 Suppl 2:22-6.

[23] Heinsohn S, Evermann U, Zur Stadt U, Bielack S, Kabisch H. Determination of the prognostic value of loss of heterozygosity at the retinoblastoma gene in osteosarcoma. *International journal of oncology* 2007;30:1205-14.

[24] Scholz RB, Kabisch H, Weber B, Roser K, Delling G, Winkler K. Studies of the RB1 gene and the p53 gene in human osteosarcomas. *Pediatric hematology and oncology* 1992;9:125-37.

[25] Weichselbaum RR, Beckett M, Diamond A. Some retinoblastomas, osteosarcomas, and soft tissue sarcomas may share a common etiology. *Proceedings of the National Academy of Sciences of the United States of America* 1988;85:2106-9.

[26] Ezhevsky SA, Ho A, Becker-Hapak M, Davis PK, Dowdy SF. Differential regulation of retinoblastoma tumor suppressor protein by G(1) cyclin-dependent kinase complexes in vivo. *Molecular and cellular biology* 2001;21:4773-84.

[27] Sengupta S, Harris CC. p53: traffic cop at the crossroads of DNA repair and recombination. *Nature reviews Molecular cell biology* 2005;6:44-55.

[28] Riley T, Sontag E, Chen P, Levine A. Transcriptional control of human p53-regulated genes. *Nature reviews Molecular cell biology* 2008;9:402-12.

[29] Hughes DP, Thomas DG, Giordano TJ, McDonagh KT, Baker LH. Essential erbB family phosphorylation in osteosarcoma as a target for CI-1033 inhibition. *Pediatric blood & cancer* 2006;46:614-23.

[30] Scotlandi K, Manara MC, Hattinger CM, et al. Prognostic and therapeutic relevance of HER2 expression in osteosarcoma and Ewing's sarcoma. *Eur. J. Cancer* 2005;41:1349-61.

[31] Huang G, Mills L, Worth LL. Expression of human glutathione S-transferase P1 mediates the chemosensitivity of osteosarcoma cells. *Molecular cancer therapeutics* 2007;6:1610-9.

[32] Link MP, Goorin AM, Miser AW, et al. The effect of adjuvant chemotherapy on relapse-free survival in patients with osteosarcoma of the extremity. *The New England journal of medicine* 1986;314:1600-6.

[33] Meyers PA, Heller G, Healey JH, et al. Osteogenic sarcoma with clinically detectable metastasis at initial presentation. *Journal of clinical oncology: official journal of the American Society of Clinical Oncology* 1993;11:449-53.

[34] Bielack SS, Kempf-Bielack B, Heise U, Schwenzer D, Winkler K. Combined modality treatment for osteosarcoma occurring as a second malignant disease. Cooperative German-Austrian-Swiss Osteosarcoma Study Group. *Journal of clinical oncology: official journal of the American Society of Clinical Oncology* 1999;17:1164.

[35] Goorin AM, Schwartzentruber DJ, Devidas M, et al. Presurgical chemotherapy compared with immediate surgery and adjuvant chemotherapy for nonmetastatic osteosarcoma: Pediatric Oncology Group Study POG-8651. *Journal of clinical oncology: official journal of the American Society of Clinical Oncology* 2003;21:1574-80.

[36] Nakajima H, Sim FH, Bond JR, Unni KK. Small cell osteosarcoma of bone. Review of 72 cases. *Cancer* 1997;79:2095-106.

[37] Harris MB, Cantor AB, Goorin AM, et al. Treatment of osteosarcoma with ifosfamide: comparison of response in pediatric patients with recurrent disease versus patients previously untreated: a Pediatric Oncology Group study. *Medical and pediatric oncology* 1995;24:87-92.

[38] Meyers PA, Schwartz CL, Krailo M, et al. Osteosarcoma: a randomized, prospective trial of the addition of ifosfamide and/or muramyl tripeptide to cisplatin, doxorubicin, and high-dose methotrexate. *Journal of clinical*

oncology: official journal of the American Society of Clinical Oncology 2005;23:2004-11.

[39] LaCasce AS. Therapeutic use and toxicity of high-dose methotrexate. In: Basow DS, ed. UpToDate. Waltham, MA: UpToDate; 2013.

[40] Leu KM, Ostruszka LJ, Shewach D, et al. Laboratory and clinical evidence of synergistic cytotoxicity of sequential treatment with gemcitabine followed by docetaxel in the treatment of sarcoma. *Journal of clinical oncology: official journal of the American Society of Clinical Oncology* 2004;22:1706-12.

[41] Navid F, Willert JR, McCarville MB, et al. Combination of gemcitabine and docetaxel in the treatment of children and young adults with refractory bone sarcoma. *Cancer* 2008;113:419-25.

[42] Zwerdling T, Krailo M, Monteleone P, et al. Phase II investigation of docetaxel in pediatric patients with recurrent solid tumors: a report from the Children's Oncology Group. *Cancer* 2006;106:1821-8.

[43] Hawkins DS, Bradfield S, Whitlock JA, et al. Topotecan by 21-day continuous infusion in children with relapsed or refractory solid tumors: a Children's Oncology Group study. *Pediatric blood & cancer* 2006; 47:790-4.

[44] Langevin AM, Bernstein M, Kuhn JG, et al. A phase II trial of rebeccamycin analogue (NSC #655649) in children with solid tumors: a Children's Oncology Group study. *Pediatric blood & cancer* 2008; 50:577-80.

[45] McGregor LM, Spunt SL, Furman WL, et al. Phase 1 study of oxaliplatin and irinotecan in pediatric patients with refractory solid tumors: a children's oncology group study. *Cancer* 2009;115:1765-75.

[46] Warren KE, Aikin AA, Libucha M, et al. Phase I study of O6-benzylguanine and temozolomide administered daily for 5 days to pediatric patients with solid tumors. *Journal of clinical oncology: official journal of the American Society of Clinical Oncology* 2005;23:7646-53.

[47] Guo W, Healey JH, Meyers PA, et al. Mechanisms of methotrexate resistance in osteosarcoma. *Clinical cancer research: an official journal of the American Association for Cancer Research* 1999;5:621-7.

[48] Shih C, Chen VJ, Gossett LS, et al. LY231514, a pyrrolo[2,3-d]pyrimidine-based antifolate that inhibits multiple folate-requiring enzymes. *Cancer research* 1997;57:1116-23.

[49] O'Keefe RJ, Guise TA. Molecular mechanisms of bone metastasis and therapeutic implications. *Clinical orthopaedics and related research* 2003:S100-4.

[50] Cheng YY, Huang L, Lee KM, Li K, Kumta SM. Alendronate regulates cell invasion and MMP-2 secretion in human osteosarcoma cell lines. *Pediatric blood & cancer* 2004;42:410-5.

[51] Ory B, Heymann MF, Kamijo A, Gouin F, Heymann D, Redini F. Zoledronic acid suppresses lung metastases and prolongs overall survival of osteosarcoma-bearing mice. *Cancer* 2005;104:2522-9.

[52] Sonnemann J, Eckervogt V, Truckenbrod B, Boos J, Winkelmann W, van Valen F. The bisphosphonate pamidronate is a potent inhibitor of human osteosarcoma cell growth in vitro. *Anti-cancer drugs* 2001;12:459-65.

[53] Meyers PA, Healey JH, Chou AJ, et al. Addition of pamidronate to chemotherapy for the treatment of osteosarcoma. *Cancer* 2011; 117: 1736-44.

[54] Chan JM, Stampfer MJ, Giovannucci E, et al. Plasma insulin-like growth factor-I and prostate cancer risk: a prospective study. *Science* 1998; 279:563-6.

[55] Hankinson SE, Willett WC, Colditz GA, et al. Circulating concentrations of insulin-like growth factor-I and risk of breast cancer. *Lancet* 1998;351:1393-6.

[56] Ma J, Pollak MN, Giovannucci E, et al. Prospective study of colorectal cancer risk in men and plasma levels of insulin-like growth factor (IGF)-I and IGF-binding protein-3. *Journal of the National Cancer Institute* 1999;91:620-5.

[57] Yu H, Spitz MR, Mistry J, Gu J, Hong WK, Wu X. Plasma levels of insulin-like growth factor-I and lung cancer risk: a case-control analysis. *Journal of the National Cancer Institute* 1999;91:151-6.

[58] Sekyi-Otu A, Bell RS, Ohashi C, Pollak M, Andrulis IL. Insulin-like growth factor 1 (IGF-1) receptors, IGF-1, and IGF-2 are expressed in primary human sarcomas. *Cancer research* 1995;55:129-34.

[59] Beevers CS, Li F, Liu L, Huang S. Curcumin inhibits the mammalian target of rapamycin-mediated signaling pathways in cancer cells. *International journal of cancer Journal international du cancer* 2006;119:757-64.

[60] Bjornsti MA, Houghton PJ. The TOR pathway: a target for cancer therapy. *Nature reviews Cancer* 2004;4:335-48.

[61] Wan X, Helman LJ. The biology behind mTOR inhibition in sarcoma. *The oncologist* 2007;12:1007-18.
[62] Tokunaga C, Yoshino K, Yonezawa K. mTOR integrates amino acid- and energy-sensing pathways. *Biochemical and biophysical research communications* 2004;313:443-6.
[63] O'Reilly KE, Rojo F, She QB, et al. mTOR inhibition induces upstream receptor tyrosine kinase signaling and activates Akt. *Cancer research* 2006;66:1500-8.
[64] Dhillon AS, Hagan S, Rath O, Kolch W. MAP kinase signalling pathways in cancer. *Oncogene* 2007;26:3279-90.
[65] Yoon SS, Segal NH, Park PJ, et al. Angiogenic profile of soft tissue sarcomas based on analysis of circulating factors and microarray gene expression. *The Journal of surgical research* 2006;135:282-90.
[66] Yamamoto T, Ebisuya M, Ashida F, Okamoto K, Yonehara S, Nishida E. Continuous ERK activation downregulates antiproliferative genes throughout G1 phase to allow cell-cycle progression. *Current biology: CB* 2006;16:1171-82.
[67] van Maldegem AM, Bhosale A, Gelderblom HJ, Hogendoorn PC, Hassan AB. Comprehensive analysis of published phase I/II clinical trials between 1990-2010 in osteosarcoma and Ewing sarcoma confirms limited outcomes and need for translational investment. *Clinical sarcoma research* 2012;2:5.
[68] Maki RG, D'Adamo DR, Keohan ML, et al. Phase II study of sorafenib in patients with metastatic or recurrent sarcomas. *Journal of clinical oncology: official journal of the American Society of Clinical Oncology* 2009;27:3133-40.
[69] DuBois S, Demetri G. Markers of angiogenesis and clinical features in patients with sarcoma. *Cancer* 2007;109:813-9.
[70] Inoue K, Ozeki Y, Suganuma T, Sugiura Y, Tanaka S. Vascular endothelial growth factor expression in primary esophageal squamous cell carcinoma. Association with angiogenesis and tumor progression. Cancer 1997;79:206-13.
[71] Ishigami SI, Arii S, Furutani M, et al. Predictive value of vascular endothelial growth factor (VEGF) in metastasis and prognosis of human colorectal cancer. *British journal of cancer* 1998;78:1379-84.
[72] Maeda K, Chung YS, Ogawa Y, et al. Prognostic value of vascular endothelial growth factor expression in gastric carcinoma. *Cancer* 1996;77:858-63.

[73] Kaya M, Wada T, Akatsuka T, et al. Vascular endothelial growth factor expression in untreated osteosarcoma is predictive of pulmonary metastasis and poor prognosis. *Clinical cancer research: an official journal of the American Association for Cancer Research* 2000;6:572-7.
[74] Charity RM, Foukas AF, Deshmukh NS, Grimer RJ. Vascular endothelial growth factor expression in osteosarcoma. *Clinical orthopaedics and related research* 2006;448:193-8.
[75] Huynh C, Poliseno L, Segura MF, et al. The novel gamma secretase inhibitor RO4929097 reduces the tumor initiating potential of melanoma. *PloS one* 2011;6:e25264.
[76] Rubin LL, de Sauvage FJ. Targeting the Hedgehog pathway in cancer. *Nature reviews Drug discovery* 2006;5:1026-33.
[77] Hocht C, Mayer M, Taira CA. Therapeutic perspectives of angiotensin-(1–7) in the treatment of cardiovascular disease. *Open Pharmacol. J.* 2009;3:21-31.
[78] Allred AJ, Diz DI, Ferrario CM, Chappell MC. Pathways for angiotensin-(1---7) metabolism in pulmonary and renal tissues. *American journal of physiology Renal physiology* 2000;279:F841-50.
[79] Rodgers KE, Ellefson DD, Espinoza T, Hsu YH, diZerega GS, Mehrian-Shai R. Expression of intracellular filament, collagen, and collagenase genes in diabetic and normal skin after injury. Wound repair and regeneration: official publication of the Wound Healing Society [and] the European Tissue Repair Society 2006;14:298-305.
[80] Oda K, Matsuoka Y, Funahashi A, Kitano H. A comprehensive pathway map of epidermal growth factor receptor signaling. *Molecular systems biology* 2005;1:2005 0010.
[81] Wright C, Angus B, Nicholson S, et al. Expression of c-erbB-2 oncoprotein: a prognostic indicator in human breast cancer. *Cancer research* 1989;49:2087-90.
[82] Gorlick R, Huvos AG, Heller G, et al. Expression of HER2/erbB-2 correlates with survival in osteosarcoma. *Journal of clinical oncology: official journal of the American Society of Clinical Oncology* 1999;17:2781-8.
[83] Zhou H, Randall RL, Brothman AR, Maxwell T, Coffin CM, Goldsby RE. Her-2/neu expression in osteosarcoma increases risk of lung metastasis and can be associated with gene amplification. *Journal of pediatric hematology/oncology* 2003;25:27-32.
[84] Somers GR, Ho M, Zielenska M, Squire JA, Thorner PS. HER2 amplification and overexpression is not present in pediatric

osteosarcoma: a tissue microarray study. *Pediatric and developmental pathology: the official journal of the Society for Pediatric Pathology and the Paediatric Pathology Society* 2005;8:525-32.

[85] Thomas DG, Giordano TJ, Sanders D, Biermann JS, Baker L. Absence of HER2/neu gene expression in osteosarcoma and skeletal Ewing's sarcoma. *Clinical cancer research: an official journal of the American Association for Cancer Research* 2002;8:788-93.

[86] Ebb D, Meyers P, Grier H, et al. Phase II trial of trastuzumab in combination with cytotoxic chemotherapy for treatment of metastatic osteosarcoma with human epidermal growth factor receptor 2 overexpression: a report from the children's oncology group. *Journal of clinical oncology: official journal of the American Society of Clinical Oncology* 2012;30:2545-51.

[87] Jakacki RI, Hamilton M, Gilbertson RJ, et al. Pediatric phase I and pharmacokinetic study of erlotinib followed by the combination of erlotinib and temozolomide: a Children's Oncology Group Phase I Consortium Study. *Journal of clinical oncology: official journal of the American Society of Clinical Oncology* 2008;26:4921-7.

[88] McGary EC, Weber K, Mills L, et al. Inhibition of platelet-derived growth factor-mediated proliferation of osteosarcoma cells by the novel tyrosine kinase inhibitor STI571. *Clinical cancer research: an official journal of the American Association for Cancer Research* 2002;8:3584-91.

[89] Sulzbacher I, Traxler M, Mosberger I, Lang S, Chott A. Platelet-derived growth factor-AA and -alpha receptor expression suggests an autocrine and/or paracrine loop in osteosarcoma. *Modern pathology: an official journal of the United States and Canadian Academy of Pathology*, Inc 2000;13:632-7.

[90] Kubo T, Piperdi S, Rosenblum J, et al. Platelet-derived growth factor receptor as a prognostic marker and a therapeutic target for imatinib mesylate therapy in osteosarcoma. *Cancer* 2008;112:2119-29.

[91] Buchdunger E, Cioffi CL, Law N, et al. Abl protein-tyrosine kinase inhibitor STI571 inhibits in vitro signal transduction mediated by c-kit and platelet-derived growth factor receptors. *The Journal of pharmacology and experimental therapeutics* 2000;295:139-45.

[92] Hingorani P, Zhang W, Gorlick R, Kolb EA. Inhibition of Src phosphorylation alters metastatic potential of osteosarcoma in vitro but not in vivo. *Clinical cancer research: an official journal of the American Association for Cancer Research* 2009;15:3416-22.

[93] Atadja PW. HDAC inhibitors and cancer therapy. Progress in drug research Fortschritte der Arzneimittelforschung Progres des recherches pharmaceutiques 2011;67:175-95.

[94] Shabason JE, Tofilon PJ, Camphausen K. HDAC inhibitors in cancer care. *Oncology* (Williston Park) 2010;24:180-5.

[95] Johnstone RW. Histone-deacetylase inhibitors: novel drugs for the treatment of cancer. *Nature reviews Drug discovery* 2002;1:287-99.

[96] Khan O, La Thangue NB. HDAC inhibitors in cancer biology: emerging mechanisms and clinical applications. *Immunology and cell biology* 2012;90:85-94.

[97] Tumber A, Collins LS, Petersen KD, et al. The histone deacetylase inhibitor PXD101 synergises with 5-fluorouracil to inhibit colon cancer cell growth in vitro and in vivo. *Cancer chemotherapy and pharmacology* 2007;60:275-83.

[98] McGlynn P, Lloyd RG. Recombinational repair and restart of damaged replication forks. *Nature reviews Molecular cell biology* 2002;3:859-70.

[99] Patel A, Kaufmann SH. Development of PARP inhibitors: an unfinished story. *Oncology* (Williston Park) 2010;24:66, 8.

[100] Buisson R, Dion-Cote AM, Coulombe Y, et al. Cooperation of breast cancer proteins PALB2 and piccolo BRCA2 in stimulating homologous recombination. *Nature structural & molecular biology* 2010;17:1247-54.

[101] Murai J, Huang SY, Das BB, et al. Trapping of PARP1 and PARP2 by Clinical PARP Inhibitors. *Cancer research* 2012;72:5588-99.

[102] Shen Y, Rehman FL, Feng Y, et al. BMN 673, a novel and highly potent PARP1/2 inhibitor for the treatment of human cancers with DNA repair deficiency. *Clinical cancer research: an official journal of the American Association for Cancer Research* 2013.

[103] Teicher BA, Ara G, Herbst R, Palombella VJ, Adams J. The proteasome inhibitor PS-341 in cancer therapy. *Clinical cancer research: an official journal of the American Association for Cancer Research* 1999;5:2638-45.

[104] Bommakanti SV, Dudek AZ, Khatri A, Kirstein MN, Gada PD. Phase 1 trial of gemcitabine with bortezomib in elderly patients with advanced solid tumors. *American journal of clinical oncology* 2011;34:597-602.

[105] Marumoto T, Honda S, Hara T, et al. Aurora-A kinase maintains the fidelity of early and late mitotic events in HeLa cells. *The Journal of biological chemistry* 2003;278:51786-95.

[106] Siggelkow W, Boehm D, Gebhard S, et al. Expression of aurora kinase A is associated with metastasis-free survival in node-negative breast cancer patients. *BMC cancer* 2012;12:562.

[107] Heiner JP, Miraldi F, Kallick S, et al. Localization of GD2-specific monoclonal antibody 3F8 in human osteosarcoma. *Cancer research* 1987;47:5377-81.

[108] Navid F, Santana VM, Barfield RC. Anti-GD2 antibody therapy for GD2-expressing tumors. *Current cancer drug targets* 2010;10:200-9.

[109] Cheresh DA, Pierschbacher MD, Herzig MA, Mujoo K. Disialogangliosides GD2 and GD3 are involved in the attachment of human melanoma and neuroblastoma cells to extracellular matrix proteins. *The Journal of cell biology* 1986;102:688-96.

[110] Roth JA, Cristiano RJ. Gene therapy for cancer: what have we done and where are we going? *Journal of the National Cancer Institute* 1997;89:21-39.

[111] Hingorani P, Zhang W, Lin J, Liu L, Guha C, Kolb EA. Systemic administration of reovirus (Reolysin) inhibits growth of human sarcoma xenografts. *Cancer* 2011;117:1764-74.

[112] Heriot AG, Marriott JB, Cookson S, Kumar D, Dalgleish AG. Reduction in cytokine production in colorectal cancer patients: association with stage and reversal by resection. *British journal of cancer* 2000;82:1009-12.

[113] Reynolds JT, Watkins JM, Dufan TA, Kubsad SS. Irradiation of donor mononuclear cells for treatment of chemorefractory metastatic solid cancers: a community-based immune transplant pilot study. *Cancer research and treatment: official journal of Korean Cancer Association* 2012;44:133-41.

[114] Dey BR, McAfee S, Colby C, et al. Anti-tumour response despite loss of donor chimaerism in patients treated with non-myeloablative conditioning and allogeneic stem cell transplantation. *British journal of haematology* 2005;128:351-9.

[115] Waller EK, Boyer M. New strategies in allogeneic stem cell transplantation: immunotherapy using irradiated allogeneic T cells. *Bone marrow transplantation* 2000;25 Suppl 2:S20-4.

[116] Kleinerman ES. Biologic therapy for osteosarcoma using liposome-encapsulated muramyl tripeptide. *Hematology/oncology clinics of North America* 1995;9:927-38.

[117] Meyers PA, Schwartz CL, Krailo MD, et al. Osteosarcoma: the addition of muramyl tripeptide to chemotherapy improves overall survival--a

report from the Children's Oncology Group. *Journal of clinical oncology: official journal of the American Society of Clinical Oncology* 2008;26:633-8.

INDEX

A

B

C

D

E

F

G

H

I

J

K

L

M

N

O

P

Q

R

S

T

U